# BEHAVIORAL ISSUES IN AUTISM

# CURRENT ISSUES IN AUTISM

Series Editors: Eric Schopler and Gary B. Mesibov
*University of North Carolina School of Medicine*
*Chapel Hill, North Carolina*

---

AUTISM IN ADOLESCENTS AND ADULTS
Edited by Eric Schopler and Gary B. Mesibov

BEHAVIORAL ISSUES IN AUTISM
Edited by Eric Schopler and Gary B. Mesibov

COMMUNICATION PROBLEMS IN AUTISM
Edited by Eric Schopler and Gary B. Mesibov

DIAGNOSIS AND ASSESSMENT IN AUTISM
Edited by Eric Schopler and Gary B. Mesibov

THE EFFECTS OF AUTISM ON THE FAMILY
Edited by Eric Schopler and Gary B. Mesibov

HIGH-FUNCTIONING INDIVIDUALS WITH AUTISM
Edited by Eric Schopler and Gary B. Mesibov

NEUROBIOLOGICAL ISSUES IN AUTISM
Edited by Eric Schopler and Gary B. Mesibov

PRESCHOOL ISSUES IN AUTISM
Edited by Eric Schopler, Mary E. Van Bourgondien, and Marie M. Bristol

SOCIAL BEHAVIOR IN AUTISM
Edited by Eric Schopler and Gary B. Mesibov

# Contributors

JENNIFER BERRYMAN, State University of New York, Binghamton, New York 13902

JOSEPH CAUTELA, Behavior Therapy Institute, 10 Phillips Road, Sudbury, Massachusetts 01776

GLEN DUNLAP, Florida Mental Health Institute, University of South Florida, Tampa, Florida 33612-2399

WILLIAM D. FREA, Autism Research Center, University of California at Santa Barbara, Santa Barbara, California 93106-9490

PETER F. GERHARDT, The Eden Services, 1 Logan Drive, Princeton, New Jersey 08540

JUNE GRODEN, The Groden Center, Inc., 86 Mount Hope Avenue, Providence, Rhode Island 02906

SANDRA L. HARRIS, Graduate School of Applied and Professional Psychology, Rutgers, The State University of New Jersey, Busch Campus, Piscataway, New Jersey 08855-0819

KATHLEEN A. HEARSEY, Division TEACCH, School of Medicine, The University of North Carolina at Chapel Hill, Chapel Hill, North Carolina 27599-7180

DAVID L. HOLMES, The Eden Services, 1 Logan Drive, Princeton, New Jersey 08540

BRIAN A. IWATA, Department of Psychology, The University of Florida, Gainesville, Florida 32611

LEE KERN, Children's Seashore House, Biobehavioral Unit, 3405 Civic Center Boulevard, Philadelphia, Pennsylvania 19104.

ROBERT L. KOEGEL, Autism Research Center, University of California at Santa Barbara, Santa Barbara, California 93106-9490

JOHNNY L. MATSON, Department of Psychology, Louisiana State University, Baton Rouge, Louisiana 70803

PATRICIA M. MEINHOLD, Department of Pediatrics, The Ohio State University, and The Children's Hospital, Columbus, Ohio 43205

GARY B. MESIBOV, Division TEACCH, School of Medicine, The University of North Carolina at Chapel Hill, Chapel Hill, North Carolina 27599-7180

JAMES A. MULICK, Department of Pediatrics, The Ohio State University, and The Children's Hospital, Columbus, Ohio 43205

MICHAEL D. POWERS, Department of Psychology, Newington Children's Hospital, Newington, Connecticut 06111

STACEY PRINCE, Center for Clinical Research, University of Washington, Seattle, Washington 98195

FRANK R. ROBBINS, Early Childhood Learning Center, 150 Fearing Street, Amherst, Massachusetts 01002

ERIC SCHOPLER, Division TEACCH, School of Medicine, The University of North Carolina at Chapel Hill, Chapel Hill, North Carolina 27599-7180

LAURA SCHREIBMAN, Department of Psychology, University of California at San Diego, La Jolla, California 92093

JAY A. SEVIN, Department of Psychology, Louisiana State University, Baton Rouge, Louisiana 70803

RICHARD G. SMITH, Department of Psychology, The University of Florida, Gainesville, Florida 32611

ALAN V. SURRATT, Center on Human Development, University of Oregon, Eugene, Oregon 97403-1235

TIMOTHY R. VOLLMER, Department of Psychology, Louisiana State University, Baton Rouge, Louisiana 70803

JENNIFER R. ZARCONE, Department of Behavioral Psychology, The Kennedy Institute, 707 North Broadway, Baltimore, Maryland 21205

# BEHAVIORAL ISSUES IN AUTISM

Edited by

## Eric Schopler

and

## Gary B. Mesibov

*University of North Carolina School of Medicine*
*Chapel Hill, North Carolina*

PLENUM PRESS • NEW YORK AND LONDON

Library of Congress Cataloging-in-Publication Data

Behavioral issues in autism / edited by Eric Schopler and Gary B.
   Mesibov.
         p.    cm. -- (Current issues in autism)
      Includes bibliographical references and index.
      ISBN 0-306-44600-6
      1. Autistic children--Rehabilitation.  2. Behavior disorders in
   children--Treatment.  3. Mentally handicapped children--Behavior
   modification.    I. Schopler, Eric.   II. Mesibov, Gary B.
   III. Series.
   RJ506.A9B343  1994
   618.92'8982--dc20                                                93-49102
                                                                        CIP

10 9 8 7 6 5 4 3

ISBN 0-306-44600-6

Printed in the United States of America

To the many families
struggling with behavioral concerns,
with the hope that this volume
will provide insight, understanding, support, and assistance

# Preface

Division TEACCH, a statewide program in North Carolina, serves people with autism and their families through the School of Medicine at the University of North Carolina at Chapel Hill. TEACCH was one of the first, and remains one of the most comprehensive and effective, programs in the world working with this population. Over the years the puzzling and unusual behavior problems these children present have been among the most interesting and challenging of the enigmas parents and professionals confront. This book is designed to provide information on these behaviors that will be relevant and useful.

As with the preceding books in our series, *Current Issues in Autism,* this volume is based in part on one of the annual TEACCH Conferences held in Chapel Hill in May. The books are not simply published proceedings of the conference papers. Instead, conference participants are asked to develop full-length chapters around their presentations. Other international experts, whose work is beyond the scope of each conference but related to its major theme, are asked to contribute chapters as well. These volumes provide the most up-to-date information on research and professional practice available on the most important issues in autism.

This volume is designed to advance the understanding of behavior problems in autism. A general perspective on major issues and strategies in the field is presented. There are also major sections devoted to assessment techniques, intervention strategies, and major controversies in the field. We expect the volume to be of interest to students, professionals, and parents concerned with understanding and managing behavior problems of individuals with autism.

ERIC SCHOPLER<br>
GARY B. MESIBOV

# Acknowledgments

A volume of this scope would be impossible without the cooperation, assistance, and support of many people. It is our great pleasure to acknowledge each of them. Our thanks go to Helen Garrison, who skillfully coordinated the TEACCH Conference on this theme. Her superb work on all aspects of these conferences has been an important aspect of the evolution of these books. Our secretarial staff, including Vickie Weaver, Jeanette Ferguson, Ann Bashford, and Amy Slaughter, handled the many typing and administrative chores with skill, competence, and good cheer. John Swetnam carefully reviewed each chapter, and his superb organizational skills kept this project moving ahead. His thoroughness and attention to detail are evident throughout the book.

As with all of our projects, these books would not be possible without our extraordinary TEACCH colleagues, too numerous to name, who provide ongoing help, insights, cooperation, and splendid work. Their understanding of people with autism and their families is extraordinary and provides the knowledge and inspiration that we try to impart through these books.

As is true for all our efforts in the TEACCH program, writing this book would not have been possible without the assistance of the families of our clients. Their energy, cooperation, and participation in our program have taught us so much about this important topic.

Finally, the University of North Carolina at Chapel Hill School of Medicine, especially the Department of Psychiatry under the capable leadership of David Janowsky, has provided the environment that cultivates and nurtures scholarly pursuits of this kind. We also are most grateful to the North Carolina State Legislature, which makes this and our many other projects possible through their continued support.

# Contents

Chapter 3

ADMINISTRATIVE ISSUES INVOLVING BEHAVIORAL
APPROACHES IN AUTISM

Michael D. Powers

Chapter 4

BEHAVIORAL PRIORITIES FOR AUTISM AND RELATED
DEVELOPMENTAL DISORDERS

Eric Schopler

**Part II: Assessment Issues**

Chapter 5

SELF-MANAGEMENT OF PROBLEMATIC SOCIAL BEHAVIOR

Robert L. Koegel, William D. Frea, and Alan V. Surratt

Chapter 6

DEVELOPMENTAL DISORDERS AND BROAD EFFECTS
OF THE ENVIRONMENT ON LEARNING AND
TREATMENT EFFECTIVENESS

James A. Mulick and Patricia M. Meinhold

**Part III: Treatment Issues**

Chapter 7

ASSESSMENT AND TREATMENT OF SELF-INJURIOUS BEHAVIOR

Brian A. Iwata, Jennifer R. Zarcone, Timothy R. Vollmer,
and Richard G. Smith

Chapter 8

TREATMENT OF FAMILY PROBLEMS IN AUTISM

Sandra L. Harris

Chapter 9

THE IMPACT OF STRESS AND ANXIETY ON INDIVIDUALS
WITH AUTISM AND DEVELOPMENTAL DISABILITIES

June Groden, Joseph Cautela, Stacey Prince, and Jennifer Berryman

Chapter 10

STRUCTURED TEACHING

Gary B. Mesibov, Eric Schopler, and Kathleen A. Hearsey

**Part IV: Special Issues**

Chapter 11

ISSUES IN THE USE OF AVERSIVES: FACTORS ASSOCIATED
WITH BEHAVIOR MODIFICATION FOR AUTISTIC AND
OTHER DEVELOPMENTALLY DISABLED PEOPLE

Johnny L. Matson and Jay A. Sevin

Chapter 12

SOME CHARACTERISTICS OF NONAVERSIVE INTERVENTION
FOR SEVERE BEHAVIOR PROBLEMS

Glen Dunlap, Frank R. Robbins, and Lee Kern

Chapter 13

THE EDEN DECISION MODEL: A DECISION MODEL WITH
PRACTICAL APPLICATIONS FOR THE DEVELOPMENT OF
BEHAVIOR DECELERATIVE STRATEGIES

Peter F. Gerhardt and David L. Holmes

# I

# Overview

# Introduction to Behavioral Issues in Autism

## ERIC SCHOPLER and GARY B. MESIBOV

Although there are many definitions of the autism syndrome (Ritvo & Freeman, 1978; Rutter & Schopler, 1992), all of them consistently identify social, communication, and behavioral peculiarities and deficits. The social deficits are often the most compelling and are the reason why Leo Kanner (1943) chose the term *autism* to describe this group of children in his seminal paper. Communication deficits typically are the most interesting because of their idiosyncrasies and deviance from normal development. Communication characteristics include such diversity as total muteness, pronoun reversals, echolalia, and repetitive statements. The behavior difficulties in autism are not as easy to characterize or describe. They can be simply humorous and trivial deviations from what we generally expect to see in others, such as enjoying the click of an automobile turn signal or loving to watch the rhythm of a garbage truck picking up its cargo. Characteristic behaviors also can be more extreme—even devastating—such as the self-injurious, destructive behaviors that sometimes dominate the lives of these children and their families. Between these two extremes are a wide range of behavior problems that emerge from frustration over problems with communication, interactions, and understanding.

ERIC SCHOPLER and GARY B. MESIBOV • Division TEACCH, School of Medicine, The University of North Carolina at Chapel Hill, Chapel Hill, North Carolina 27599-7180.

*Behavioral Issues in Autism*, edited by Eric Schopler and Gary B. Mesibov. New York, Plenum Press, 1994.

## INTRODUCTION

These behavioral characteristics of autism are the focus of this book. Because so much of the time and energy used in helping people with autism is consumed by issues related to behavior problems, this is a most appropriate and necessary area of specialization. Behavioral difficulties also have triggered some of the major controversies in the field of autism. Questions about the use of aversives, the tendency of children with autism to imitate others, and whether or not placements in classrooms with nonhandicapped peers are the most appropriate have interested and confounded professionals for many years.

It is hard to know why the behavior problems in autism arouse so much interest and controversy. It is partly, no doubt, the uniqueness of these behaviors, the seriousness of their difficulties, their parents' advocacy, and the anxieties and fears they generate in many members of the community. Some behavior problems are dangerous and require careful attention and consideration to protect autistic clients, their families, and coworkers. These behaviors often separate people with autism from their nonhandicapped peers and local communities.

In this book we will try to present a comprehensive and balanced approach to issues in this area. Leading experts will apply state-of-the-art concepts to this important and controversial area. Although we might not resolve the major controversies that have divided the field, we hope to provide a broad perspective and reasonable dialogue about the questions under identification. Our book is divided into four parts: an overview, a discussion of assessment, a focus on treatment, and a final section describing major issues in the field.

## OVERVIEW

The overview chapters describe basic issues and principles that will be covered throughout the book. The chapter by Laura Schreibman reviews behavioral principles. Representing only one of many different approaches to behavioral difficulties in autism, these principles were the early alternative to the destructive psychoanalytic approaches (Schopler, 1971) and form the basis of most current intervention techniques. Schreibman's description of behavioral techniques is clear, comprehensive, thoughtful, and precise. Even readers with considerable expertise in this area will find her synthesis helpful.

After reviewing the major behavioral principles, Schreibman concludes her chapter with a discussion of important issues in the field. Questions about aversives, generalization, and behavioral assessment are followed-up in this book by other authors. Schreibman's brief introduction to these complex questions will whet readers' appetites for what follows.

The chapter by Michael Powers reminds us that intervention principles for managing behavior must be seen in the larger context of a program and its administration; behavior management techniques do not occur in a vacuum. According to Powers, organizational processes can resolve impediments to effective behavioral programming and uncover potential remediation strategies. Powers begins his chapter with a discussion of the organizational constraints of limited resources, the perception of inflexibility, sensitivity to external pressures, multiple constituencies, and problems with communication. According to Powers, flexibility is an important priority, although programs must be careful not to compromise essential aspects of their intervention techniques. Powers describes several strategies programs can use: technology, coordination, utilization, the criteria of ultimate functioning, and the assumption of educability.

In concluding, Powers argues that administrative impediments to successful behavioral intervention generally involve either a lack of technically sophisticated behavioral programs or not embedding them in relevant social contexts. Clinical failures have resulted from inattention to one of these factors or their interrelationships. He outlines specific procedures that can overcome these obstacles.

Eric Schopler concludes the overview with a summary of how administrative structure can facilitate effective interventions. He outlines the program features essential for accomplishing program goals. Schopler's summary highlights major points that successful programs should address.

Schopler's chapter is based on his experience in developing North Carolina's statewide program for people with autism and related communications handicaps (Division TEACCH: Treatment and Education of Autistic and related Communication handicapped Children). It is the only program in the United States that provides comprehensive service, research, and multidisciplinary training on behalf of people with autism and related disorders. For Schopler, this program offers a unique perspective for discussing the issue of behavioral treatment models.

After reviewing the TEACCH Program, Schopler discusses enduring treatment principles and concepts that have been viable over the 25 years that his program has been serving North Carolina families. These include improving adaptation between the clients and their communities, emphasizing the process of assessment for individualized treatment, using structure as the core of intervention techniques, focusing on skill enhancement, combining cognitive and behavioral approaches, and using a generalist training model. Schopler's insights from so many years of effective service should be interesting and thought-provoking for most parents and professionals.

## ASSESSMENT ISSUES

The section on assessment issues begins with a chapter by Koegel and his colleagues addressing exciting new developments in the area of self-management of problematic social behaviors. Promoting self-management skills is consistent with the increased emphasis on independent functioning and community-based approaches. Clients with strong self-management skills require less supervision and can adapt more easily to their community-based settings. The implications of this approach could be far reaching.

After describing common sources of behavioral difficulties in autism, the authors outline their treatment procedures. The pretraining stage identifies targeted behaviors. Therapists then develop measurement techniques and initiate the treatment phase. Creating independence is the unique focal aspect of this approach. It is what transfers typical behavioral programs into ones that each client controls and maintains. The authors provide provocative examples of their approach with problems such as responsivity to peer initiation, reducing stereotypies, and verbal initiations.

The section on assessment ends with Mulick and Meinhold's chapter describing the broad effects of the environment on learning and treatment effectiveness. All of us know how much we are influenced by environmental factors, yet these factors have not received adequate attention in the behavioral literature because of an emphasis on individual clients and their responses. The authors identify and describe setting factors such as incentives and motivation; alternative actions; social ecology; and generally accepted customs, rules, and regulations. By focusing on the environmental impact of common treatment approaches and interventions, these authors offer a much broader perspective than is typically found in the literature.

## TREATMENT ISSUES

Chapters in the third section of this book focus on treatment issues. Iwata and his colleagues offer a well-organized, articulate, and productive discussion of self-injurious behaviors and how they might be assessed and treated. Among the most frightening and difficult of the behavior problems in autism, self-injurious behaviors are poorly understood and inadequately managed. The authors start with a discussion of critical variables, showing how both biological factors and principles of learning can cause and maintain these strong and destructive behavioral difficulties. The authors then outline pretreatment considerations and what is involved in performing a careful assessment.

The bulk of this chapter describes intervention strategies. Ways of modifying antecedent conditions, discontinuing reinforcements, offering differential reinforcements, using punishments, and experimenting with pharmacologic interventions are clearly and comprehensively reviewed. Iwata and his colleagues' systematic approach will be helpful to anyone dealing with these difficult problems by suggesting consistent strategies and offering rich new ideas and insights.

Harris discusses treatment issues involving families of people with autism. She describes how family dynamics can influence a child with autism as well as how the child can influence a family. These dynamic family–child interactions can have a dramatic effect on the child's functioning.

Harris begins with a discussion of how children with autism impact their families. The literature on mother versus father reactions is reviewed in detail. Siblings also are an important part of the family, and Harris reviews the developing literature on their role and possible contributions to more effective interactions and family functioning. After reviewing this developing literature, Harris describes some of the important aspects that determine outcome: coping strategies, stress, social support, family training, marital disharmony, and family cohesion.

Readers of this chapter will find both a good overview of relevant literature and new ideas for family interventions. Harris's integration of the literature and clinical possibilities is especially helpful.

Groden and colleagues present a new and creative way to deal with behavior difficulties through progressive relaxation. Their straightforward style will appeal to most readers of this volume. The authors begin with a discussion demonstrating how stress and anxiety are crucial factors in many behavioral difficulties of people with autism. They then introduce their relaxation program in the context of techniques to improve self-management and skill enhancement. The program helps people with autism make a relaxation response to stress, replacing their typically maladaptive behaviors. The authors' data demonstrate that 44% of their clients learn to relax with a verbal cue and an additional 31% learn to relax independently. Their strategies for adapting traditional relaxation techniques to people with autism and their excellent case examples are of great interest and significance.

The final chapter in the treatment section introduces the TEACCH techniques for structured teaching. Although most educational programs for people with autism emphasize structure, Division TEACCH has defined, elaborated, and implemented this concept in greater detail than is commonly seen. The chapter by Schopler and his colleagues describes how Division TEACCH accomplishes this.

Structured teaching begins with a clear and minimally distracting physical environment. Schedules, work systems, and clear visual tasks are an important part of this approach. The authors describe these aspects in detail, using many case examples from their rich clinical experiences. Ways of using structure to minimize the cognitive learning impairments characteristic of autism, and capitalizing on the autistic students' strengths in visual processing, desire for sameness, and special interests also are introduced and described. The TEACCH structure is adapted to variations in developmental functions and individual learning needs. The reader will find these structure principles and their adaptations thought-provoking and useful. The authors offer many examples of the use of these techniques in a wide variety of classroom situations.

## SPECIAL ISSUES

The final section of the book is on special issues and programs. Recently there has been considerable discussion and debate about the role, if any, of aversives in programming for people with autism. Most of this discussion has been emotional, rather than research-based. Because the use of aversives is an issue of great concern, it is crucial that both parents and professionals review the considerable accumulated evidence about aversives and that alternative strategies be identified and implemented.

Matson and Sevin offer a comprehensive review of the literature on aversives. Their chapter provides a rational basis for discussions that have not always been reasonable. This chapter is required reading for anyone who has argued strongly about aversives, whether for or against.

Matson and Sevin begin with a definition of major terms and concepts, then trace the history of the debate over aversives, and finally describe how advocates developed ideas independent of professional practice. They show how emotion-laden terms, misleading arguments, and inaccurate references to data have dominated discussions about aversives. Of particular concern to the authors is the argument that nonaversive procedures are unnecessary because the data clearly demonstrate the effectiveness of aversive procedures in several well-controlled studies when positive procedures alone had previously failed in treating life-threatening behaviors. The authors also refute the arguments that aversives have more side effects, do not lead to generalization, are inconsistent with community-based standards, and that there is no support for their use among parent and professional groups.

The authors conclude by urging the need for treatment options, especially with severe and debilitating behaviors. Although they argue that developing prosocial behaviors, self-control, and manipulating environmental antecedents can reduce the need for aversive interventions, they do not foresee the total elimination of aversives. If clients are to receive the best treatments available, especially when their behaviors are life-threatening, professionals and advocates will have to evaluate the professional literature more rationally and according to empirical evidence, rather than appealing to testimonials and emotional, value-laden arguments.

Though Matson and Sevin do not find data to support the extreme position against all aversives, they do not argue for an increase in aversives or even for their widespread use. Instead, they urge professionals and advocates to maintain this as a treatment option, especially for severe behavior difficulties. While arguing for the continued availability of aversives as a treatment option, they fully support the use of more positive treatment approaches when appropriate.

The chapter by Dunlap and colleagues describes and defines the nonaversive treatment options that are evolving. They begin with a helpful discussion of the definition and applications of nonaversive interventions. This comprehensive review will help readers understand the range of possible positive interventions. They then describe functional assessment procedures and the importance of hypothesis-driven interventions. While presenting strategies and procedures clearly and directly, the authors also communicate that the process is generally not simple or straightforward. Once again, parents and professionals in the field are given the important message that there are no simple or easy cures.

Consistent with Matson and Sevin, the authors describe the growing interest in changing antecedent stimuli that might trigger inappropriate behaviors. As examples, they discuss noise level, instructional commands, crowding, task materials, and schedule unpredictability. They cite some interesting and important studies showing that identifying and manipulating antecedent variables can reduce or eliminate behavior problems. This is an important new emphasis gaining in popularity because of its effectiveness. It shows that preventing the occurrence of problem behaviors is a more effective long-term strategy than dealing with them by manipulating their consequences after they occur.

Curriculum-based interventions are similar to manipulating antecedent events. The goal here is to change what the client is doing instructionally to minimize behavioral difficulties. Altering instructional demands, task difficulty, instructional materials, or instructional responses can strengthen alternative behaviors, and minimize inappropriate responses. These techniques also help to avoid inappropriate outbursts.

The authors also argue for increasing personal control and choice. This is consistent with techniques presented by Matson and Sevin and by Koegel et al. Although we sometimes do not recognize the importance of the human need for choice and control in handicapped people, these needs can be powerful motivators. The challenge often is to find ways for severely handicapped people to satisfactorily control their environments by making meaningful choices.

Communication is an essential skill, and the lack of this ability can trigger many behavioral difficulties. Improving the ability to communicate is another way of helping severely handicapped clients. The authors describe this intervention technique and how it can be applied to clients at many different developmental levels.

This book concludes with a description by Gerhardt and Holmes of the Eden Decision Model.This is a concrete and practical statement of how to make decisions about using strategies to decrease problem behaviors. For those who think that scholarly articles often do not fully capture real-life problems, this chapter will be a refreshing change.

The Eden process starts with a careful analysis of client needs. This is done by recording data, analyzing environmental conditions, examining the curriculum, and identifying sources of reinforcement. Once these steps are taken, a procedure to decrease inappropriate behaviors is developed. This program is based on the belief that a thorough analysis of the client's environment can maximize the chances that the environment will meet the client's individual needs. Aversives are used in this system, but only after all other possibilities have been explored and exhausted.

The model presented here offers a practical guide for making critical yet difficult decisions. The authors explain their process through several well-chosen case studies. These examples of the use of behavioral principles in a community-based program demonstrate the application of many of the techniques in the book.

Our brief summary has only touched on some of the many ideas, procedures, issues, and debates presented in the chapters that follow. Our introductory comments cannot cover them all. We are pleased that our volume has accomplished our goal of providing the most scholarly, accurate, and comprehensive discussion of behavior problems to date. We hope it will have a major effect on the understanding and treatment of these fascinating and compelling difficulties.

## REFERENCES

Kanner, L. (1943). Autistic disturbances of affective contact. *Nervous Child, 2,* 217–250.
Ritvo, E. R., & Freeman, B. J. (1978). National Society for Autistic Children definition of the syndrome of autism. *Journal of Autism and Childhood Schizophrenia, 8,* 162–167.
Rutter, M., & Schopler, E. (1992). Classification of pervasive developmental disorders: Some concepts and practical considerations. *Journal of Autism and Developmental Disorders, 22*(4), 459–482.
Schopler, E. (1971). Parents of psychotic children as scapegoats. *Journal of Contemporary Psychotherapy, 4,* 17–22.

# 2

# General Principles of Behavior Management

## LAURA SCHREIBMAN

Few individuals responsible for the care and/or treatment of children with autism would dispute the fact that these children present one of the toughest challenges we have faced. Everyone is challenged: the family, the schools, treatment specialists, and the entire community. Over the years since autism was first described by Leo Kanner (1943), a number of treatment approaches have been proposed and implemented, only to lead to limited and/or disappointing results. However, treatment from a behavioral perspective, that is, treatment based upon the principles of learning, has proven to have particular promise as a means of helping this severely handicapped population.

The purpose of this chapter is to acquaint the reader with the general principles involved in the application of behavior therapy to children with autism. After an orientation to the behavioral perspective and behavioral assessment, specific treatment procedures are presented. These include procedures involving the manipulation of behavioral consequences and procedures involving the manipulation of behavioral antecedents. Following this is a discussion of procedures designed to facilitate the generality and maintenance of our treatment effects. Finally, we will look at current issues and trends in the treatment of children with autism, including a discussion of the use of aversive procedures, promising new approaches to accomplishing widespread behavior change, and the expanding role of behavioral assessment.

LAURA SCHREIBMAN • Department of Psychology, University of California at San Diego, La Jolla, California 92093.

*Behavioral Issues in Autism*, edited by Eric Schopler and Gary B. Mesibov. New York, Plenum Press, 1994.

To begin, let us look at how the behavioral approach to the treatment of autism has come to be the dominant treatment approach for these children. The current dominance of the behavioral approach to the treatment of autism can be viewed as due to several factors.

First, the failure of the previously dominant approach, the application of psychodynamic theory, opened the door for a different form of treatment. The psychodynamic approach, whose major proponent was Bruno Bettelheim (e.g., 1967), was based upon the erroneous assumption that autism was due to faulty parenting and psychopathology of the parents. The prescribed treatment was to remove the children from the harmful environment provided by the parents and put the child in a permissive, accepting environment within which the child could emerge from the autistic "fortress." To make a very long story short, this did not work. In fact there are no empirically substantiated data to suggest that treatment based upon this model is effective.

Second, although we are well convinced that autism is an organically based disorder, we as yet do not know the precise etiological factor or factors responsible. Without more precise knowledge of the physiological correlates of autism we do not at this time have available any medical preventative nor medical treatment regimens for the syndrome of autism (although there are some pharmacological agents used for various specific behaviors).

A third factor responsible for the dominance of the behavioral approach is its basis in experimental psychology, with its emphasis on systematic replication and objective assessment of effectiveness. This has allowed the delineation of the relationship between an individual's behavior and his/her environment, and this in turn has allowed us to identify the principles of learning. In contrast to psychoanalytic theory with its highly complex and subjective features, the application of learning principles is very straightforward and relatively easy to understand. Accordingly these principles can be taught to a wide range of potential treatment providers, including both professionals and lay individuals. In fact we know that a wide variety of individuals including teachers (e.g., Horner, Meyer, & Fredericks, 1986; Koegel, Rincover, & Egel, 1982; Koegel, Russo, & Rincover, 1977; Koegel, Russo, Rincover, & Schreibman, 1982), parents (e.g., Dangel & Poster, 1984; Koegel, Schreibman, Britten, Burke, & O'Neill, 1982; O'Dell, 1985; Schreibman, Koegel, Mills, & Burke, 1984), siblings (e.g., Schreibman, O'Neill, & Koegel, 1983), and peers (e.g., Oke & Schreibman, 1990; Strain & Fox, 1981) can use these principles and be effective therapists for children with autism.

A fourth factor, and obviously the most important, is that it works. In fact, treatment based upon learning theory is the form of treatment with the most empirical substantiation for effectiveness with this population (e.g., Schreibman, 1988). Not only has it been demonstrated to be effective, but its reliance on the principles of experimental psychology and its emphasis on replication ensure that it is a progressive field, always evaluating itself and refining its techniques to be more and more effective and efficient.

## THE BEHAVIORAL PERSPECTIVE

One major advantage of the behavioral approach to the treatment of autism is that its use does not depend upon a knowledge of the etiology of the disorder nor does it view autism as a unitary "disease." From a behavioral standpoint, autism is viewed as a *syndrome* comprised of specific behavioral excesses and deficits. Excesses are behaviors that occur at an intensity or frequency that is inappropriate or those behaviors that are inappropriate at any intensity. Examples of behavioral excesses in autism include self-stimulation, self-injury (SIB), and compulsions. Behavioral deficits are those behaviors that do not occur at adequate strength or those that are not exhibited and whose absence is inappropriate. Examples of behavioral deficits in autism are language, social deficits, and inappropriate patterns of attention. Each of these excesses and deficits can be studied and understood in relationship to the environmental factors that serve to control it. Once this relationship is studied, demonstrated, and understood, the environment is manipulated in such a way as to increase, decrease, or maintain the specific behavior (e.g., Dunlap, Koegel, O'Neill, 1985; Schreibman, 1988; Schreibman & Koegel, 1981). A child's treatment program is comprised of that set of procedures designed to address the specific behavioral excesses and deficits exhibited by that specific child.

Fortunately, there already exists a rather extensive literature on many of the specific behavioral excesses and deficits seen in autism, and a clinician can access this literature to identify potentially effective treatment procedures for the case at hand. However, in some instances the clinician may find him/herself confronted with a specific behavior for which the controlling variables are not known, and in these cases the clinician must attempt to find the controlling variables. This is usually accomplished by observing events immediately preceding the behavior (the antecedents) and the events immediately following the behavior (the consequences) and looking for some reliable pattern. This is sometimes referred to as the **ABC** (Antecedent→Behavior→Consequence) pattern of behavior, and it can be extremely useful to a treatment provider, be it a trained professional or a layperson such as a parent. Let us consider the example of a mother who is frustrated by the fact that her child with autism, George, requires over an hour to eat dinner because he keeps getting up from the table and has to be enticed back to the table several times within the hour. Because the mother is sure that the child wants the dinner, she cannot understand why he continually gets up from the table. The mother begins to record the ABC pattern, and what she finds is that just prior to getting up from the table George is usually eating a less preferred food item (e.g., broccoli). Just after he gets up, someone in the family entices him back to the table by offering a preferred food item (e.g., spaghetti). Looking at this pattern over several instances suggests that the child has learned that if he does not like a particular food, he can obtain a preferred food by getting up from the table. Now the relationship between the behavior and the environment is rather clear, and the environment may be manipulated to change the behavior. In this case the mother may decide that if her son gets up from the table she will remove all of his food and he will get nothing else to eat until the next scheduled meal time. If her interpretation of the ABC pattern is correct, George should learn that leaving the table means that *no* food is forthcoming, and thus he might be expected to remain at the table.

For behavioral researchers it is not enough to observe and speculate on a functional relationship between behavior and environmental events. Rather they follow-up these speculations with systematic verification of the hypothesis. Thus they will manipulate the environment in order to determine what effect this manipulation has on the behavior. For example, Iwata, Dorsey, Slifer, Bauman, and Richman (1982) conducted a functional analysis of SIB. These investigators systematically manipulated aspects of the environment of self-injurious children and found that the effects were highly individualized. Thus, for example, one child's SIB might serve the function of avoiding task demands (i.e., it was an avoidance behavior) whereas another child's SIB served the function of getting attention. The sometimes highly idiosyncratic functional relationship between behavior and environmental events emphasizes the importance of assessing these relationships on a case-by-case basis if necessary. The accumulation of information from these analyses is very important for the continual improvement of behavioral treatment techniques because it provides an informed basis for identifying potential treatments. To illustrate, the accumulated literature on SIB suggests that there are three well-established learned motivations for the behavior: positive attention, escape/avoidance, and self-stimulation (e.g., Carr, 1977; Iwata et al., 1982). (It should also be acknowledged, however, that reduction of SIB resulting from administration of pharmacological agents [e.g., opiate antagonists such as naltrexone] suggests the possibility of organic factors in the manifestation of SIB in some cases.)

## BEHAVIORAL ASSESSMENT

As might be expected, in order to determine the important functional relationships between behavior and environmental events, the behavioral approach is very dependent upon accurate and reliable assessment of both behaviors and the specific environmental events to be studied. Behaviors must be defined in an objective, behavioral, observable manner such that there is no doubt whether or not the behavior occurred and at what strength. Thus, rather than say a child is "highly aggressive," we would specifically define "aggression" as "child hits, kicks other children, or pulls another child's hair." We would then be interested in the frequency with which these aggressive behaviors occurred. For example, do they occur three times an hour, or four times a week, and so forth? Other behaviors might be measured in terms of their duration (e.g., length of tantrum), or latency (number of seconds that elapse between presentation of broccoli and child leaving the table). Similarly, we require the same objective assessment for environmental events. Saying that Johnny gets "attention" for throwing a tantrum is not adequate. "Attention" may be behaviorally defined as "mother verbally soothes the child ("Don't be upset, Johnny") and/or gives the child a preferred item such as a cookie or access to the backyard.

Careful and accurate assessment is a hallmark feature of behavioral treatment. We are not only dependent upon such assessment for the determination of our behaviors and environmental events but also for our determination of the effectiveness of our intervention. For this reason behavioral researchers and clinicians continuously monitor behavior in order to determine if the treatment we are using is having the desired effect. By obtaining an objective measure of the behavior, we are not likely to be influenced by subjective judgments. Thus, no matter what we think or what we want to occur, the data will tell us if our treatments are leading to increases in positive behavior, decreases in inappropriate behavior, no change in behavior, changes in nontreatment environments, maintenance of behavior over time, and the like. This prevents us from coming to the wrong conclusion and continuing to implement an ineffective treatment or prematurely abandoning an effective one.

## SPECIFIC BEHAVIORAL PROCEDURES

Remediating the specific behavioral excesses and deficits exhibited by children with autism has typically involved utilizing those learning principles known to affect the strength of operant (voluntary) behavior. Specifically, behavioral excesses are treated using principles known to decrease the strength of operants, and behavioral deficits are treated using principles known to establish and increase the strength of operants. When we wish to address a particular behavior we can do so from two sides. We can alter the consequences of the behavior, or we can alter the preceding events that serve as a cue for the behavior. To relate this to our discussion above, we can manipulate the *antecedents* (known as discriminative stimuli), or we can manipulate the *consequences*. Although the majority of the established behavioral techniques focus on the alteration of consequent events, there is a growing body of very important literature addressing the alteration of antecedents. We will address both of these approaches.

## Manipulating Consequences

There are several ways in which one can change the strength of a behavior by manipulating the consequences. If one wishes to *establish* a behavior of *increase* its strength, one may use positive reinforcement or negative reinforcement. Let us look at some examples of the use of these procedures with the autistic population.

### Positive Reinforcement

This refers to the strengthening of an operant behavior by following that behavior with a positive event (positive reinforcer). For example, Lovaas, Berberich, Perloff, and Schaeffer (1966) demonstrated that they could teach nonverbal children with autism a therapist's vocalization by providing a bit of favored food immediately after (and contingent upon) the child's correct response. As the investigators continued reinforcing the vocal imitation in this manner, the children became more and more adept at imitation. Once established, this imitation served as the cornerstone in building more complex language functions, such as semantics and syntax (Lovaas, 1966, 1977; Risley & Wolf, 1967).

### Negative Reinforcement

This refers to the strengthening of an operant behavior by following that behavior with the escape or avoidance of a negative event (negative reinforcer). Carr, Newsom, and Binkoff (1976) demonstrated that one child's SIB was strengthened by negative reinforcement. Specifically, the child did not like to be confronted with task demands such as those presented by a teacher. The child learned that if he hit himself the teacher stopped the demands. Carr et al. (1976) showed that for this child the escape or avoidance of an aversive event (demands) served to strengthen the SIB.

### Prompting

Although the procedures above can strengthen an existing behavior, sometimes the behavior does not exist at all in the child's repertoire and must first be established. There are several ways in which reinforcement can be used to establish new behaviors. Prompting refers to a procedure where the individual is guided to perform the response. This can be done by physically manipulating the individual such as holding the lips together to help form the "mm" sound during language training or assisting the child in pulling up her pants when teaching dressing skills. Other forms of prompts include such techniques as pointing to the correct answer in a discrimination task or exaggerating the size of the correct stimulus when teaching the task "circle" versus "square." The only requirement for prompts is that they be functional in leading to the correct performance of the behavior (i.e., they must work) and that they ultimately be removed or "faded" so that the individual can perform the response unprompted.

## Shaping

Another procedure commonly used to teach a new response is shaping. Basically, shaping involves reinforcing successive approximations to the target response until the response is established. The Lovaas (1966) study cited above is a good example of the use of shaping. In teaching the mute children to imitate vocal responses, the investigators first reinforced any sound made by the child immediately following the model of the therapist. As the children became more reliable in making sounds at the right time, the therapist waited until the sound was a little more like the modeled sound. Gradually, the therapist reinforced sounds that more and more closely approximated the target sound until the child was reliably imitating the correct sound. Later, the individual sounds were put together to form words. Shaping was used here because the therapist might have had to wait forever for the child to spontaneously say the word so that it could be strengthened by positive reinforcement. Using shaping, however, the therapist was able to establish the target response.

## Chaining

Yet another way in which a complex target behavior can be established is by chaining. In this procedure, the desired behavior is broken down into individual steps, and the steps are taught one by one, in sequence, until the complex behavior occurs. For example, if one wishes to teach a child to pull up his pants when told "pants up," it is much easier and more reliable to use chaining than to wait for the child to spontaneously emit the sequence so that it can be reinforced. Thus, a therapist might first teach the child to hold onto a pair of pants when told "pants up" and reinforce this response. When the child will reliably do this, the therapist might move on to teach the second step in the sequence. The child might be required to hold the pants and to put them down by his feet. This two-step sequence is now reinforced. Once established, the therapist moves on to the third step and requires the child to hold the pants, put them by his feet, and put one foot through one leg hole, etc. This process is continued until the child has completed the entire sequence and puts on the pants when instructed to do so. This example describes *forward* chaining in which the first response in the sequence is taught first and the last step is taught last. One might also choose to employ *backward* shaping wherein the last step in the sequence is taught first and the sequence is taught backward. Both forms of chaining are effective.

Although the above procedures are aimed at establishing new behaviors or strengthening existing ones, there are other uses of consequences designed to *decrease* and/or *eliminate* behaviors that are undesirable. These include extinction, punishment, and response cost.

## Extinction

Probably the most commonly used procedure to decrease a behavior is extinction wherein a behavior that has previously been followed by positive reinforcement is no longer followed by the positive event. For example, many children (with or without autism) learn to throw tantrums to gain attention or to otherwise manipulate the adults around them. A child might cry and scream for mother's attention or perhaps to get her to give in when she has said "no" to a request for a cookie or perhaps to get people to leave him alone. Typically the tantrum behavior is reinforced by the consequence the environment provides (e.g., attention, a cookie, being left alone). Using extinction, the parent or other care-giver ensures that the reinforcement is no longer provided. Thus the mother does not attend to the child, or give the cookie, or leave the child alone. Under these circumstances we would expect to see the behavior decrease. Two characteristics of extinction are important. First, at the onset of the extinction procedure there will be a temporary increase in the strength of the behavior (called an extinction "burst") as the child tries harder to reinstate the reinforcement. But after this temporary increase the behavior will decrease. Second, with extinction the behavior does not decrease immediately, but does so gradually. Lovaas and Simmons (1969) clearly demonstrated the effectiveness of extinction to decrease SIB. Two boys engaged in high rates of self-injury and had done so for many years. Typically, the environment of these boys (state institutions) treated the SIB by putting the children in restraints and providing attention in the form of soothing comments. Lovaas and Simmons used extinction wherein each boy was allowed to engage in the SIB and no one provided attention of any kind. The children were alone in a room (although constantly under observation). These investigators demonstrated that under the extinction procedure the boys gradually ceased to hit themselves. (It should be noted here that the investigators had established that during the extinction procedure the children would not do serious harm to them-selves). In another study, cited earlier, Carr et al. (1976) demonstrated that one child's SIB was maintained by the escape or avoidance of aversive stimuli. The child had learned that if he hit himself when presented with a demand (e.g., a teacher's instruction) the demand situation would be terminated or avoided (i.e., negative reinforcement). Because the SIB was reinforced by the removal of the demand, extinction could have been implemented by continuing to present the demands even though the child was engaging in SIB.

## Punishment

Although extinction is often the method of choice to reduce behavior, it is sometimes the case that extinction cannot be arranged or that the behavior is too dangerous or detrimental to allow to decrease gradually. In these cases one will typically use a form of punishment. Punishment is a rather unfortunate term in learning theory because it really just describes a procedure in learning yet it does have a rather unpleasant colloquial meaning. When behavior modifiers speak of punishment, they are merely describing a situation where the occurrence of an undesirable behavior is followed by an event the individual finds aversive. This event can be anything from a frown or gentle "no" to more severe aversives such as a loud "NO" or a spank, and so forth. In fact anything can be a punisher if the individual does not like it. If a child hates candy, then candy could serve as a punisher.

## Punishment by Application

One common form of punishment is a situation in which a behavior is followed by the presentation of an aversive stimulus. This is sometimes referred to as punishment by application. For example, in the Lovaas and Simmons (1969) study cited above, these investigators demonstrated how punishment in the form of a brief, localized, contingent electric shock rapidly suppressed SIB in three children who had extensive histories of self-injury and who had not responded to other treatments. Immediately after the occurrence of an SIB act, a therapist said "No!", and the child received a brief shock to the leg. It took only one or two of these shocks to completely suppress the behavior. The suppressive effect of the treatment did not spontaneously generalize across people or environments, and the investigators had to program shock in different environments and by different people, but the suppression of the SIB allowed these children to be free of mechanical restraints and to learn alternative, more appropriate behaviors with which to manipulate their environment. Although this study clearly illustrates the effective use of a punishment procedure, it is important to emphasize that much less severe forms of aversive stimuli in a punishment paradigm have been used, and in fact these milder forms of punishment are the more common. To illustrate,

SIB has been effectively treated using water mist (Dorsey, Iwata, Ong, & McSween, 1980) and aversive odors (Tanner & Zeiler, 1975) as the contingent aversive stimulus.

## Overcorrection

Another form of punishment, called overcorrection, has also been used effectively with a variety of populations including children with autism (Azrin, Gotlieb, Hughart, Wesolowski, & Rahn, 1975; Azrin, Kaplan, & Foxx, 1973). This procedure also uses presentation of a contingent aversive stimulus, although it avoids physical aversives. Briefly, this procedure involves having the child engage in effortful behavior (aversive stimulus) contingent upon the target behavior excess. For example, a child who engages in self-stimulatory arm movements might be required to spend 15 minutes practicing exercises with his/her hands such as holding them up, holding them down, holding them out to the side, and repeating this sequence. This procedure involves an aversive event but also can be seen as teaching the child other, more appropriate, arm movements.

## Punishment by Withdrawal

Although the above forms of punishment involve the application of an aversive stimulus, another form of punishment involves the contingent removal or avoidance of a positive stimulus. This is sometimes referred to as punishment by withdrawal or response cost. Probably an example that is familiar to most of us if the mother who sends her child to bed without dinner after the child has committed some offense. Contingent upon an inappropriate behavior the child loses positive reinforcers that were otherwise available (i.e., dinner and various afterdinner activities such as TV, etc.).

## Time-Out

This is another example of this type of punishment, and it is one of the most frequently used procedures to decrease behavior. With time-out the occurrence of inappropriate behavior is followed by the removal of the child from an opportunity to receive any positive reinforcement for a period of time (White, Nielsen, & Johnson, 1972). It is an effective, but relatively mild, punishment technique. Wolf, Risley, and Mees (1964) provided an early example of the use of this procedure. They worked with a child with autism who exhibited tantrums and SIB. These disruptive behaviors were effectively reduced by placing the child alone in a room each time the behavior occurred. Two points are very important to remember when using time-out. First, one must pay attention to the duration of the time-out period. Although durations of 2 minutes (Bostow & Bailey, 1969) to 3 hours (Burchard & Tyler, 1965) have been used successfully, durations in the range of 5 to 20 minutes are most often used. Second (and this is a point many people forget) is that time-out is only likely to be effective if the "time-in" setting is more reinforcing than the time-out setting (Solnick, Rincover, & Peterson, 1977). Thus it may be the case that sending a child to her room may not be an effective procedure if the child does not enjoy being with the family. This child may actually prefer the solitude of the room in which case it would not be an effective punisher.

## Manipulating Antecedents

As mentioned earlier, it is also possible, and in some cases more efficient, to change behaviors by altering their antecedents instead of their consequences. This, of course, obviates the necessity of applying aversive consequences. Antecedents are stimulus events (discriminative stimuli) that function to control behavior because they promise particular consequences for responding. For example, a ringing telephone is an antecedent (discriminative stimulus) for picking up the instrument and saying "Hello" because of the promised consequences of someone talking to us on the other end of the line. We would be unlikely to pick up a phone and say "Hello" if the phone were not ringing because a silent phone does not promise the consequence of someone talking to us. Similarly, all of our operant behavior is under the control of these antecedents and by manipulating them, we can alter the behavior.

Touchette, MacDonald, and Langer (1985) provided an excellent and important example of how the severely aggressive and self-injurious behavior of developmentally disabled individuals could be effectively controlled and eliminated by manipulating antecedents. These investigators pointed out that the disruptive behavior of these individuals occurred under some stimulus conditions but not under others. Thus, the child might engage in aggression or SIB when demands are placed upon him but almost never engage in these severe behaviors while watching television, eating, or bathing. Touchette et al. (1985) propose that certain stimulus conditions become discriminative (i.e., cues) for disruptive behavior, and other stimulus conditions do not. With this being the case, the clinician or researcher can immediately reduce the frequency of the disruptive behavior to zero (or near zero) by programming events such that none of the cues for the behavior are presented. Thus, to continue our example, the child's day could be filled with watching TV, bathing, and eating, and be devoid of situations where demands were made on him. Such a program should lead to long periods of no disruptive behavior. Situations that once led to SIB and aggression (e.g., demands) would then be gradually reintroduced in such a way that they no longer evoke the disruptive behavior. The obvious advantage of this treatment approach is that it may be possible to immediately gain control over severely disruptive behavior without the use of a contingent aversive stimulus. The potential limitations to this approach are (1) it is not always feasible to program an individual's environment such that cues for the disruptive behavior are never provided and only cues for nondisruptive behaviors are provided, (2) it may not always be possible to identify the functional environmental cues, and (3) individuals might not always respond to the same cues in the same manner. Yet, the technique obviously holds great promise as a means of achieving immediate control over behavior.

Carr et al. (1976) provided another example of the use of altering antecedents to change behavior. These investigators were working with Tim, a child with autism whose face slapping was reliably cued by teaching situations in which demands (e.g., "Touch your shoe," "Point to the window") were made. The investigators first established that demands were discriminative for the SIB by showing that SIB reliably followed demands and did not follow nondemand vocalizations such as "The walls are white" or "It's sunny today." Next, the investigators altered the demands such that they no longer were presented in the same manner as before. Rather, the experimenter told short stories to the child and occasionally stopped and presented a demand, then began telling the story again. Embedding the demand in a positive context effectively led to Tim's compliance with the demand and greatly reduced his SIB. Because the demands were normally presented in a teaching situation where they were presented one after another, this embedding the demands within nondemands effectively changed the stimulus situation such that it did not cue the SIB. To follow up the Carr et al. (1976) study, one would probably design a treatment procedure in which the teacher would *gradually* introduce more demands between nondemands until the child would tolerate an appropriate teaching situation.

## Programming Generalization and Maintenance of Behavior Change

One characteristic of children with autism that is not surprising is that it is extremely difficult to teach them new behaviors. Over the years behavioral treatment has demonstrated an admirable ability to decrease behavioral excesses and to establish and increase new behaviors and behaviors that occur at a deficient level. As a matter of fact, much of the early work in the behavioral arena was focused on establishing these behavior changes, and we were quite busy patting ourselves on the back for our success and ingenuity in accomplishing these goals. Unfortunately, however, our early successes had one important limitation. When behavioral researchers broadened their assessments to look at generalization and maintenance of the treatment effects, the results were disappointing. All too often these generalization effects were minimal or nonexistent.

Children with autism are notorious for displaying problems in generalization, and one need only ask a teacher or parent for examples of this failure to generalize. Typically the child will learn a behavior such as labeling body parts and perform this perfectly at school but will fail to label body parts when the parents ask at home. All types of generalization are affected. The child fails to show *stimulus generalization* in a situation such as that described above when a behavior (e.g., labeling body parts) is learned in one setting (e.g., school) but fails to be exhibited in another setting (e.g., home) or with other people (e.g., parents). Failure of *response generalization* is evident when the child learns a specific behavior (e.g., walk across the street when the signal is green) but fails to generalize to another related behavior (e.g., ride the bike across the street when the signal is green). Problems in *temporal generalization,* or maintenance, are evident when the child learns a behavior but will not exhibit the behavior after a period of time.

As soon as the problems of generalization of treatment effects with these children became evident, behavioral researchers began to address the problem. The first approach adopted was to incorporate those procedures known to enhance generalization with nonautistic populations into treatment programs for individuals with autism. Although a discussion of the many, many generalization strategies that have employed with individuals with autism is beyond the scope of this chapter, some of the most commonly used strategies can be briefly described here. For more discussion of generalization strategies with autistic individuals, the interested reader is referred to Horner, Dunlap, and Koegel (1988), Schreibman (1988), Schreibman (1990), and Stokes and Baer (1977).

One strategy for facilitating generalization of behavior change is to make the treatment environment similar to the natural (generalization) environment (Stokes & Baer, 1977). One way to accomplish this is to use *intermittent schedules of reinforcement* during the treatment. This presents an atmosphere that is more like the natural environment where behaviors are seldom reinforced on a continuous reinforcement schedule. In such cases, the new behavior may be established using continuous reinforcement but is then gradually shifted to an intermittent schedule (where every response is not reinforced) so that it is more difficult for the child to discriminate the treatment from the nontreatment environment. This enhances stimulus generalization (e.g., Koegel & Rincover, 1977) and maintenance of treatment gains, allowing naturally occurring intermittent reinforcers to "take over" in natural environments.

Using *naturally maintaining contingencies* (natural reinforcers) during treatment will also make the treatment resemble nontreatment settings (e.g., Stokes & Baer, 1977). Here it is important that the reinforcers used in the training setting are similar to those that are available in generalization settings and that the behaviors taught are those likely to earn these reinforcers. For example, Carr

(1980) taught children with autism to use sign language to request items they were likely to find outside the treatment environment and that had reinforcing value to them (e.g., food and toys). This resulted in the generalization of spontaneous signing for these items because signing was reinforced in the natural environment by the presentation of the preferred items.

One can also enhance generalization by directly training generalized responding. *Sequential modification* is a procedure in which generalization is programmed in every situation where it does not spontaneously occur. Nordquist and Wahler (1973) trained the parents of a child with autism in a clinic setting to increase the child's compliance and teach imitative skills. Once the behaviors were trained in the clinic setting and it was determined that the skills had not generalized to the home, the parents implemented their trained skills in the home. Treatment gains then generalized from the clinic to the home environment. A related procedure, *training sufficient exemplars,* involves training sufficient behavior examples or in sufficient settings to lead to generalization across other, untrained, examples. Schreibman and Carr (1978) taught children who exhibited echolalia to use the generalized response "I don't know" when confronted with a verbal stimulus to which they could not respond. These investigators trained several examples of such stimuli (e.g., "Where is Cincinnati?", "What is a zebra?") until the children would answer "I don't know" to new, untrained examples.

In addition, researchers and clinicians have found that generalization can be enhanced by incorporating treatment in extended settings. Thus, providing treatment via *classroom settings* and *parent training* has had a major and positive impact on the effectiveness and generalization of treatment effects. Although these means of facilitating generalization have been widely addressed in the literature, their discussion is beyond the scope of this chapter, and the interested reader is referred to Dangel and Poster (1984), Horner et al. (1986), Koegel, Rincover, and Egel (1982), and Schreibman (1988).

## Formulating Treatment Combinations

In order to clearly present the basic behavioral principles, the examples described above have typically involved only one procedure. In reality, as is probably apparent, treatment usually involves combinations of the above procedures. Thus punishment procedures should never be used in the absence of positive programming to teach alternative behaviors. As mentioned above, when Lovaas and Simmons (1969) effectively reduced the SIB in their subjects the children could now learn other, more appropriate, ways to manipulate their environment. Language training was begun to teach the children to communicate their desires in a more acceptable fashion. This is a good example of procedures working hand in hand. The language training could not have been conducted unless the SIB was stopped, and the SIB will only remain suppressed if the children can communicate their desires in a non-SIB manner.

The development of a treatment plan for an individual child or adult with autism involves the identification of behavioral excesses and deficits, an analysis of environmental determinants of the behaviors, decisions on the various techniques to be used to address these excesses and deficits, and continual monitoring of treatment effects. The effectiveness of the entire intervention plan depends on the skill of the treatment provider in effectively using all of these aspects of treatment.

## CURRENT ISSUES AND TRENDS IN THE BEHAVIORAL TREATMENT OF AUTISM

As mentioned at the beginning of this chapter, the effectiveness of behavioral treatment for the autistic population is not really in doubt. Over 30 years of empirical support testify to the effectiveness of this form of treatment. However, true to its basis in experimental psychology and its reliance on continual assessment and evaluation of effects, behavioral treatment has identified areas in need of further research and clarification. The identification of areas in which we require further information is the first step in focusing our research efforts on further improving and refining the treatments that we can make available to these severely handicapped children and their families. The issues to be discussed below are three of the areas receiving the most attention at the current time. Although there are other issues being addressed by behavioral researchers, the following are particularly timely.

### Use of Aversive Procedures

Although punishment procedures are effective for reducing or eliminating a variety of inappropriate and disruptive behaviors, the fact remains that the issue of punishment is a rather emotionally charged one. It is important to emphasize again that when a behavioral clinician or researcher uses the term *punishment,* he/she is referring to a particular relationship between behavior and the contingent environmental event. The nature of the event does not have to be a physical aversive; rather the only quality it must have is that the individual to whom it is presented finds it aversive. In fact, for a child with autism it may well be that a kiss, hug, or caress is a punisher because the child may find each of these aversive.

The issue of using aversives in treatment programs for autistic and other populations is an emotional one and one that has very vocal proponents on both sides. Some question the ethics of imposing any form of aversive procedure to these individuals, whereas others hold the position that it would be unethical to withhold effective treatments involving aversives, particularly if no nonaversive procedure is available or if nonaversive procedures have failed to reduce a severely disruptive behavior. The basic issue is further complicated by smaller issues such as the definition of "aversive." Do we mean only physical aversives such as contingent electric shock, a spank, contingent restraint? Do we mean anything that the individual might find aversive such as a frown, being told "no," time-out? Obviously some stimuli and procedures are more acceptable than others, but the more global issue of causing the individual to experience some form of unpleasantness remains.

There are other issues of which one must be aware when considering the use of punishment. First, punishment serves only to suppress, not eliminate, a behavior. It is therefore very important to teach the child another behavior to replace the inappropriate behavior if one wishes the suppression to be maintained. For example, if a child has been engaging in SIB for the positive attention it provides, one might consider using the punishment procedure to gain temporary control over this serious behavior and during the suppression period teach the child another, more appropriate, behavior for attention (e.g., talking, playing). Second, there has been an increasing focus in recent years on the promotion of nonaversive interventions in the treatment of autistic and other individuals (Horner, Dunlap, Koegel, Carr, Sailor, Anderson, Albin, & O'Neill, 1990). As noted above, punishment is defined functionally so that whether a stimulus is aversive or not is determined by its effect on the behavior upon which it is contingent. There is nothing inherent in the technical definition of punishment that denotes pain. When considering interventions, the rule of thumb is that the least intrusive effective treatment should be employed. One needs to respect the dignity of the client and choose those procedures likely to facilitate the individual's integration into society, as opposed to segregating him/her by instituting an aversive procedure that serves to stigmatize or to reduce the opportunities to participate in society. Third, although punishment procedures have been shown to be effective, issues relating to the use of these procedures in community settings have not been adequately addressed to date, and we must do so if we are to provide our most effective treatments in such settings.

Unfortunately, the bottom line is that we do not yet have a complete technology of nonaversive procedures (e.g., NIH, 1989). Although this is the ultimate goal toward which behavioral researchers strive, the fact remains that there are some behavior problems in certain situations that can only be effectively treated using some form of aversive procedure (e.g., Linsheid, Iwata, Ricketts, Williams, & Griffin, 1990). The fact also remains, however, that some of these procedures cannot be arranged in some treatment settings (e.g., some community or school placements), and thus the need to develop alternative treatments becomes even more pressing. Importantly, if one looks at the behavioral literature over the past 30 years, one can see that the continual refinement of techniques has to a large extent involved the development of less aversive procedures and the concomitant development of nonaversive techniques. The work on altering antecedents (Touchette et al., 1985; Carr et al., 1976) provides an excellent example of work along these lines. Similarly, one is less likely to find studies using electric shock or other strong aversive stimuli. Instead, studies addressing some of the more severe behavior excesses exhibited by autistic and other handicapped populations are now more likely to investigate more "mild" aversives or nonaversives. These very same severe behaviors in the past might have been treated using much stronger aversives.

It is the goal of every behavioral researcher to avoid the use of aversives whenever possible and to strive toward the development of nonaversive treatments. One must be concerned with preserving the rights and the dignity of the individual. However, we must also be concerned with maximizing the opportunities available for the individual to participate as fully as possible in the community and society. It may be the case that if the only currently effective treatment for a behavior involves an aversive, and we do not make the treatment available, we may be denying the individual their right to a full and happy life in society.

## Current Issues in Generalization

Earlier in this chapter we briefly discussed characteristic problems in generalization often exhibited in autism and the application of behavioral procedures to enhance generalization effects. Although these procedures are the same as those used with any populations, recently new techniques have been developed that hold promise for enhancing generalization and greatly broadening our treatment effects. Let us look at these new strategies.

Focusing on response generalization, Carr and his colleagues have emphasized looking at the function of aggressive and other disruptive behavior on the child's environment (e.g., Carr, 1988). These investigators have speculated that for autistic and other severely language-impaired children, disruptive behaviors may have a communicative function. There are a number of ways in which a person can communicate needs and wishes, and only some of these involve language as we normally consider it. Carr and Durand (1985a) suggest there is a relationship between disruptive behaviors and the person's ability to communicate and further suggest that it may be useful to view behavior problems as a primitive form of communication. Following a functional analysis of the behavior, the treatment provider may proceed to teach verbal skills designed to communicate the same meaning as the problem behavior. To illustrate, Carr, Schreibman, and Lovaas (1975) demonstrated that one apparent function of immediate echolalia was to communicate that the child did not have a response to the verbal stimulus presented by another person. When asked "What's your name?", the child might correctly say "Rita," but if asked "Who's the President?", the child would likely echo the question because the President's name was unknown or the child did not comprehend what was being asked. In a subsequent investigation, Schreibman and Carr (1978) taught children a verbal skill (saying "I don't know") when confronted with a verbal stimulus to which they had no response. This effectively replaced the echolalic responding to unknown stimuli. Response generalization was accomplished because the echolalia decreased with the "I-don't-know" training even though echolalia was not directly treated. Carr and Durand (1985b) in a rather remarkable demonstration, showed that a child's aggressive behavior could be conceptualized as the child's way of communicating that he did not wish to engage in a particular activity, that the activity was too difficult, and so on. By teaching the child to say "Help me," the child's communicative intent was achieved in a more appropriate manner, and the reinforcement he received for the speech maintained the language skill. The aggressive behavior decreased although it was never directly targeted. Thus the problem behavior and communicative intent were *functionally equivalent,* and one response could be replaced by another. This area of *functional equivalence training* is a particularly exciting line of research and one holding great promise for the development of treatment procedures to enhance generalization.

Another new strategy and one that may hold promise for extensive and effective generalization is the teaching of *"pivotal" target behaviors.* Pivotal behaviors are ones that affect widespread changes in other behaviors. It is obvious that treatment of children with autism would be more effective and efficient it if focused on a few of these pivotal behaviors instead of a myriad of individual target behaviors. A substantial body of research (Koegel & Mentis, 1985; Lovaas, Koegel, & Schreibman, 1979) has implicated two such central behaviors in the failure of treatment gains to generalize. These two behaviors are *motivation* and *responsivity to multiple cues.*

Anyone who works with children with autism is familiar with their severe problems in motivation. They are rarely motivated to learn new behaviors nor to generalize those behaviors that they have learned. Because of this motivation problem, and the failure of these children to respond to such "normal" reinforcers as affection and the approval of others, researchers have in the past had to resort to artificial reinforcers such as food and avoidance of pain (Schreibman, 1988). We know that if we can increase the children's motivation (even if we must use these artificial reinforcers), we do see an increase in learning and performance. Thus, it seems reasonable to expect that increases in motivation will lead to improvement over a broad range of behaviors.

Children with autism are also well known for their attention deficits, specifically their failure to respond to simultaneous multiple cues (e.g., Schreibman, 1988; Lovaas et al., 1979). Many of these youngsters exhibit *stimulus overselectivity,* responding to an overly restricted range of cues in the environment. It is certainly not surprising that a child who has difficulty responding to simultaneous input would exhibit severe problems in learning and generalization. Rincover and Koegel (1975) presented a dramatic illustration of this problem. These investigators had therapists teach children to perform simple responses such as touching "nose" when so directed. After the children learned the response, a different therapist was brought in and asked the child to perform the same response. Several of the children failed to perform the behavior when asked by the new therapist. Subsequent analysis revealed that these children's responses had come under control of a very limited, and usually irrelevant, stimulus in the original teaching situation. For example, one child's responses came under the control of a particular hand movement of the original therapist. Because the new (generalization) therapist did not use this idiosyncratic movement, the cue controlling the behavior was absent, and the child did not perform the response. Basically the child had not learned to respond to the verbal instruction "touch your nose" but rather to a particular, irrelevant, hand movement that accompanied the instruction.

Based on the findings described above, it is apparent that problems in motivation and responsivity may be responsible for a variety of the behavioral deficits seen in autism. Accordingly, it seems reasonable to assume that a treatment package comprised of specific procedures previously identified as effective in increasing motivation and procedures shown to increase the children's responsivity to multiple cues might lead to widespread generalization and maintenance of treatment effects. Recent research has indeed focused on training these pivotal target behaviors.

Schreibman, Koegel, and their colleagues (Koegel, Koegel, & Schreibman, 1991; Koegel & Schreibman, 1977; Koegel, O'Dell, & Koegel, 1987; Laski, Charlop, & Schreibman, 1988; Schreibman, Charlop, & Koegel, 1982; Schreibman, Koegel, & Koegel, 1989) have demonstrated that utilization of these motivation- and responsivity-enhancing procedures does lead to increased learning, more positive collateral behavior change, and increased generalization of learned behavior. Some of the procedures to enhance motivation include (1) allowing the child a good deal of control over the activities involved in training; (2) frequent variation of the learning tasks; (3) using direct (as opposed to indirect) reinforcers; (4) varying the reinforcers; and (5) reinforcing the child's attempts to respond (rather than only reinforcing correct responses). Koegel et al. (1987) found that a language training paradigm incorporating these elements was superior to a more structured, repetitive-practice, language training program in several dimensions of generalization, including increased use of appropriate, spontaneous, and generalized speech. In addition, we have developed procedures that are effective in teaching many children with autism to successfully utilize simultaneous multiple cues and thus improve their learning and generalization of acquired behavior. Basically, this is accomplished by training the child on a series of conditional discriminations (discriminations requiring response to simultaneous multiple cues) and after training on several of these tasks, the child begins to approach new discriminations by attending to multiple cues (Koegel & Schreibman, 1977; Schreibman et al., 1982). The findings from the studies cited above has allowed the development of a pivotal response training package (Koegel, Schreibman, Good, Cerniglia, Murphy, & Koegel, 1989) that focuses upon both increasing motivation and increasing responsivity to multiple cues.

Another relatively recent behavioral procedure to address the problem of generalization is training the children in *self-management* skills. By teaching the children to monitor, evaluate, and reinforce their own behavior we are placing the responsibility of treatment on the child (or adult) with autism rather than on the care provider. The child can thereby provide his/her own treatment in any environment he/she may enter. This certainly holds great potential for enhancing generalization. In addition, the acquisition of self-management skills serves to help the individual be more independent of other caretakers and increases the likelihood that he or she will be able to function independently in the community.

Using self-management procedures, the individual first learns to discriminate appropriate behavior from inappropriate behavior. Once this discrimination is established, the individual is taught to monitor the occurrence of his/her own appropriate (or inappropriate) behavior during a specified time interval. This may be done by having the person count the frequency of the behavior on a wrist counter or use a watch with a chronograph alarm that signals the passage of the interval and then record whether or not he or she has engaged in the behavior. Reinforcement is available for correct monitoring and correct responding. Intervals are gradually extended, and the treatment provider gradually fades him/herself from the setting until the child (or adult) can maintain his/her own behavior for long periods of time in the absence of supervision.

Self-management has been demonstrated to be effective in reducing the aberrant and stigmatizing behavior of people with mild to severe cognitive impairment (e.g., Dunlap, Dunlap, Koegel, & Koegel, 1991; Grace, Cowart, & Matson, 1988). In recent demonstrations with children with autism, it has been shown to be useful in accomplishing long-term and generalized reductions in self-stimulatory behavior (Koegel & Koegel, 1990), increasing appropriate play in unsupervised settings (Stahmer & Schreibman, 1992), improving social and disruptive behavior (Koegel, Koegel, Hurley, & Frea, 1992), teaching unsupervised performance of daily living skills (Pierce & Schreibman, in press), and increasing participation in family activities (Krantz, MacDuff, & McClannahan, 1993).

## The Expanding Role of Assessment

The behavioral approach to treatment has always emphasized the importance of careful and thorough assessment. As discussed at the beginning of this chapter, such assessment is crucial in the objective quantification of behaviors under study, functional analysis of important environmental variables, and for ongoing evaluation of treatment effectiveness. In recent years the area of assessment has been expanded to include a wide range of techniques that allow us to more accurately assess different types of behavior and to assess in more applied (as opposed to controlled experimental) environments. A particularly important innovation is a specific type of assessment that allows for increased information and for incorporating the values and perspective of the community within which we operate.

In taking responsibility for providing treatment to someone, there is an implicit set of decisions that are made. Behavioral practitioners, and indeed all treatment providers, end up making decisions as to what behaviors need to be changed, how they will be changed, and what criteria are used for determining treatment effectiveness. Because behavioral treatments have become so popular and because many severely handicapped populations receive such treatment, it stands to reason that one might question on what basis these decisions are made. Can a particular therapist determine what should be changed, how it will be changed, and whether the outcome of the treatment is successful? Does this particular therapist have the "right" to make these decisions? Does this particular therapist adhere to the same value system as the community when making such decisions? These are important questions and as behaviorists became more and more successful in changing behavior and as the techniques became more widespread, behavioral researchers and practitioners have developed a technology to gather information about the social acceptability of their efforts.

The behavioral treatment of autism has typically been considered successful if it can be shown that specific, objectively measured target behaviors change in a positive direction as a function of the treatment. Thus, we may measure treatment gains in terms of changes in the number of observed intervals in which a child engages in self-stimulation, psychotic speech, appropriate play, appropriate speech, and the like. We may also have information on changes in the frequency of SIB acts or aggressive episodes. Although we may be able to produce consistent and reliable changes in these specific behaviors, one can also ask just what is the significance of these behavioral changes in terms of more global judgment of the child's progress. After treatment is the child judged as more "normal," more "likable," less likely to be institutionalized, etc.? That is, can our objective measures of behavior change be correlated with subjective judgments of change provided by members of the community? Obviously, any form of treatment that cannot produce changes that are apparent to others cannot be said to be truly effective. In addition, what do members of the child's community feel are important behaviors to target for change? Also, how do members of the community feel about the procedures we use in our treatment? It is certainly the case that some treatments are more socially acceptable than others. The assessment of the social acceptability and significance of treatment effects, treatment targets, and treatment procedures is called *social validation* and has become an increasingly useful adjunct to objective assessment in evaluating and planning behavioral treatment programs (e.g., Kazdin, 1977; Schwartz & Baer, 1991; Wolf, 1978).

In the first of a series of investigations aimed at socially validating the effects of behavioral treatment of children with autism, Schreibman, Koegel, Mills, and Burke (1981) sought to determine the relationship between objective, observational measures of pre–post treatment change in the children and the subjective judgments of change formed of those children by untrained, naive observers. First, undergraduate college students viewed segments of videotapes showing the children interacting with their mothers in a room full of toys. These students were asked to write descriptions of the children. A rating scale consisting of 19 Likert-type items was derived from these descriptions encompassing the areas of language, social interactions, play, and behaviors such as restlessness, wandering attention, and repetitive behaviors. Following the development of the scale, five more groups of undergraduate students were asked to view (in randomized order) 5-minute videotape segments of 14 children with autism taken before behavioral treatment and after 6 months of treatment and to rate the children on the Likert-item scale. This scale provided a measure of the subjective impressions of the children.

To obtain the objective measures, two trained observers scored the same segments of videotape for the percentage of occurrence (across continuous 10-second intervals) of eight behaviors that are typically regarded as clinically important. These included self-stimulation, play, tantrums, appropriate language, psychotic language (e.g., echolalia), social nonverbal behavior, and noncooperation.

When the judges' subjective ratings were then correlated with the objective scoring by the trained observers, the investigators found a strong relationship between the two. That is, when looking at children who showed improvement on the behavioral measures from pre- to posttreatment, there was a significant corresponding increase in the judges' subjective impressions. On these measures, these children were seen as significantly more skilled in language, more socially desirable, and more likable at posttreatment than at pretreatment. In contrast, those children who showed very little or no gains in appropriate behavior on the behavioral measures were seen by the judges as unchanged or worse. In addition to this global result (that judges subjectively saw the changes in the children's behavior), it was found that there were high correlations between measured objective behaviors (e.g., "self-stimulation") and specific items on the Likert-type questionnaire (e.g., "Child engages in repetitious behavior"). These results clearly argue that the objectively measured changes in the behavior of the children are apparent to naive judges and that the specific behaviors focused upon for treatment are socially important.

The above study served as a demonstration that social validation technology could be a very useful and informative way to obtain information on the social significance of treatment outcome. However, further assessments were required because one could certainly argue that college undergraduate students are not the most relevant consumers of the treatment of children with autism. Using the same basic methodology as in the study cited above, Schreibman, Runco, Mills, and Koegel (1982) replicated the social validation of treatment with teachers making the subjective judgments. Elementary-school teachers perceived the efficacy of the behavioral treatment and, as with the undergraduate judges in the Schreibman et al. (1981) study, viewed the specific and global behaviors in a way that was similar to that of the trained observers using the objective scoring system. Another interesting finding of this second study was that certain behaviors (i.e., social behavior, cooperation) seemed to be especially significant in influencing the teachers' judgments about the children. Hence, these behaviors might be especially important treatment targets for change if we wish to influence the children's placement in educational settings.

Utilizing two extremely important groups of consumers of treatment for children with autism, parents and normal peers, Runco and Schreibman (1983, 1988) replicated these social validation assessments. Adapting the questionnaire and procedures according to the judges (parents or normal peers), these investigations found that (1) these groups rated the children as improved after treatment, and (2) the judges indicated more of a willingness to be close to, and to interact with, the child with autism after, as opposed to before, treatment.

Looking at another important aspect of social validation assessment, Runco and Schreibman (1987) focused on the social importance of various behaviors as *targets* of treatment. These investigators found that parents differed from teachers in those behaviors they viewed as most in need of change. The parents, for example, did not consider aberrant speech to be a very important focus of treatment as compared to other behaviors. However, teachers rated speech as a more important target for treatment. Because we know that language skill is highly correlated with treatment prognosis, Runco and Schreibman's (1987) finding might indicate the importance of educating the parents about the significance of certain behaviors.

Social validation technology has also allowed us to determine other aspects of treatment effects, such as the affect of the treatment recipients and the treatment providers. Koegel, O'Dell, and Dunlap (1988) found that children with autism were judged to exhibit more positive affect (interest, enthusiasm, and happiness) when being taught language skills using a procedure to enhance motivation than they did when being taught the same skills using a more standard repetitive-practice procedure. Similarly, Schreibman, Kaneko, and Koegel (1991) found that parents exhibited more positive affect when using a pivotal response training package, as opposed to a repetitive practice program, when teaching their own children.

As can be seen, social validation can be extremely useful in determining the social significance of our treatments. In addition, it can be used as a guide to the development of treatment plans. Thus if we know which behaviors seem to be important in the judgments of those people who make major decisions about the autistic child's life, such as teachers and parents, we can direct our treatment efforts toward changing the behaviors. But perhaps the most critical aspect of social validation assessment is that it ensures that our efforts remain responsive to, and dictated by, the community within which we want these children to live.

## CONCLUDING COMMENTS

The goal of this chapter has been to familiarize the reader with some of the basic principles involved in the behavioral treatment of children with autism. The greatest strength of the behavioral approach is its foundation in, and emphasis on, objective empirical support for its direction. The principles involved have been derived from many years of extensive experimentation both in laboratory and applied settings. The continual testing has allowed for the refinement of techniques and guarantees that the field will move forward, increasing in efficacy and efficiency. This should put to rest the old arguments that behavioral treatments are simplistic and are only effective in changing relatively isolated behaviors. The breadth of the behaviors addressed in the behavioral approach and the increasing emphasis on more global behaviors (e.g., pivotal behaviors and generalization) well illustrate the comprehensive nature of the treatment targets and the treatment procedures now available and under study. Our discussion of current issues in the behavioral treatment of autism demonstrates the cutting edge today. There is likely to be major research in these areas, and the "cutting edge" of tomorrow will probably be very different. This is the mark of a dynamic, active, and progressive treatment modality.

ACKNOWLEDGMENT

Preparation of this chapter was facilitated by U.S.P.H.S. Research Grants MH 39434 and MH 28210 from the National Institute of Mental Health.

## REFERENCES

Azrin, N. J., Gottlieb, L., Weslowski, M. D., & Rahn, T. (1975). Eliminating self-injurious behavior by educative procedures. *Behaviour Research and Therapy, 13,* 110–111.
Azrin, N. J., Kaplan, S. J., & Foxx, R. H. (1973). Autism reversal: Eliminating stereotyped self-stimulation of retarded individuals. *American Journal of Mental Deficiency, 18,* 241–248.
Bettelheim, B. (1967). *The empty fortress.* New York: Free Press.

Bostow, D. E., & Bailey, J. B. (1969). Modification of severe disruptive and aggressive behavior using brief timeout and reinforcement procedures. *Journal of Applied Behavior Analysis, 2,* 31–38.

Burchard, J. D., & Tyler, V. O., Jr. (1965). The modification of delinquent behavior through operant conditioning. *Behaviour Research and Therapy, 2,* 245–250.

Carr, E. G. (1977). The motivation of self-injurious behavior: A review of some hypotheses. *Psychological Bulletin, 84,* 800–816.

Carr, E. G. (1979). Teaching autistic children to use sign language: Some research issues. *Journal of Autism and Developmental Disorders, 9,* 345–359.

Carr, E. G. (1979, November). Generalization of treatment effects following educational intervention with autistic children and youth. In B. Wilcox & A. Thompson (Eds.), *Critical issues in educating autistic children and youth* (pp. 118–134). U.S. Department of Education, Office of Special Education.

Carr, E. G. (1980). Sign Language. In O. I. Lovaas, A. Ackerman, D. Alexander, P. Firestone, M. Perkins, & D. Young (Eds.), *The me book: Teaching manual for parents and teachers of developmentally disabled children.* Baltimore: University Park.

Carr, E. G. (1988). Functional equivalence as a mechanism of response generalization. In R. H. Horner, G. Dunlap, & R. L. Koegel (Eds.), *Generalization and maintenance: Lifestyle changes in applied settings* (pp. 221–241). Baltimore: Paul H. Brookes.

Carr, E. G., & Durand, V. M. (1985a). The social-communicative basis of severe behavior problems in children. In S. Reiss & R. Bootzin (Eds.), *Theoretical issues in behavior therapy* (pp. 219–254). New York: Academic.

Carr, E. G., & Durand, V. M. (1985b). Reducing behavior problems through functional communication training. *Journal of Applied Behavior Analysis, 18,* 111–126.

Carr, E. G., Newsom, C. D., & Binkoff, J. A. (1976). Stimulus control of self-destructive behavior in a psychotic child. *Journal of Abnormal Child Psychology, 4,* 139–153.

Carr, E. G., Schreibman, L., & Lovaas, O. I. (1975). Control of echolalic speech in psychotic children. *Journal of Abnormal Child Psychology, 3,* 331–351.

Dangel, R. F., & Polster, R. A. (1984). *Parent training: Foundations of research and practice.* New York: Guilford.

Dorsey, M. F., Iwata, B. A., Ong, P., & McSween, T. E. (1980). Treatment of self-injurious behavior using a water mist: Initial response suppression and generalization. *Journal of Applied Behavior Analysis, 13,* 343–353.

Dunlap, G., Koegel, R. L., & O'Neill, R. E. (1985). Pervasive developmental disorders. In P. H. Bornstein & A. E. Kazdin (Eds.), *Handbook of clinical behavior therapy with children* (pp. 499–540). Homewood, IL: Dorsey.

Dunlap, L. K., Dunlap, G., Koegel, L. K., & Koegel, R. L. (1991). Using self-monitoring to increase students' success and independence. *Teaching Exceptional Children, 23,* 17–22.

Grace, N., Cowart, C., & Matson, J. L. (1988). Reinforcement and self-control for treating a chronic case of self-injury in Lesch-Nyhan Syndrome. *Journal of the Multihandicapped Person, 1,* 53–59.

Horner, R. H., Dunlap, G., & Koegel, R. L. (Eds.). (1988). *Generalization and maintenance: Lifestyle changes in applied settings.* Baltimore: Paul H. Brookes.

Horner, R. H., Dunlap, G., Koegel, R. L., Carr, E. G., Sailor, W., Anderson, J., Albin, R. W., & O'Neill, R. E. (1990). Toward a technology of "nonaversive" behavioral support. *The Journal of the Association for the Severely Handicapped, 15,* 125–132.

Horner, R. H., Meyer, L. H., & Fredericks, H. D. (Eds.). (1986). *Education of learners with severe handicaps: Exemplary service strategies.* Baltimore: Paul H. Brookes.

Iwata, B. A., Dorsey, M. F., Slifer, K. J., Bauman, K. E., & Richman, G. S. (1982). Toward a functional analysis of self-injury. *Analysis and Intervention in Developmental Disabilities, 2,* 3–20.

Kanner, L. (1943). Autistic disturbances of affective contact. *Nervous Child, 2,* 217–250.

Kazdin, A. E. (1977). Assessing the clinical or applied importance of behavior change through social validation. *Behavior Modification, 1,* 427–451.

Koegel, L. K., Koegel, R. L., Hurley, C., & Frea, W. D. (1992). Improving social and disruptive behavior in children with autism through self-management. *Journal of Applied Behavior Analysis, 25,* 341–354.

Koegel, R. L., & Koegel, L. K. (1990). Extended reductions in stereotypic behavior of students with autism through a self-management treatment package. *Journal of Applied Behavior Analysis, 23,* 119–127.

Koegel, R. L., Koegel, L. K., & Schreibman, L. (1991). Assessing and training parents in teaching pivotal behaviors. In R. J. Prinz (Ed.), *Advances in behavioral assessment of children and families* (pp. 65–82). Greenwich: JAI.

Koegel, R. L., & Mentis, M. (1985). Motivation in childhood autism: Can they or won't they? *Journal of Child Psychology and Psychiatry and Allied Disciplines, 26,* 185–191.

Koegel, R. L., O'Dell, M. C., & Dunlap, G. (1988). Producing speech use in nonverbal autistic children by reinforcing attempts. *Journal of Autism and Developmental Disorders, 18,* 525–538.

Koegel, R. L., O'Dell, M. C., & Koegel, L. K. (1987). A natural language teaching paradigm for nonverbal autistic children. *Journal of Autism and Developmental Disorders, 17,* 187–200.

Koegel, R. L., & Rincover, A. (1977). Research on the difference between generalization and maintenance in extra-therapy responding. *Journal of Applied Behavior Analysis, 10,* 1–12.

Koegel, R. L., Rincover, A., & Egel, A. L. (1982). *Educating and understanding autistic children.* Houston: College Hill.

Koegel, R. L., Russo, D. C., & Rincover, A. (1977). Assessing and training teachers in the generalized use of behavior modification with autistic children. *Journal of Applied Behavior Analysis, 10,* 197–205.

Koegel, R. L., Russo, D. C., Rincover, A., & Schreibman, L. (1982). Assessing and training teachers. In R. L. Koegel, A. Rincover, & A. L. Egel (Eds.), *Educating and understanding autistic children* (pp. 178–202). Houston: College Hill.

Koegel, R. L., & Schreibman, L. (1977). Teaching autistic children to respond to simultaneous multiple cues. *Journal of Experimental Child Psychology, 24,* 299–311.

Koegel, R. L., Schreibman, L., Britten, K. R., Burke, J. C., & O'Neill, R. E. (1982). A comparison of parent training to direct clinic treatment. In R. L. Koegel, A. Rincover, & A. L. Egel (Eds.), *Educating and understanding autistic children* (pp. 260–279). Houston: College Hill.

Koegel, R. L., Schreibman, L., Good, A. B., Cerniglia, L., Murphy, C., & Koegel, L. K. (1989). *How to teach pivotal behaviors to autistic children.* Santa Barbara: University of California.

Krantz, P. J., MacDuff, M. T., & McClannahan, L. E. (1993). Programming participation in family activities for children with autism: Parents' use of photographic activity schedules. *Journal of Applied Behavior Analysis, 26,* 137–138.

Laski, K. E., Charlop, M. H., & Schreibman, L. (1988). Training parents to use the Natural Language Paradigm to increase their autistic children's speech. *Journal of Applied Behavior Analysis, 21,* 391–400.

Linscheid, T. R., Iwata, B. A., Ricketts, R. W., Williams, D. E., & Griffin, J. C. (1990). Clinical evaluation of the Self-Injurious Behavior Inhibiting System (SIBIS). *Journal of Applied Behavior Analysis, 23,* 53–78.

Lovaas, O. I. (1966). A program for the establishment of speech in psychotic children. In J. K. Wing (Ed.), *Early childhood autism* (pp. 115–144). London: Pergamon.

Lovaas, O. I. (1977). *The autistic child.* New York: Irvington.

Lovaas, O. I., Berberich, J. P., Perloff, B. F., & Schaeffer, B. (1966). Acquisition of imitative speech in schizophrenic children. *Science, 151,* 705–707.

Lovaas, O. I., Koegel, R. L., & Schreibman, L. (1979). Stimulus overselectivity in autism: A review of research. *Psychological Bulletin, 86,* 1236–1254.

Lovaas, O. I., & Simmons, J. Q. (1969). Manipulation of self-destruction in three retarded children. *Journal of Applied Behavior Analysis, 2,* 143–157.

National Institutes of Health (1989). Treatment of destructive behaviors in persons with developmental disabilities. *Consensus Development Conference Statement,* September 11–13, 1989.

Nordquist, V. M., & Wahler, R. G. (1973). Naturalistic treatment of an autistic child. *Journal of Applied Behavior Analysis, 6,* 79–87.

O'Dell, S. L. (1985). Progress in parent training. In M. Hersen, R. M. Eisler, & P. M. Miller (Eds.), *Progress in behavior modification* (Vol. 19; pp. 57–108). New York: Academic.

Oke, N. J., & Schreibman, L. (1990). Training social initiations to a high-functioning autistic child: Assessment of collateral change and generalization in a case study. *Journal of Autism and Developmental Disorders, 20,* 479–497.

Pierce, K., & Schreibman, L. (in press). Teaching children with autism daily living skills in unsupervised settings through pictorial self-management. *Journal of Applied Behavior Analysis.*

Rincover, A., & Koegel, R. L. (1975). Setting generality and stimulus control in autistic children. *Journal of Applied Behavior Analysis, 8,* 235–246.

Risley, T. R., & Wolf, M. M. (1967). Establishing functional speech in echolalic children. *Behaviour Research and Therapy, 5,* 73–88.

Runco, M. A., & Schreibman, L. (1983). Parental judgments of behavior therapy efficacy with autistic children: A social validation. *Journal of Autism and Developmental Disorders, 13,* 237–248.

Runco, M. A., & Schreibman, L. (1987). Brief report: Socially validating behavioral objectives in the treatment of autistic children. *Journal of Autism and Developmental Disorders, 17,* 141–147.

Runco, M. A., & Schreibman, L. (1988). Children's judgments of autism and social validation of behavior therapy efficacy. *Behavior Therapy, 19,* 565–576.

Schreibman, L. (1988). *Autism.* Newbury Park, CA: Sage.

Schreibman, L. (1990). Autism: Issues in the generalization of treatment effects. In G. Mayfield & T. H. Ollendick (Eds.), *Postgraduate advances in autism disorder* (pp. 1–40). Berryville, VA: Forum Medicum.

Schreibman, L., & Carr, E. G. (1978). Elimination of echolalic responding to questions through the training of a generalized verbal response. *Journal of Applied Behavior Analysis, 11,* 453–463.

Schreibman, L., Charlop, M. H., & Koegel, R. L. (1982). Teaching autistic children to use extra stimulus prompts. *Journal of Experimental Child Psychology, 33,* 475–491.

Schreibman, L., Kaneko, W. M., & Koegel, R. L. (1991). Positive affect of parents of autistic children: A comparison across two teaching techniques. *Behavior Therapy, 22,* 479–490.

Schreibman, L., & Koegel, R. L. (1981). A guideline for planning behavior modification programs for autistic children. In S. M. Turner, K. S. Calhoun, & H. E. Adams (Eds.), *Handbook of clinical behavior therapy* (pp. 500–526). New York: Wiley.

Schreibman, L., Koegel, R. L., & Koegel, L. K. (1989). Autism. In M. Hersen (Ed.), *Innovations in child behavior therapy* (pp. 395–428). New York: Springer.

Schreibman, L., Koegel, R. L., Mills, D. L., & Burke, J. C. (1984). Training parent-child interactions. In E. Schopler & G. B. Mesibov (Eds.), *The effects of autism on the family* (pp. 187–205). New York: Plenum.

Schreibman, L., Koegel, R. L., Mills, J. I., & Burke, J. C. (1981). The social validation of behavior therapy with autistic children. *Behavior Therapy, 12,* 610–624.

Schreibman, L., O'Neill, R. I., & Koegel, R. L. (1983). Behavioral training for siblings of autistic children. *Journal of Applied Behavior Analysis, 16,* 129–138.

Schreibman, L., Runco, M. A., Mills, J. I., & Koegel, R. L. (1982). Teachers' judgments of improvements in autistic children in behavior therapy: A social validation. In R. L. Koegel, A. Rincover, & A. L. Egel (Eds.), *Educating and understanding autistic children* (pp. 78–87). Houston: College Hill Press.

Schwartz, E. F., & Baer, D. M. (1991). Social validity assessment: Is current practice state of the art? *Journal of Applied Behavior Analysis, 24,* 289–204.

Solnick, J. V., Rincover, A., & Peterson, C. R. (1977). Determinants of the reinforcing and punishing effects of time-out. *Journal of Applied Behavior Analysis, 10,* 415–428.

Stahmer, A. C., & Schreibman, L. (1992). Teaching children with autism appropriate play in unsupervised environments using a self-management treatment package. *Journal of Applied Behavior Analysis, 25,* 447–459.

Stokes, T. F., & Baer, D. M. (1977). An implicit technology of generalization. *Journal of Applied Behavior Analysis, 10,* 349–368.

Strain, P. S., & Fox, J. J. (1981). Peers as behavior change agents for withdrawn classmates. In B. B. Lahey & A. E. Kazdin (Eds.), *Advances in clinical child psychology* (vol. 4, pp. 167–198). New York: Plenum Press.

Tanner, B. A., & Zeiler, M. (1975). Punishment of self-injurious behavior using aromatic ammonia as the aversive stimulus. *Journal of Applied Behavior Analysis, 8,* 53–57.

Touchette, P. E., MacDonald, R. F., & Langer, S. N. (1985). A scatter plot for identifying stimulus control of problem behavior. *Journal of Applied Behavior Analysis, 18,* 343–351.

White, G. D., Nielsen, G., & Johnson, S. M. (1972). Time-out duration and the suppression of deviant behavior in children. *Journal of Applied Behavior Analysis, 5,* 111–120.

Wolf, M. M. (1978). Social validity: The case for subjective measurement or how applied behavior analysis is finding its heart. *Journal of Applied Behavior Analysis, 11,* 203–214.

Wolf, M. M., Risley, T. R., & Mees, H. (1964). Applications of operant conditioning procedures to the behavior problems of an autistic child. *Behaviour Research and Therapy, 1,* 305–312.

# 3

# Administrative Issues Involving Behavioral Approaches in Autism

## MICHAEL D. POWERS

Administrators and clinicians are becoming more aware that reliable, sophisticated, and effective behavior management technologies often are insufficient to implement and maintain changes in the challenging behavior of individuals with autism. As interventions have moved from highly controlled settings to the community, research and practice have been both expanded and complicated (Rappaport, 1977). Several writers have argued that attention to the organizational system with recognition of the social, cultural, political, and economic forces impacting those in the system is essential (Fisher, 1983; Greenblatt, 1983; Powers & Franks, 1988). Although it seems obvious that scientific inquiries in the applied arena must always be cognizant of these forces, it is more typically the case that such factors are systematically ignored. Sarason (1981) notes that the theories of individual change to which most human service professionals are exposed in their own training are insufficient for developing a coherent theory of systemic change.

Thus, the challenge for program administrators is to recognize and address the equivocal results of apparently sound intervention plans at the individual level and the organizational level by scrutinizing more closely the systemic factors interfering with effective intervention for challenging behavior in persons with autism. This chapter will describe administrative issues for consideration in

---

MICHAEL D. POWERS • Department of Psychology, Newington Children's Hospital, Newington, Connecticut 06111.

*Behavioral Issues in Autism*, edited by Eric Schopler and Gary B. Mesibov. New York, Plenum Press, 1994.

implementing behavior management programs to treat challenging behavior that address these systemic forces. Clinical and social considerations that guide intervention efforts will be described, and guidelines for promoting systemic change to support the responsive administration of intervention efforts will be provided.

## ADMINISTRATIVE CONSIDERATIONS IN IMPLEMENTING BEHAVIORAL PROGRAMS TO TREAT CHALLENGING BEHAVIOR

Service delivery settings for individuals with autism both generate and respond to social forces that must be considered if behavioral treatment of challenging behavior is to proceed successfully. Several authors (Liberman, 1979; Powers & Franks, 1988; Reppucci, 1973; Reppucci & Saunders, 1974) have described administrative problems confronting behavior therapists trying to establish and maintain behavioral programs in organizations. Each of these organizational constraints can impede the optional implementation of behavioral interventions to treat challenging problems in persons with autism. These issues include institutional constraints, limited resources, perceived inflexibility, external pressure, two populations, language, labeling, compromise, port-of-entry, existing staff, and political realities. Attention to organizational issues such as these facilitates consideration of impediments to the effective administration of behavioral programs, as well as insight into possible strategies to remediate these obstacles. Each impediment is discussed below.

### Institutional Constraints

Organizations, as living systems (Miller, 1978; Powers, 1988) operate with an implicit or explicit charter that has been established to guide decision making and behavior. In many human service organizations, the components or mandates within the charter are implicit and only broadly described in written policy statements. In others the organization's philosophy is well-articulated to its members and the public, both in writing and in practice. Where interventions for challenging behavior are congruent with implicit or explicit policies, little disruption occurs. When client needs or interventions proposed extend beyond those considered appropriate by the organization, constraints may be imposed administratively or procedurally by the organization to preserve those boundaries defined in the operating charter. In the latter case, negative effects on the intervention and outcomes may be evident.

## Limited Resources

Resource constraints on organizations are an all-too-familiar reality in human services. Although we typically think first of financial resources, it is important to consider others, including physical, personnel, and technological resources. For a long time it was assumed (erroneously) that an increase in financial resources was the solution to most problems concerning the treatment of children with autism. The theory that one can buy what one needs fails on three levels. First, it assumes incorrectly that superior resources (e.g., better teachers, better materials, better language simulators) exist within the marketplace in sufficient quantities to meet all needs. Second, it fails to account for administrative realities that govern competing requests for fiscal resource allocation including those from teacher unions or PTAs, or from existing physical-space constraints and institutional mandates that may override special education expenditures. Third, even when those new resources can be made available, administrative structures must be established to support and maintain their use. For example, the ability to hire a teacher specially trained in autism does not necessarily guarantee program success. That new teacher enters an existing organizational system that may value strategies different from his/her repertoire. For example, the author has been involved in school programs where teachers of typical children and other special needs' youngsters were personally challenged by the consistency and contingency of the teaching, behavior management, and data collection methods used by the newly arrived teacher of children with autism. If a teacher entering an existing organizational system is to succeed, administrative support in entering the system is essential.

## Perception of Inflexibility

Behavioral technology for treating challenging behavior has come a long way in a short time, and progress is evident in many areas. For most practitioners, however, the conflict between maintaining technological integrity or procedural fidelity and the organization's demands for compromise is a vexing problem. Behavioral consultants will often speak of consultees who complain that they have no time to gather formative or summative data. The resulting perceived inflexibility of behavior analysts (who reiterate the need for data) by others may stem from the behavior analyst's unwillingness to support intervention compromises that may dilute the desired outcome, or from perceived arrogance of the consultant by program staff. Although the former is understandable (perhaps even audible in certain circumstances), the latter is not. Realistic recognition by consultants of an organization's pace for change, and subsequent acceptance of successive approximations toward the intervention goal must be counterbalanced with the behavioral consultant's mandate to provide treatment that is empirically sound and carefully monitored.

## External Pressure

Organizations do not exist in a vacuum. Historical, political, and social interrelationships determine the particular ecology for the program, and by extension for the behavioral intervention. Although some organizations are sufficiently well-defined to have many constituencies and many views but one agenda, this is by no means the norm. Perhaps the sheer magnitude of problems presented by children with autism, coupled with the absence of any cure, promotes forceful exposition of different points of view. Although external *input* is valuable, even essential, to the development of a high-quality service system, external pressure can distract the organization from its stated purposes.

Behavioral interventions for challenging behavior have received substantial external scrutiny of late in two areas: (a) the extent to which the interventions use procedures considered "aversive," punishing, or nonfunctional, and (b) the extent to which the interventions promote or take place in community-integrated environments. External pressures in these two areas have both benefitted and harmed individuals with autism. The benefit of public scrutiny and defacto consumer evaluation by the community has led to more substantial research efforts in the stimulus control of challenging behavior. As a result an empirically based behavioral technology of positive behavior management is being defined and put into practice. The negative effects result from premature wholesale endorsement of an evolving technology not yet capable of meeting the needs of every child with a challenging behavior. The same arguments hold for community-based intervention.

On balance, we are better off for the external pressure inasmuch as it has served to promote growth within organizations serving children with autism. Runaway polemics not in synchrony with available data are destructive to the process of administering programs and supporting effective interventions. Attention to external forces, and consideration of external input, is most prudent.

## Two Populations

One would be hard-pressed to describe a treatment millieu for an individual with autism that involved one and only one intervention agent. Due to the massive problems generalizing behavior across people and settings, single-agent interventions would actually constitute poor practice. Yet, adherence to best-practice standards for training generalization and maintenance (see Stokes & Osnes, 1988) by employing multiple trainers can create an administrative problem affecting intervention outcome: The behavioral consultant must rely on someone else (e.g., parent, staff, teachers' aide) to control the contingencies. Considerable research on training staff in institutions (Reid, Parsons, & Green, 1989), community-based settings (McClannahan, 1991) and training parents (Egel & Powers, 1989) has clarified issues and strategies for establishing and maintaining effective and reliable behavioral interventions for challenging behavior. Widespread application of these strategies will reduce the administrative problem caused by multiple intervention agents.

## Language

All professional disciplines have evolved their own lexicon and "culture of communication." In this regard behavior analysis is not alone. Common referents are like communicative shorthand; they succinctly express a term or process in an unambiguous way (at least for those initiated into the discipline). To the extent that interventions for challenging behavior describe physical cues as "setting events," rewards as "reinforcers," and the stimulus that occasions behavioral performance as a "discriminative stimulus," problems of communication are relatively straightforward, as are solutions; either use nontechnical language or teach others to understand and use the terms.

The language of behavioral intervention is not always so unambiguous, however. Two constructs come to mind by way of examples: *Aversives/nonaversives* and *integration*. Behavioral interventions for challenging behavior are at greatest risk administratively when language and meanings are ambiguous or not defined functionally. In human communication, there often is a tendency to define a thing by dichotomizing it with its (supposed) opposite. Thus, integration is the absence of segregation. Positive behavior management procedures entail the absence of any negative (i.e., aversive) procedures. Although this is a tempting strategy, it is an oversimplification.

Language is only as precise as the social-communicative context within which it occurs. Thus, terms like *punishment* can be defined functionally as "stimulus events that, when applied following a behavior, decrease the likelihood of future occurrence of that behavior." The same term, however, can be defined in a sociopolitical context, as in "stimulus events that reduce the human dignity and choice-making opportunities of people with disabilities." The debate concerning aversive procedures is an excellent example of the problems of language in the treatment of challenging behavior (Repp & Singh, 1990, offer an outstanding review of this issue). Its importance here is as an example of an administrative issue that may compromise a behavioral intervention because the vocabulary is either not common to all participants, or not sanctioned, or defined from a different perspective. Amelioration of this type of problem may involve training intervenors in the terms, defining them functionally or with greater precision, or developing a consensual position on the social, political, and communicative context of the behavioral intervention in question.

## Labeling

Related to language are problems with labels. If the precision with which we speak facilitates communication, then the precision we bring to bear to the assessment and treatment process contributes significantly to the reduction of challenging behavior. This is especially important when we consider situations or activities that appear to reliably precede problem behavior. Clinical decision making must be based on functional relationships. Such relationships include the effects of a teaching strategy on child outcome, and the effect of a child's curriculum on his or her behavior, as well as the effect of particular activities, demands, or constraints on behavior. Without an understanding of these functional relationships, program staff and managers more easily fall prey to using vague labels to describe problems. For example, the presence of self-abuse while at school can too easily be blamed on "the school" or "swimming class" or "the teacher." More careful analysis might determine that episodes of self-abuse are more likely to occur on Mondays and Tuesdays when swimming class begins at 9 A.M., days on which the regular teacher's free period coincides with swimming (as well as days on which the pool water is colder in the morning because the heater has been turned off for the weekend). With vague labels, the forgoing problem (i.e., the class itself or the teacher's absence) would likely have been poorly defined with subsequent less-than-optional outcomes. Greater specificity in problem analysis would have expanded the range of options for manipulating antecedent conditions and potentially increased the likelihood that self-abuse would be reduced.

## Compromise

Flexibility is a hallmark of effective management of human service programs. The exigencies of life for many people with autism and their families are such that unexpected problems and crises do occur, often demanding a fresh look at old issues. Over time, however, the same conditions that created the initial demand for flexibility may lead to excessive compromise on important clinical issues. If, for example, a client's aggressive behavior results in less demanding educational programming during the afternoon hours followed by a commensurate reduction in aggressive outbursts, the staff may be highly (negatively) reinforced. It may not be evident that reduced demands contributed to the reduction in the target behavior. If they fail to recognize the importance of teaching alternative, more acceptable communicative behaviors to replace the aggression, the clinical compromise would be excessive. Program administrators must know their customers: They must understand the organizational constraints and demands that exist and that may mitigate against systematic interventions for challenging behavior. They must also be sufficiently skilled in behavior analysis (or delegate to someone who is) to recognize the differences between rigidity, arrogance, and organizational realities.

To be sure, it is sometimes important to take a firm stand, to set a "behavioral bottom line" that will not be crossed. But it is also important to appreciate successive approximations toward the goal by staff and to work with awareness of organizational process, historical and organizational interrelationships, and with sensitivity to the organization's ecology (e.g., past and current practices, perception of efficacy, ability to generate and respond positively to self-criticism). The reader interested in more detail is referred to Powers (1988).

## Port-of-Entry

When a new intervention for challenging behavior is to be implemented, administrative and clinical staff must determine where in the organization the intervention will have the greatest sanction, and thereby greatest likelihood for success and maintenance. Several factors may influence this decision. Where behavioral intensity is a factor and behavioral interventions are well-accepted, administrators/clinicians may choose to proceed to the most troublesome situation first, recognizing that direct-care staff commitment and experience will support a successful implementation effort. However, where direct-care staff are inexperienced, suspicious of the clinical or administrative staff, or hostile toward behavioral interventions, a more cautious approach may be warranted. In this latter scenario the administrator or clinician may judiciously choose to begin intervention where there is the greatest (and quickest) chance of success and where staff can be most closely involved with the treatment program and its success. In this latter case "winning their hearts and minds" (through success) and promoting ownership of the success (through active participation in program design and delivery) will augur well for future intervention efforts.

## Existing Staff

New behavioral interventions are not proposed and implemented in a vacuum. Just as the program site, existing physical resources (e.g., space, materials) and technological resources (e.g., computer hardware and software for data collection and analysis) are important variables, human resources also must be considered. It is often the case that new interventions are proposed for implementation by existing staff, including direct-care personnel, professional staff, and consultants. Initiators of new interventions must recognize that all staff will implicitly and explicitly evaluate the "worthiness" of the new treatment plan on clinical and subclinical levels. As such, commitment of existing staff to correct implementation will not only be due to the technical sophistication of the treatment plan but also to such factors as how well the initiator entered the system, the perceived competence of the initiator, and the perceived potential impact of the intervention both in terms of client habilitation and the removal/reduction of aversive contingencies from the staff.

Existing staff can become allies or nemeses and often cannot be replaced if inefficient. A concerted effort at working with staff to promote a sense of ownership of the treatment plan and a sense of personal responsibility for its success may provide the critical element of support for program maintenance. Reid, Parsons, and Green (1989) provide a comprehensive review of issues and strategies for training staff to implement behavioral interventions.

## Political Realities

The late Thomas P. (Tip) O'Neill, former speaker of the U.S. House of Representatives, was known to remind his colleagues that "all politics are local." Any behavioral consultant who has tried unsuccessfully to transfer a successful intervention from a tightly controlled clinical setting to the community will immediately appreciate the wisdom behind the speaker's words. Political realities impacting effective intervention for challenging behavior include union work rules, internal program politics, state policies concerning the use of restrictive procedures, community standards, the social validity of the treatment plan to consumers and other constituencies, and the interface of social norms and technology. Awareness of, and attention to, these issues often is positively related to intervention acceptance and outcome.

## CLINICAL AND SOCIAL CONSIDERATIONS GUIDING INTERVENTION EFFORTS

Successful administration of behavioral interventions for challenging behavior is dependent upon the effective use of existing technology within the social context of the family, community, or agency. In the past, many program administrators and behavior therapists have given insufficient attention to the interface between clinical decision making and social values supporting an expanded view of the rights of individuals with disabilities. Although some have argued that behavioral technology is "value-free," it is increasingly clear that *application* of this technology occurs in value-laden environments. As a result, intervenors must at least be cognizant of these values and the sociopolitical forces that define the issues if effective implementation of behavioral interventions is to be achieved.

This section will describe three issues that should be addressed in the planning, implementation, and evaluation of interventions for challenging behavior: technology use and coordination, the criterion of ultimate functioning, and the assumption of educability. These issues were selected because they have contributed significantly to the development and refinement of two key issues facing families, clinicians, and educators today: the concept of affirmative, effective treatment and the integration of people with autism into the mainstream of society.

## Technology–Coordination–Utilization: The Essential Triad

Although the behavioral management concerns administrators confront with clients under their care present challenges of varying degrees, it can safely be said that many of the impediments to skill building and the deceleration of unwanted behavior are least likely due to the unavailability of an effective technology of behavior change. In recent years, important advances have been made in the description of technologies of behavior management (Harris & Handleman, 1990; *Journal of Applied Behavior Analysis,* 1968–present; LaVigna & Donnellan, 1986; Repp & Singh, 1990), generalization and maintenance (Horner, Dunlap, & Koegel, 1988) and systematic instruction (Snell, 1987).

Each of these technologies, separately and together, afford the clinician a set of assessment and treatment options unavailable even 15 years ago. This is not to imply that the problems in technology utilization are related solely to issues of training and administrative support. Indeed, in our rush to identify specific techniques, clinicians and researchers have sometimes underemphasized the use of behavioral assessment data to predict and subsequently verify functional relationships between target behaviors and treatments.

As the empirical foundation for these procedures continued to evolve, the sophistication with which severe behavior problems can be treated effectively and maintained under conditions occurring in the community will be enhanced even further. Yet the degree to which *currently* available procedures are used appropriately remains a significant empirical, social, political, and administrative problem.

Problems with technology acceptance and use, coordination of treatment efforts, and utilization of human, technological, or physical resources all can negatively impact behavioral interventions for challenging behavior. Conversely, effective outcomes (defined as outcomes producing clinically significant, empirically validated, socially valid, sustained changes) can be attributed to success within each area of this triad. Each is defined below briefly.

*Technology* refers to procedures for positive programming, restrictive procedures, reinforcer assessment, applied behavior analysis, generalization and maintenance, curriculum development, and instructional methods. By *coordination,* we refer to consistency of application of appropriate technologies both across and within staff, as well as the congruence of technology use and implementation strategies with an organization's policies, history, or mandates. In short, technology use must be coordinated with the organization's and community's social norms. *Utilization* refers to the fact that good technology is nonfunctional unless implemented appropriately. This implies a need for staff training and ongoing supervision in technology utilization (cf. Reed, McCarn, & Green, 1988; Reid, Parsons, & Green, 1989).

By way of example, it is no less acceptable for an agency using only positive procedures to fail to document the rate of reinforcement delivered by staff in compliance with a procedure to reduce aggression by differentially reinforcing incompatible, alternative behavior than it is for an agency to fail to document staff compliance with established policy governing the use of a restrictive procedure. Both fail the client in that both have a high likelihood of procedural unreliability. Unfortunately, organizations, human rights committees, and state or federal monitoring agencies are more likely to request, require, and review data documenting reliable implementation of behavior-reduction procedures than to investigate data on the reliable implementation of reinforcement contingencies. This underemphasis has a high likelihood of restricting a client's right to effective treatment.

It can be argued that the greatest obstacle to effective intervention for challenging behavior is the lack of coordination and underutilization of existing technologies of behavior change. The complexity of this apparently simple problem is at once evident. Any action initiated and/or supported by a system with more than one member must account for the interdependence of the other members of the system. To the extent that administrative, clinical, and program governance (e.g., boards of directors, departments of mental retardation/developmental disabilities) priorities and policies differ, technology coordination and utilization are affected. Resolution of discrepancies between administrative, clinical, and governance constituencies becomes an important focus for intervention. Maher and Bennett (1984), Powers (1988), and Powers and Handleman (1984) provide guidelines for addressing systems issues in program planning and evaluation efforts with agencies serving individuals with severe disabilities.

## The Criterion of Ultimate Functioning

The assumption that clients with challenging behavior will successfully adapt to life in the community is diminished in the absence of systematic instruction in specific skills that are necessary and valued by the community. Brown and his colleagues (Brown, Nietupski, & Hamre-Nietupski, 1976) use the term *criterion of ultimate functioning* to describe the benchmark against which all interventions applied to a person with a disability must be judged. This term is applied individually to describe the environment the client will ultimately be capable of functioning in. Although it is assumed that these environments will vary across people with disabilities, it is inherent in this framework that at the very least, the environment should be integrated with nondisabled, same-age individuals to the maximum extent possible.

The importance of this concept cannot be overstated. If we believe that a client can ultimately succeed in a competitive job and live in a supervised apartment, then all intervention efforts must be directed toward that goal. Assessment of relevant next environments must be undertaken and the client's behavioral strengths, deficits, and abilities must be evaluated against that idiographic standard. Skills and behaviors targeted to be taught must be functional to that next environment and evaluated within the context of the environment (as opposed to evaluated only in an analog setting). The clinical significance of behavior change must be evaluated within the context of the appropriate next environment.

Such a position has clear implications for assessment, intervention, and evaluation efforts by clinicians and administrators. Administrative and clinical staff decision making must support and enable assessment and treatment procedures that target those ultimate environments as well as intermediate environments along the way. Further, staff training and monitoring take on added emphasis given the need for reliable and systematic implementation of instructional objectives. Although the implementation of this concept will vary somewhat for school-age individuals with autism (Christian & Luce, 1985) and preschoolers with autism (Powers, 1992), the administrative mandate remains constant.

## The Assumption of Educability

Will all individuals with autism benefit from the application of behavioral technology to their learning and behavioral needs, or do limits to habilitation exist? This question has been the subject of debate for years, moreso in recent times because of the fiscal constraints faced by states and agencies. Not surprisingly, the passage of PL 94-142 in 1975 and PL 99-457 in 1986 added another dimension to the discussion as children previously seen as poor learning risks were placed into programs with the charge that they receive an affirmative educational effort. To the benefit of all children with disabilities, researchers from education, psychology, and speech/language pathology recognized the need to develop new technologies of assessment and instruction to meet the unique learning challenges imposed by autism. The net effect has been the development of sophisticated technologies of behavioral assessment, systematic instruction, generalization, and behavior management that, taken together, provide empirical support for an affirmative answer to the question of habilitation.

Educability, however, is a legal term. Martin (1981) notes that educability implies a potential for positive change in the learner and that the courts have required evidence of documented, evaluable, sustained, and appropriate attempts to remediate learning and behavioral excesses and deficits. Given their emphasis on careful assessment, procedurally reliable interventions, and evaluation methodologies that demonstrate the functional relationship between assessment data, treatment plan, and intervention outcomes, behavioral approaches to teaching children with autism have provided substantial supportive data for the legal definition of effective education as well.

"Failures" are still, and unfortunately will always be, identified by educators and clinicians. It is imperative, however, that we appreciate the failures of people with autism to learn as failures in teaching technology utilization and coordination. One could argue that individuals with autism do not fail; we fail to understand their unique learning styles and to individualize our teaching methods sufficiently so that they can learn. This is not to say simply that any skill can be acquired if properly taught. The profound deficits of autism exercise a limiting effect on the acquisition of many social and communicative behaviors. For the present, however, it is empirically (and therefore legally) unclear where these limitations exist, and whether they exist for all people with autism or only for certain subgroups.

Given this uncertainty the following recommendations appear prudent:

1. The relationship between psychophysiological conditions and learning in people with autism are only recently receiving empirical attention (Romanczyk, Lockshin & O'Connor, 1993). Additional efforts are needed to develop instructional technologies that will be responsive to individual conditions such as anxiety, attention, and arousal as they impact the acquisition of new skills.
2. Efforts to define and assess antecedent stimulus conditions and setting events that effect learning should be increased, with special attention to task demands, curricula, physical space constraints, and competing stimuli. Schrader and Gaylord-Ross (1990) provide a comprehensive model for the assessment of these and other conditions.
3. We should adopt a pragmatic approach regarding the extent of community involvement to which a person with a severe challenging behavior is exposed. This approach should balance the individual's right to effective

treatment (Van Houten, Axelrod, Favell, Foxx, Iwata, & Lovaas, 1988), the right to effective education (Barrett, Beck, Binder, Cook, Engleman, Greer, Kyrklund, Johnson, Maloney, McCorkle, Vargas, & Watkins, 1991), and the person's right to participate in environments that are the least restrictive. This balance must not only consider the empirical validity of the intervention and its outcome, but the social validity of the target behavior, intervention, and proposed outcome as well.

4. Where limiting conditions to habilitation are encountered, they should be specified with precision. Moreover, as Favell, Risley, Wolfe, Riddle, and Rasmussen (1981) suggest, changes in conditions should be identified so that, if evidenced at a later point in the client's life, these changes will signal the necessity of reanalyzing discontinued or deferred habilitation objectives.

5. Increased emphasis should be placed on the use of functional analysis of behavior problem for clinical decision making (cf. Iwata, Vollmer, & Zarcone, 1990). Bailey and Pyles (1989) provide a particularly useful assessment framework for this purpose.

## GUIDELINES FOR PROMOTING SYSTEMIC CHANGE

Impediments to effective administration of behavioral interventions for individuals with autism require solutions that are both technologically sophisticated and clearly embedded in a relevant social context. Historically, many administrative and clinical failures have been due to overattention to one or the other of these factors. Even where both are addressed, impediments may remain because of a failure to account for the interrelationship between social and clinical factors in treatment planning and evaluation.

An appreciation of the systemic forces impacting administrative decision making for individuals with autism displaying challenging behavior argues for a planned, strategic approach to organizational change. Several writers (Greenblatt, 1983; Reppucci, 1973) have proposed guidelines for organizational change that have relevance to programs serving individuals with autism who exhibit challenging behavior. These include:

1. A philosophy guiding behavioral interventions must be developed with the participation of the members of the organization.

2. Administrative involvement and support must be evident from the earliest stages of intervention planning, through all phases of implementation and evaluation.

3. The support and involvement of other relevant constituencies (school PTA, local ASA chapter) should be sought and developed as appropriate.

4. The cultivation of optimism and a "we-can-do-it" attitude in administrative, clinical, teaching, and paraprofessional staff at all levels is essential.

5. Administrative structures should promote cooperation, communication, and consistency between administrative, clinical, teaching, and paraprofessional staff.

6. Employee skills should be utilized in implementing and evaluating the intervention plan without regard to job specification.

7. Resistance to behavioral interventions by some members of the organization can be overcome by education, ingenuity, and efforts to include the resistant individuals in the planning and evaluation process. Obtaining the support and commitment of a few key staff members may start a grassroots effort that will, over time, become a force for change.

8. Rewards for staff compliance with the intervention, goal attainment, and innovation must be incorporated into the administrative structure.

9. A corps of promising staff must be cultivated as "backup leaders" for the future. In this way, stability and long-term continuity of administrative philosophy for behavioral assessment and intervention is enhanced.

10. Active involvement of higher-level organizations (e.g., disability rights groups, state departments of mental retardation and developmental disabilities, professional associations) is necessary to develop a broad base of support and to ensure accountability.

11. The effects of the behavioral intervention should be formally evaluated. Promising data can be invaluable in convincing recalcitrant members of the organization of the importance of treatment continuation, and for enlisting the interest and assistance of community members.

These guidelines serve to underscore the need to attend to the process of change even as administrators and clinicians attempt to better address the behavioral and habilitation needs of individuals with autism. Superior content (e.g., innovative ideas, effective new intervention techniques) will likely be less efficient over time in the absence of a dynamic, supportive organizational process.

## CONCLUSION

The purpose of this chapter has been to provide a framework for understanding administrative issues confronting professionals treating challenging behavior in persons with autism. As administrators, parents, and clinicians become more aware of systemic impediments to change, new ways of confronting these barriers and promoting effective, socially valid interventions will be possible. Further, by acknowledging the interdependence of technological, social, political, and fiscal realities the effectiveness of service delivery will be enhanced.

# REFERENCES

Bailey, J. S., & Pyles, D. A. (1989). Behavioral diagnostics. In E. Cipani (Ed.), *The treatment of severe behavior disorders* (pp. 85–107). Washington, DC: AAMR.

Barlow, D. H., & Hersen, M. (1984). *Single case experimental designs.* New York: Plenum Press.

Barrett, B. H., Beck, R., Binder, C., Cook, D. A., Englemann, S., Greer, R. D., Kyrklund, S. J., Johnson, K. R., Maloney, M., McCorkle, N., Vargas, J. S., & Watkins, C. L. (1990). The right to effective education. *The Behavior Analyst, 14,* 79–82.

Brown, L., Nietupski, J., & Hamre-Nietupski, S. (1976). The criterion of ultimate functioning and public school services for severely handicapped students. In M. A. Thomas (Ed.), *Hey, don't forget about me! Education's investment in the severely, profoundly, and multiply handicapped* (pp. 2–15). Reston, VA: Council for Exceptional Children.

Campbell, D. T., & Stanley, J. C. (1966). *Experimental and quasi-experimental designs for research.* Chicago: Rand-McNally.

Christian, W. P., & Luce, S. C. (1985). Behavioral self-help training for developmentally disabled individuals. *School Psychology Review, 14,* 177–181.

Egel, A. L., & Powers, M. D. (1989). Behavioral parent training: A view of the past and suggestions for the future. In E. Cipani (Ed.), *Treatment of severe behavior disorders* (pp. 153–173). Washington, DC: AAMR.

Favell, J. E., Risley, T. R., Wolfe, A. F., Riddle, J. I., & Rasmussen, P. R. (1981). The limits of habilitation: How can we identify them and how can we manage them? *Analysis and Intervention in Developmental Disabilities, 1,* 37–44.

Fisher, D. (1983). The going gets tough when we descend from the ivory tower. *Analysis and Intervention in Developmental Disabilities, 3,* 249–255.

Greenblatt, M. (1983). Some principles guiding institutional change. *Analysis and Intervention in Developmental Disabilities, 3,* 257–259.

Harris, S. L., & Handleman, J. S. (1990). (Eds.). *Aversive and nonaversive interventions: Controlling life-threatening behavior of the developmentally disabled.* New York: Springer.

Horner, R. L., Dunlap, G., & Koegel, R. L. (1988). (Eds.). *Generalization and maintenance.* Baltimore: Paul Brookes.

Iwata, B. A., Vollmer, T. R., & Zarcone, J. R. (1990). The experimental (functional) analysis of behavior disorders: Methodology, applications and limitations. In A. C. Repp & N. N. Singh (Eds.), *Perspectives on the use of nonaversive and aversive interventions for persons with developmental disabilities* (pp. 301–330). Sycamore, IL: Sycamore Publishing Co.

*Journal of Applied Behavior Analysis.* (1968–present).

LaVigna, G. W., & Donnellan, A. M. (1986). *Alternatives to punishment: Solving behavior problems with nonaversive strategies.* New York: Irvington.

Liberman, R. P. (1979). Social and political challenges to the development of behavioral programs in organizations. In P. Sjoden, S. Bates, & W. S. Docken (Eds.), *Trends in behavior therapy* (pp. 369–398). New York: Academic Press.

Maher, C. A., & Bennett, R. E. (1984). *Planning and evaluating special education services.* Englewood Cliffs, NJ: Prentice Hall.

Martin, R. (1981). All handicapped children are educable. *Analysis and Intervention in Developmental Disabilities, 1,* 5–12.

McClannahan, L. E. (1991, May). *Key issues in staff training.* Invited address presented at the annual conference of the Association for Behavior Analysis, Atlanta.

Miller, J. S. (1978). *Living systems.* New York: McGraw-Hill.

Powers, M. D. (1988). A systems approach to serving persons with developmental disabilities. In M. D. Powers (Ed.), *Expanding systems of service delivery for persons with developmental disabilities* (pp. 1–14). Baltimore: Paul Brookes.

Powers, M. D. (1988). (Ed.). *Expanding systems of service delivery for persons with developmental disabilities.* Baltimore: Paul H. Brookes.

Powers, M. D. (1992). Early intervention for children with autism. In D. Berkell (Ed.), *Autism: Assessment, diagnosis and treatment* (pp. 225–252). Hillside, NJ: Lawrence Erlbaum.

Powers, M. D., & Franks, C. M. (1988). Behavior therapy and the educative process. In J. C. Witt, S. N. Elliott, & F. M. Gresham (Eds.), *Handbook of behavior therapy in education* (pp. 3–36). New York: Plenum Press.

Powers, M. D., & Handleman, J. S. (1984). *Behavioral assessment of severe developmental disabilities.* Rockville, MD: Aspen.

Rappaport, J. (1977). *Community psychology: Values, research and action.* New York: Holt, Rinehart & Winston.

Reid, D. H., McCarn, J. E., & Green, C. W. (1988). Staff training and management in school programs for severely developmentally disabled students. In M. D. Powers (Ed.), *Expanding systems of service delivery for persons with developmental disabilities* (pp. 199–215). Baltimore: Paul H. Brookes.

Reid, D. H., Parsons, M. B., & Green, C. W. (1989). Treating aberrant behavior through effective self-management. In E. Cipani (Ed.), *Treatment of severe behavior disorders* (pp. 175–190). Washington, DC: AAMR.

Repp, A. C., & Singh, N. N. (1990). (Eds.). *Perspectives on the use of nonaversive and aversive interventions for persons with developmental disabilities.* Sycamore, IL: Sycamore Publishing Co.

Reppucci, N. D. (1973). Social psychology of institutional change: General issues for intervention. *American Journal of Community Psychology, 1,* 330–341.

Reppucci, N. D., & Saunders, J. T. (1983). Focal issues for institutional change. *Professional Psychology: Research and Practice, 14,* 514–528.

Romanczyk, R. G., Lochskin, S., & O'Connor, J. (1993). Psychophysiology and issues of anxiety and arousal. In J. K. Luiselli, J. K. Matson, & N. N. Singh (Eds.), *Assessment, analysis and treatment of self-injury.* New York: Springer-Verlag.

Sarason, S. B. (1981). *Psychology misdirected.* New York: Free Press.

Schrader, C., & Gaylord-Ross, R. (1990). The eclipse of aversive technology: A triadic approach to assessment and treatment. In A. Repp & N. N. Singh (Eds.), *Nonaversive and aversive interventions for persons with developmental disabilities* (pp. 403–417). Sycamore, IL: Sycamore Publishing Co.

Snell, M. (1987). *Systematic instruction for persons with severe handicaps.* Columbus, OH: Merrill.

Stokes, T. F., & Osnes, P.G. (1988). The developing applied technology of generalization and maintenance. In R. H. Horner, G. Dunlap, & R. L. Koegel (Eds.), *Generalization and maintenance* (pp. 5–19). Baltimore: Paul Brookes.

Van Houten, R., Axelrod, S., Bailey, J. S., Favell, J. E., Foxx, R. M., Iwata, B. A., & Lovaas, O. I. (1988). The right to effective behavioral treatment. *The Behavior Analyst, 11,* 111–114.

# 4

# Behavioral Priorities for Autism and Related Developmental Disorders

## ERIC SCHOPLER

## INTRODUCTION

This chapter is based on our experience in developing North Carolina's statewide program for the *T*reatment and *E*ducation of *A*utistic and related *C*ommunication handicapped *CH*ildren (Division TEACCH). It is the only statewide program, mandated by state law to provide service, research, and multidisciplinary training in behalf of autism and related developmental disorders. As both the oldest and only comprehensive university program of this kind, it provides a unique source of clinical and research data to discuss the broader issue of behavioral treatment models.

In this chapter I briefly describe the scope of North Carolina's TEACCH model and some of the historical factors providing program structure and direction. This is followed by a description of obstacles in the form of misapplied treatment concepts and specific treatment techniques. These are offset by assigning priority to nonspecific treatment factors used for finding optimum individual treatment and education techniques. From this perspective, the second part of the chapter involves the discussion of enduring treatment principles and concepts shown to be viable over time. Selected for their usefulness in guiding both empirical research and accountable intervention, they offer a viable alternative to uncritically embracing specific treatment models and techniques. Finally, implications for future treatment development are discussed.

ERIC SCHOPLER • Division TEACCH, School of Medicine, The University of North Carolina at Chapel Hill, Chapel Hill, North Carolina 27599-7180.

*Behavioral Issues in Autism*, edited by Eric Schopler and Gary B. Mesibov. New York, Plenum Press, 1994.

## NORTH CAROLINA'S TEACCH MODEL

### Background

Historically, the social treatment of autism and related developmental disorders has cycled from infanticide and inhuman abuse to institutional neglect, and from benign neglect to special education and community inclusion (Schopler & Hennike, 1990). However, autism was not identified by name until World War II (Kanner, 1943). At that time, psychoanalytic theory was the primary and mistaken basis for explaining and treating autism. The erroneous overextension of Freudian theory was especially popular in the United States at that time and was applied to many states of disease and unhappiness indiscriminately without rational and empirical research support.

Autistic children were said to be reacting with social withdrawal from pathologic parents—"refrigerator mothers," whose negative and rejecting unconscious attitudes and wishes produced the autistic symptoms. Treatment was primarily by parentectomy or placement away from parents in a residential institution (Bettelheim, 1967), but no empirical support for these psychogenic theories was found (Cantwell & Baker, 1984; Rimland, 1964), although the resulting scapegoating (Schopler, 1971) produced needless misunderstanding and suffering for both children and their parents. During subsequent years, an empirical basis for the understanding and treatment of both physical and mental health problems was increasingly adopted.

The TEACCH Program began with a small number of children and their parents, whose plight we attempted to improve in the clinic (Schopler & Reichler, 1971). However, I first became alerted to the misunderstanding they were exposed to from the hostile and the dramatic Freudian preoccupation taught by Bruno Bettelheim (Schopler, 1993). It was seeing the relationship between the psychoanalytic caricature taught by Bettelheim and the demoralizing effects on individual families with autistic children that led us to establish a program based on the opposite formulation that families were not the cause of the disorder but the cause of the rehabilitation. The empirical verification of this assumption enabled us to remain client-centered, even after our program grew to statewide and comprehensive coverage.

### Program Description

After the initial research grant from NIMH demonstrated that parents could collaborate effectively in a cotherapy role (Schopler & Reichler, 1971), the state passed legislation establishing the program on a permanent basis. Program priorities included services for autistic children via parent involvement from preschool to adulthood, conducting related empirical research, and offering multi-disciplinary training. The mandate was to provide help in the three main areas of each client's life including home adjustment, education, and community advocacy, and to do so via relevant organizational structures (Reichler & Schopler, 1976).

## Home Adjustment

Helping families cope with the special needs presented by their child was facilitated by the establishment of six regional TEACCH Centers, each located in a city also housing one of the branches of our state university, thus facilitating research, training, and staff development. The centers are involved with diagnostic assessment, parent training and support, consultation, and professional training.

## Education

Autistic children could be moved from psychiatric facilities to public schools if some of their needs for special education in the areas of social skills, communication, and behavior management were met through structured teaching. Starting with 10 classrooms, there are now over 160 TEACCH-affiliated classrooms according to contracts made with each school. Such a contract typically calls for the hiring of teachers jointly between TEACCH Center staff and the school, training teachers to understand and manage the special problems of autism in an intensive 1-week training, the diagnostic assessment of each child at a center, and subsequent placement in an optimum classroom. This usually includes a special classroom of 6 to 8 children with a teacher, an assistant teacher, and opportunities for mainstream and community teaching experiences. Consultation is provided either for individual children or the school systems, and continuing education presentations are offered throughout the year.

## Community Advocacy

The third area in addition to family adjustment and education is the relationship between the client and the community-at-large. The main purpose of this aspect of the parent–professional collaboration is twofold: (1) to increase public understanding of autism and its manifestations and (2) to develop cost-effective services not currently available. These objectives are attained via parent groups. Each classroom and each regional center has its own parent group. Each of these is represented in both the state and national autism societies.

In this role, parent–professional collaboration first produced enabling program legislation in 1971. The main need at that time was to have children accurately diagnosed and then allowed access to public schools, using individualized educational programs developed with the involvement of parents. Once these objectives were supported federally by PL 94-142, the next advocacy issue was services for adolescents and adults. These included earlier transition from school curriculum to vocational training and opportunities, as well as supported employment with job coaches. It also included group home development, respite care for families, social skills groups, summer camp programs, and a residential living and learning center located on university land with a wide range of vocational training opportunities.

I have reviewed briefly the program structure we developed for understanding and intervention in behalf of autism and related disorders. The inclusion of service with university-based research priority provided a mechanism for contributing to new knowledge, while reviewing both old and new treatment techniques and for making tested changes with minimum bureaucratic delay.

Before reviewing some of the principles and concepts generalizing to other locations and developmental disorders, it may be helpful to review some of the main obstacles to long-term program viability we have experienced during the past two decades.

## OBSTACLES TO OPTIMUM INDIVIDUALIZED TREATMENT

A great many specific therapies or treatment concepts for autism and related developmental problems have appeared in the public press and professional journals during the past few decades (see Table 1). Table 1 lists more than two dozen of such techniques without suggestion that these are all inclusive. These techniques are frequently heralded with great excitement either by parents who are convinced they have witnessed the miraculous improvement they are searching for, or by professionals believing or hoping for the fame and rewards of finding a cure. On the face of it, this appears to be the road to scientific progress, but with excessive media hype and extension beyond reasonable data, it often leads to unnecessary costs and unexpected disappointments. For a parent overwhelmed by the diagnosis of autism, heard for the first time to characterize the newest member of the family, the possible choices of available treatment techniques can represent confusing and costly options. Moreover, the most serious obstacles to the optimum individualized treatment is the excitement and hype without reasonable evaluation that usually occurs with the overextension of a treatment concept or technique beyond the data supporting its hoped for usefulness. A few representative samples include the following:

Table 1. Specific Therapies with Autism

| | |
|---|---|
| Aversive | Mainstreaming |
| Auditory training | Megavitamin |
| Dance | Music |
| Deinstitutionalization | Patterning |
| Developmental | Pharmocotherapy |
| Dolphin | Phenothiazine |
| Electroconvulsive | Physical |
| Facilitated communication | Play |
| Feingold diet | Pony |
| Fenfluramine | Psychogenesis |
| Holding | Sensory integration |
| Intensive behavior | Signing |
| Interactive | Speech |
| Logo | |

1. *Psychoanalytic therapy.* I have already mentioned the misunderstanding and suffering produced by psychoanalytic explanations of autism. Autistic children were believed to be socially withdrawn from rejecting parents, whereas subsequent empirical research showed that the causes involved various biological processes summarized in Rutter and Schopler (1978) and Schopler and Mesibov (1987). Mothers were blamed for the children's symptoms and assigned derogatory descriptors such as "refrigerator mothers." Subsequently, research evidence accumulated that mothers did not cause these symptoms by pathologic parenting. However, they did have their maternal role frustrated by their child's lack of responsiveness. So like their children, the mothers were victims of autism. Freudian professionals claimed that autistic children were untestable because of their social withdrawal but assumed the children had normal mental endowment. Subsequent research showed that autism and mental retardation could and did coexist in the majority of children across a continuum ranging from severe to normal functioning. Moreover, with appropriate testing, these children were not "untestable" (Alpern, 1967; Schopler & Mesibov, 1988).

According to psychogenic theory, separation from the parents with residential treatment was the therapy of choice, whereas empirical research showed that parents could function as cotherapists, and it was best for autistic children to be included in community public schools. There have been many other unhappy consequences that can be attributed to the misunderstanding of autism from psychoanalytic theories, needlessly increasing the stresses and burdens for autistic children and their parents. The primary reason was that Freudian concepts were theoretical explanations and assumptions for which empirical evidence was not sought nor required by true believers. It was, therefore, rather difficult for clinicians to distinguish the apparent benefits of psychoanalysis for middle-class neurotics, from an extension of such theories to developmental disorders like autism. Although the misapplication of psychoanalytic theory to autism is by now widely accepted in the field of mental health, the tendency for overextending the use of specific treatment concepts and techniques beyond the supporting data is remarkably common.

2. *Pharmacotherapy*. It is generally agreed, at this time, that no one drug can be used for the treatment of autism (Gualtieri, Evans, & Patterson, 1987). Long-term use of the neuroleptic group has been shown to have variable effects, including the long-term negative side effects of tardive dyskinesia.

Fenfluramine seemed an attractive alternative to the standard neuroleptics and was unveiled to the autism community with a dramatic flourish, reporting the unprecedented therapeutic effect of "almost doubling (one of three hospitalized young children) IQ during the course of the experiment" (Geller, Ritvo, Freeman, & Yuwiller, 1982). Moreover, a rational basis for fenfluramine treatment known to lower serotonin levels in the brain was suggested. Some autistic children were known to have low blood levels of serotonin, whereas others seemed to have excessively high levels. If this was the primary mechanism in the development of autism, fenfluramine could be a corrective for children with high serotonin levels, whereas megavitamins might be able to increase low levels of this neurotransmitter.

The dramatic IQ increase in one subject was heralded, not only in the most prestigious *New England Journal of Medicine* (Ciaranello, 1982), but also on television and in influential newspapers like the *New York Times*. This resulted in thousands of parents calling in to request that their autistic child be treated with fenfluramine. Morris Lipton, John Werry, Thomas Gualtieri, and I wrote a letter (1982) to the *New England Journal of Medicine* objecting to the premature publicity on methodological grounds, including small numbers of subjects subjected to simultaneous treatments of fenfluramine and hospitalization, with IQ results known to be unstable, especially in young children. The letter with these objections was not published.

However, on the basis of the excited publicity, a costly multicenter grant was funded with predictably ambiguous results. Beneficial effects, when they occurred, appeared only in a small proportion of the subjects and had no correlation with the treatment levels of blood serotonin. In most studies, many subjects showed negative or no effects, and in not a single case was the "near doubling" of IQ effect replicated. In a review of drug therapy, Campbell (1989) concluded that fenfluramine may be helpful for an individual autistic child, but cannot be recommended for the group, whereas in a similar review, Gualtieri et al. (1987) recommended that human trials of fenfluramine be delayed until the questions of long-term neurotoxicity already reported in laboratory animals was tested more thoroughly.

It is clear that research on the effectiveness of other drugs such as naltrexone, buspirone, stimulants, and even neuroleptics needs to be continued in order to improve predictions of positive cost–benefit ratios for responses to particular problems with individual children. For autism, no specific drug has been demonstrated as effective with the group, and drug therapy with autism is still an art rather than a science.

The experience with fenfluramine brought needless disappointment and cost to many desperate for effective treatment because the dissemination of news far exceeded the pilot data. This error can be avoided in the future with more timely drug research.

3. *Normalization and deinstitutionalization.* Normalization was imported from Scandinavia where it was intended to obtain "an existence as close to normal as possible" (Nirje, 1969) for handicapped citizens. The principle was popularized in the United States by Wolfensberger (1972) and his colleagues. It became the rallying slogan for "deinstitutionalization" and for the educational technique of mainstreaming students with autism in classrooms of nonhandicapped students.

The "normalization" principle became a rallying cry for calling attention to the mentally retarded and others housed in large, inadequate, impersonal institutional settings with few opportunities for program rehabilitation and change. It provided a focus for the indignation over conditions considered dehumanizing and uncivilized by many professionals, families, and concerned citizens.

However, like the psychoanalytic theory, the normalization principle became a theory unto itself, unrelated to either the Scandinavian caveat of as close to normal "as possible" or empirical accountability. Instead, many normalization advocates insisted on a literal and unqualified interpretation of the concept. As the unqualified normalization process was translated into social policy, negative side effects were gradually discovered (Mesibov, 1990). "Normal" was interpreted in a frequently arbitrary fashion by policymaking advocates. Group homes in urban settings were given preference over group homes in the country, though in many regions of the country, rural life is more "normal" than urban. Diversity of special services is often discouraged by bureaucrats using the normalization principle for denying special needs and individual differences. Experience with mainstreaming has shown it useful for some, but a burden for others. When the educational need of the autistic child is sufficiently different from that of the nonhandicapped student, the accommodations needed for mainstreaming such a child in a "normal" classroom may be sufficiently great to compromise the learning situations for both children. Even educators initially enthusiastic about "mainstreaming" have become critical after extended experience and research (Strain, 1989).

The negative side effects of normalization by "deinstitutionalization" can be substantial both for the deinstitutionalized client and the community. There are growing numbers of streetpeople in most American cities, many of whom had better shelter before the institutions were shut down. The ideologues advocating for unconditional "normalization" have usually been less noticeable when the unanticipated consequences of their ideological fervor needed attending. The cost of overextending this principle is likely to continue to grow in proportion to how this specific treatment concept is over extended.

4. *Behavior management.* Behavior theory became important for autism and mental retardation. It has been an alternate theory for explaining human personality contemporaneous with Freudian theory. However, it was the pioneering of Lovaas (1973) who first demonstrated the implications of behavior theory for intervention with autistic children. Unlike psychoanalytic intervention, behavior therapy was targeted at specific behaviors, and its effects could be observed. Behavior therapy first exploded onto the public attention when *Life* ran a feature story on Lovaas's bold experimentation with conditioning behavior (Lovaas, Schaeffer, & Simmons, 1965). Following the principle that rewarded behavior increases in frequency while punished behavior decreases, he placed socially withdrawn children on an electric grid, while their caretakers waited on the side. While the children avoided contact with adults, a shock was administered to their feet. When they ran to the caretaker's embrace off the grid, the electric shock ceased. Although this experiment was not replicated extensively, it did have the effect of jolting both public and professional attention to the powerful potential of behavioral techniques. These have since then been studied extensively and frequently demonstrated to have positive therapeutic effects. A more detailed discussion of just two specific behavior therapies follows.

5. *Aversive therapy.* The notions of using both punishment and rewards in the child-rearing process is familiar to all either as former children or parents. Both have been studied and used with behavior modification. The use of aversives for reducing undesirable behaviors was often reported as effective, especially with one of the most difficult of problems, severe self-injurious behavior. Aversives such as electric shock, noxious fumes, restraints, helmets, and white noise were used in some facilities, especially at the Behavior Institute in Massachusetts, specializing in the treatment of this problem. However, pressure against the use of aversives increased as several deaths were reported at this facility and the possible use of aversive behavior reduction methods were implicated.

The concept of aversive therapy became increasingly politicized, and certain professional groups, perhaps wanting to use specific treatment techniques consistent with the civil rights movement, advocated for its complete abolishment. As with the normalization concept discussed above, distinctions between rewards and punishment were made arbitrarily. Hugging an autistic person could be experienced by him as aversive, yet in the popular usage, hugging is considered rewarding. At the other extreme, and equally oversimplified, was the advocacy for using only nonaversives.

The polarization of these behavioral techniques became so extreme and strident that in 1989 the National Institutes of Health (NIH, 1990) sponsored a consensus development conference on the treatment of destructive behavior. A consensus group of 14 members heard a presentation of a review of the research literature by 15 professionals. The consensus panel's task of evaluating the evidence was complicated by the presence of political ideologues demonstrating against the use of all behavioral aversives in favor of the completely nonaversive techniques used by them. Although a research review conference had been reduced to a political rally, members of the Consensus Development Conference were able to sign and agree to a preliminary report (NIH, 1990), recommending the extension of positive reinforcement methods for eliminating destructive behaviors, and that aversives or "behavior reduction procedures" be restricted to short-term use, only after appropriate review and consent had been obtained. Although this preliminary report had been published, the final report has not at this time. Apparently advocates for "nonaversive" therapy have succeeded in delaying or suppressing it. Here then is nonaversive therapy, a specific behavior therapy for reducing destructive behavior, a technique shown to be useful under some conditions with some individuals, now extended beyond supporting data and presented as a politically correct category. It is well under way to becoming a short-lived fad.

6. *Intensive behavior therapy.* When reviewing the early results of his behavioral therapy with autistic children, Lovaas, Koegel, Simmons, and Long (1973) concluded that treatment gains were often situation-specific and temporary, but lasted better with children who continued to live with their parents, than with those who went to untrained foster parents or institutions. In response to this evaluation, Lovaas initiated an intensive behavior therapy program involving parents and children (Lovaas, 1978). Parents, usually mothers, were expected to work with the child for most of the day and for at least a year with supervision and help from graduate students. This treatment technique required a major commitment from parents. If both worked, one of them was expected to stop working, and they were expected to sign a legal contract to this commitment. Initial anecdotal reports from several parents indicated important gains made during this treatment period. The formal report was not published until 1987 (Lovaas, 1987). However this report made claims for treatment for a group of preschool autistic children with IQs approximated in the severe range of retardation, 45% were claimed as mainstreamed and for all practical purposes, cured of their autism. This report was instantly picked up by television and newspapers and became another media celebration of the latest therapy miracle. Subsequently, a number of methodological flaws in Lovaas's report were identified. These contributed to the overestimation of this reported treatment success (Schopler, Short, & Mesibov, 1989). For a brief period, some believed that school systems should install intensive behavior therapy, but it became clear to many professionals and laypeople that the media hype had once again helped to produce a technique extended beyond the supporting data.

7. *Facilitated communication.|* Facilitated communication is another ex-

ample of a specific treatment technique for autism. It was developed 8 years ago in Australia by Rosemary Crossley with a girl with cerebral palsy who was thought to be mentally retarded. The technique involves a keyboard with the alphabet. A therapist or a facilitator steadies the client's hand while the client spells out the message to be communicated. Crossley, armed with this technique, brought a young woman named Annie, out of a snake-pit-like institution and obtained permission to raise the girl in her home. Through the facilitated communication method, it was claimed that Annie was far more intelligent than had previously been reported. Moreover, it was accepted that an unknown number of other residents, believed to be mentally retarded, could actually be shown to have sound intelligence through the use of facilitated communication. The success with Annie provided the impetus for removing other clients from some custodial institutions and to pressure for global reforms. During this period, professional colleagues staffed a review panel to examine claims that facilitated communication could reveal an unexpected high intellectual functioning for nonspeaking individuals classified as mentally retarded.

The review panel raised many questions (Bettison, 1991). They were unable to obtain validation of high intellectual functioning reported via facilitated communication in individuals with cerebral palsy. They questioned whether facilitated communication originated with the facilitator or with the client previously regarded as retarded. They did not find independent evidence for high intellectual functioning in individuals with CP. Their doubts were even greater for people with different communication disorders as in autism. At a time when Australians had developed a more balanced perspective on facilitated communication, an American educator visited there and became mightily impressed with facilitated communication. On his return to the United States, he published his enthusiastic theories (Biklen, 1991) in the *Harvard Educational Review,* a publication unrestrained by either data or acceptance of any reservations expressed by the Australian review panel. Propelled by the anachronistically high status of the Harvard prestige, this set off a surge of therapeutic enthusiasm and replication unprecedented in my recollection of American media hype. Some parents heard their autistic child for the first time proclaim love for them or express poetic sentiments about the isolation of autism.

Biklen's followers report his generous estimate that more than 90% of autistic children will be able to communicate with facilitated communication. When asked how children with autism, defined as a communication disorder usually involving concrete thinking, can often produce poetic metaphors with facilitated communication, the facilitated communication convert blithely advises that we must now rethink all we know about autism. When experiments are suggested for testing the validity of facilitated communication by blindfolding the facilitator or using earphones for screening questions, these are dismissed as pointless because they will disrupt the trust and faith in the relationship taught by Biklen as the foundation of successful facilitated communication. Likewise, prospective facilitated communication therapists are taught that they can facilitate successfully only if they have trust and faith. This would appear to place an unusual amount of pressure to "facilitate" a meaningful message on students applying for a therapist position. Such emotional pressure is often reported for novices considering admission to a religious cult, but not in my experience with students at a major university.

As facilitated workshops proliferated across schools of education and related state agencies, skepticism began to spread with new evidence. The *Harvard Educational Review* turns out not to be a peer-reviewed journal. Instead, it is a student journal by and large shunning faculty input and indulging the students' publication whims. Where Diane Sawyer's *Prime Time* program endorsed facilitated communication as the latest miracle, a message bound to please her commercial sponsors, Canadian television ran a program in which the interviewer tried some experiments. When she showed flash card pictures visible to the facilitator and the client, the typed answers were always correct. This was not the case when the cards were shown only to the client. A series of studies has since been completed (Cummins & Prior, 1992; Prior & Cummins, 1992; Eberlin, McConnachie, Ibel, & Volpe, 1993), all showing that the communication was not maintained when the facilitator was blind to the questions asked.

In the meantime, a more ominous development occurred with the overextended, overhyped facilitated communication technique. In Denmark, Australia, and the United States a growing number of cases were brought to court in which a mentally handicapped person, through a facilitator, accused parents or group home staff of sexual abuse and rape. In every case, the evidence was thrown out of court. On the other hand, in Australia facilitated communication was said to be on trial instead and reported as having failed.

The case of facilitated communication has attracted more converts and advocates than have other recent treatment techniques. The deep appeal of facilitated communication for parents is easy to understand. For the first time, their child's communication block has appeared to be removed, even if the facilitator has supplied in varying degrees the missing language. At least there now is an advocate attached to their offspring. Possible explanations for the wave of teacher and professional enthusiasm seems less direct. It occurred during a period when health care systems and techniques were criticized increasingly for excessive cost and questionable service. Here then is a relatively simple technique, as simple to learn, Biklen explained in a television interview, as eating. Moreover, young teachers and speech pathologists in Biklen's workshops are taught that the most important element in facilitation communication is faith. Most youngsters have easier access to their reservoir of faith than to the discipline needed to study and learn new skills. It is unnecessary to consider the reinforcing power of news coverage and grateful parents to understand the appeal of such an easy miracle.

Unfortunately, the cost of a hopeful theory shielded from empirical testing and accountability is likely to be high. In the category of autism, the number of cases for which facilitated communication is the treatment of choice is probably less than 5%, rather than the 90% estimated by Biklen. At the present time, a large undifferentiated group of children are being enlisted in facilitated communication. I have seen included those who were able to speak, yet attached to a facilitator, whereas a mute boy, capable of typing independently, had to do so through a facilitator. The cost of using inappropriate educational techniques is high to any child required to follow an educational ideology; the cost to society is equally great when the technique of an ideology lacking empirical research accountability is used in an effort to deprive an accused person of liberty and justice (Prior & Cummins, 1992).

In the previous section, I have reviewed a basic dilemma in the development of the optimum and least restrictive treatment modality for developmental disorders like autism and mental retardation. These examples, along with the other techniques listed in Table 1 share the following characteristics.

1. Each seemed like a reasonably good idea to the initiator. Sometimes the technique had been known to correct a similar problem or to add a corrective element with another technique. But regardless of source, the initiator was convinced it was responsible to try this technique with others in this clinical population.

2. There are usually one or a few cases that appear to show striking improvement, sometimes even referred to as a cure. This improvement is usually convincing to one or two observers. But because it was a single-case anecdote, the reason for the observed improvement could not be demonstrated with adequate certainty. It could have been due to any number of factors shaping an individual's responses, including spontaneous fluctuation of behavior. However, such pilot success stories find early dissemination in the news-hungry media, popular magazines, and professional journals. The resulting excitement promotes premature use of the technique and excessive support for pilot research.

3. Excessive support for pilot research tends to inflate the number of researchers flocking for available funds to replicate the advertised miracle. These replications are often based on a low probability hypothesis, without adequate theoretical justification, but promoted by media hype and hopes of desperate parents. Regardless of the replication method, none of the specific techniques has been found to be effective with either most or all autistic children.

4. Moreover, continued use also shows that each technique has costs and negative side effects, not usually considered or predicted by the initiators in the flush of pilot study drama. The specific treatment concept or

technique in question too often becomes a short-lived fad, producing unnecessary disappointment and wasted resources.

In the quarter-century Division TEACCH has been serving North Carolina statewide, we have evolved a viable policy for program structure. First we become familiar with all available information on existing or newly developing treatment techniques, and we avoid assigning program priority to any one specific treatment technique or concept. Instead we have maintained priority for the effects of nonspecific treatment factors. Frank (1961) and Schopler (1987) remind us that the patient's faith has always been fostered by the doctor–patient relationship, a socially sanctioned relationship now extended to teacher–student and parent–child. It is the relationship in which the partner, socially sanctioned with responsibilities for the less knowledgeable partner, is in the best position to understand the more dependent individual's problems and learning difficulties, along with the best knowledge of the currently available intervention techniques. It is the therapeutic or helpful aspirations of this nonspecific relationship that enables parents with professional collaboration to identify the optimum treatment techniques, including cost–benefit considerations for each individual involved. This delineation is finally less a scientific decision than one based on the art of treatment or education; that is, knowing the individual with his unique and complex history, then matching him with the best available intervention techniques.

In our years of developing the TEACCH system, we were often pressed to overextend one or the other of the relevant treatment concepts discussed in the previous section. However, I am pleased to report that with the TEACCH system, so far we have avoided, better resisted, this fad development by adhering to the nonspecific intervention priorities (Schopler, 1987). This enabled us to develop viable and lasting principles of treatment and education. Our first administrative priority grew out of our commitment to parent–professional collaboration. It required providing the treatment and education permitted by the state of the art. Concurrently, we made a commitment to study and support research into problems that were obstacles to understanding the disorder or to improve the child's adaptation. In case of conflict between these two priorities, we were inclined to resist having research interfere with treatment. Our next priority was to develop multidisciplinary training and staff to implement program priorities.

Given these priorities, it is not surprising that the most enduring principles and concepts identified from our program are those capable of generating both clinical and empirical research data. These principles, discussed below, evolved over the two decades when the accumulation of research demonstrated that autism was not a single-cause emotional illness induced by parental pathology. Instead, it was a multiply-caused chronic developmental disorder. Although biologically based, the adaptation of individuals could best be enhanced through parent–professional collaboration and special education.

## ENDURING TREATMENT PRINCIPLES AND CONCEPTS

In this section I will discuss the seven principles or concepts most viable for both program stability and for flexibility to change with the cutting edge of the field. These will be discussed both for their research and clinical implications.

1. *Improved adaptation.* The first principle is that the child's adaptation is improved in two ways. The first and generally most effective is by increasing the child's living skills and knowledge. However, when a deficit from the developmental disorder prevents the acquisition of a new skill, then the environment can be modified to accommodate the deficit. Either of these two ways will improve the child's adaptation.

This principle is listed first as it is the broadest. It offers a direction for the entire community-based enterprise, including the many diverse specific program components. With this population it is especially important to recognize and implement both of these components, as in the United States, especially, there is an inclination to look for specific treatment techniques that promise to cure the condition. Many government grants for developmental disabilities are postulated on such a promised expectation in the grant application, thus forgetting that the population by definition includes individuals with a chronic developmental disability. Improving their skill levels along with social acceptance and environmental accommodation to current deficits is the foundation of cost-effective community programming. This principle also highlights the recognition that even without the elation of expecting a cure, optimism of concerned family and professionals can be maintained more easily, because several intervention approaches are available that will improve adaptation, rather than only one. The handicapping condition can be improved while the search for a cure continues without premature and misleading hype.

The effectiveness of this principle was supported by our outcome studies (Schopler, Mesibov, & Baker, 1982). A comparison of seven follow-up studies from 1963–1982 showed that when they reached adulthood, between 40% and 78% of the autistic population was institutionalized. Whereas in the North Carolina TEACCH Program only 8% had to be institutionalized, the rest remained in the community, in school, in supported employment, in group homes, and at home. This study supported this first principle for developing and maintaining this statewide program system.

2. *Parents as cotherapists.* From the outset, having discovered that parents of autistic children were systematically misunderstood and scapegoated (Schopler, 1971) our efforts at improving both our understanding and treatment of autism involved working with parents as cotherapists or collaborators with professionals. At the clinical level, this principle has had too many applications to summarize easily. However, structural reinforcement of this principle can be found readily in

our program organization, clinical procedures, and parent–professional relation-ships (Schopler, 1987; Schopler, Mesibov, Shigley, & Bashford, 1984).

Central to our clinical operation is the one-way observation room and diag-nostic procedures, used in all six regional TEACCH Centers. After completing a child's evaluation, the therapist demonstrates certain teaching of behavior man-agement techniques to the observing parent. These are written up in a home teaching program and implemented by parents or siblings at home for brief daily sessions. Parents frequently introduce new procedures from their own observa-tions and demonstrate these to the observing therapist. Through a dialogue of mutual observation and work with the child, parents and therapists evolve the optimum individualized teaching program. A collection of such individualized teaching programs was compiled and indexed by Schopler, Lansing, and Waters (1983).

When the child is at the preschool level, the greatest need for most parents is to learn what went wrong with this child and how best to reverse or minimize any handicaps. Collaboration is primarily between the child's parents and clinic staff. After the child reaches school age the-parents-as-cotherapist model is ex-tended and shifted to the parent–teacher relationship. This, more than any other single factor helps overcome a major problem in developmental disabilities, the child's difficulty in generalizing information learned in one context to another.

Parent–teacher collaboration is encouraged along a continuum of intensity, ranging from the intense end a parent functioning regularly as an assistant to the teacher in the classroom, to special demonstration of teaching or behavioral techniques. Such demonstrations are usually initiated by the teacher, but may be brought in by the parent for the teacher. It can include parents in the classroom for occasional fieldtrips or with birthday celebrations, to monthly phone calls and home–school diary exchanges, enabling parents and teachers to coordinate the understanding and interventions with the child. After the child passes through adolescence to adulthood, the collaboration is extended through supported em-ployment and job coaches to a parent–employer collaboration to facilitate job placement and training.

Two types of parent–professional role variations have been used tradition-ally. One used most frequently within medicine is when the physician is the authority on the diagnosis and treatment of a child's disease, and the patient or the parent is primarily a passive participant. In the behavioral model, the behaviorist is the expert on the most recent scientific technology for behavior modification. The parent is trained in behavioral methodology in an active role as a trainee.

We have found neither of these two parent–professional role models adequate to the task of delivering modern, cost-effective, and comprehensive service with the autism problems. Our parent–professional collaboration involves many levels and can best be summarized in four distinct forms of relationships. When this collaborative relationship is characterized by mutual respect between professionals and parents, they are each able to shift to the appropriate role as needed.

(a) *Parent as trainees and professionals as trainer* is consistent with the traditional parent–professional roles discussed above. It is effective insofar as it is based on the recognition that professionals have seen many more similar children than the parents have and also have access to the most recent information on and evaluation of developments in new treatment techniques. The parent needs this information to better understand the child and how to foster his or her development. It is the dominant emphasis during the diagnostic evaluation and teaching demonstration.

(b) *Parent as trainer and professional as trainee* is the reversal of the previous form and is less familiar. It is based on the recognition that parents, in most cases, are the foremost experts on their own child's behavior with higher motivation than others have for living in some degree of grace and harmony with their child. This form of relationship is used when parents provide assessment information to staff, demonstrate to the staff effective interventions they developed, and also when they assist in training new staff or talk to legislators.

(c) *Emotional support* represents a form of the relationship realized in mutual emotional support between professionals and parents. This need for support becomes clear when new staff see that these parents have the same stresses endured by everyone else, but with the addition that they also have a handicapped child, a child that does not learn at the same rate as other children. This results in frustration and disappointments to which the family must adjust. If the parent role is challenged by the autism, so is the professional role for similar reasons. Once they both understand this, their mutual support for each other is usually spontaneous and survives various technical differences over treatment and management.

(d) *Community advocacy* is a form of parent–professional collaboration in which the objective is to develop community understanding and acceptance of the child's special problems and also to develop needed, cost-effective services. A common front is developed from the other three aspects of the relationship, and social-role differences are at a minimum in this role. The collaboration here is more difficult to specify than in the other forms demonstrated above. Parents' contributions are as versatile as their careers, be it writer, lawyer, or politician. However, parents, more than professionals, are considered to represent a political constituency, while professionals, on the other hand, are often thought of as those who meet that constituent's needs, similar to the politician's social role (the similarity is noticeable when both are functioning well).

Empirical research consistent with the principles of parent–professional collaboration included disproving the psychodynamic notion that parents produce their children's autistic symptoms with their own disordered thinking. Our studies showed that such parents displayed no more thought disorder than other kinds of parents and that thought-disordered responses could be produced by anxiety from professionals, negative, psychodynamic judgments (Schopler & Loftin, 1969). We also tested professional wisdom that parents misunderstand their children in major ways. However, we learned that parents' estimates of their child's developmental level correlated positively with formal test results (Schopler & Reichler, 1972). Not only were parents able to estimate their child's level of functioning reasonably well, they were also effective trainers and cotherapists (Marcus, Lansing, Andrews, & Schopler, 1978) who produced changes that carried over into the home (Short, 1984).

3. *Assessment for individualized treatment.* The third enduring principle is that individualized educational programming and treatment are based on developmental diagnostic evaluation and assessment. The importance of this concept comes from the frequently systematic professional misunderstanding of autistic children. During the early history of the autism syndrome, professionals frequently considered these children untestable (Alpern, 1967). Moreover, some behaviorists have deemphasized or ignored assessment or testing of autistic children for the purpose of distinguishing the differences between behaviors that can be shaped and modified, versus those whose rigidity was linked to a developmental deficit. More recently, one of the new treatment ideologies had emerged under the banner of "mainstreaming." Some of the fervent mainstream enthusiasts advocate that all handicapped individuals are habilitated by placement in a "normal" environment without appropriate education and assessment.

In the TEACCH system, we have found that both formal and informal diagnosis and assessment are needed in order to determine an individual's educational program, implemented in the least restrictive environment, and safeguarding each individual's right to optimum treatment. At the clinical level, this has meant training staff and students in naturalistic observation and how to make informal assessments of each client in different life contexts (Mesibov, Troxler, & Boswell, 1988).

Empirical research involved the development of a number of formal assessment instruments, counteracting past claims that such children are "untestable." These have included the Childhood Autism Rating Scale (CARS) (Schopler, Reichler, & Renner, 1988). This instrument is used for making the diagnosis of autism from systematic observation. This diagnosis, however, is not sufficient for the individual assessment needed for defining an optimum treatment program. To accomplish this, we developed the *Psychoeducational Profile (PEP)* (Schopler & Reichler, 1979), for evaluating all the other characteristics of the child, not necessarily part of the diagnostic criteria. It was recently revised for a more thorough inclusion of the preschool population (Schopler, Reichler, Bashford, Lansing, & Marcus, 1990). This assessment instrument was extended to the adolescent and adult population with the *Adolescent and Adult Psychoeducational Profile (AAPEP),* by Mesibov, Schopler, Schaffer, & Landrus (1988) for the purpose of evaluating the client with autism for the best vocational and living arrangement possible.

4. *Teaching structures.* Our fourth principle is that education is based on structured teaching. Clinically, the importance of this concept was repeatedly observed and reported during the 1960s and 1970s when autistic children were primarily treated in nondirective (Axline, 1947) and psychodynamic (Ekstein, 1954) play therapy. These frequently seemed to result in a lack of progress and a need for residential treatment, thus giving impetus to the more structured treatment of operant conditioning, and the educational program developed in our system (Lansing & Schopler, 1978).

At the level of empirical research, we were able to demonstrate that autistic children functioned better under structured conditions than they did under unstructured conditions, and that individual variations in response to structure correlated with developmental levels. Children of lower levels of developmental function benefitted more from structure than did children at higher levels (Schopler, Brehm, Kinsbourne, & Reichler, 1971). This study demonstrated a finding that has become more viable with subsequent experience. Since then, we have evolved more sophisticated teaching structures for different levels of function. These have been applied to public school classrooms throughout our TEACCH system in North Carolina. This system has been taught in a finely tuned training program, and has been applied in different cultures including Japan, Belgium, and France. The importance of structured teaching is now widely recognized, as discussed in the last chapter of this volume.

5. *Skill enhancement.* Our fifth principle underscores that the most effective approach is to enhance skills of children and parents and to recognize and accept their shortcomings. This concept follows along with our assessment emphasis. One of the primary purposes of the assessment instruments is to distinguish between emerging skills that can be enhanced immediately, and the deficit areas for which training is better delayed or treated with environment structures. The emphasis on working with existing and emerging skills while accepting relative weaknesses has been reaffirmed by clinical experience for the past 20 years. In fact, it is fair to say that this emphasis has been effective not only with children and parents, but also with staff and trainees.

The suggestion is sometimes made that such skill development emphasis is most effective with more able children and their parents. Our experience has been to the contrary. For example, recently a schizophrenic mother of an autistic child was referred to us after being released from 6 months of inpatient treatment. She had improved during hospitalization but felt unable to resume caring for her family and household. After assessment, it was found that she had some recollection of making Jello, a favorite family dessert. After a week of intensive training in Jello making, she was able to prepare it on her own. This gave her the necessary impetus to begin cooking and preparing other meals she had cooked in the past. Skill emphasis did not cure her schizophrenia but enhanced her adaptation.

At the empirical research level, we completed a study of parents' perception of program helpfulness (Schopler, Mesibov, De Vellis, & Short, 1981). Parents reported most program helpfulness with problems in their child's social relationships, motor skills, self-help skills, and communication. Children with higher IQs improved more in language and self-help skills than did children with lower IQs. In pre- and posttreatment studies based on observations of children in their own homes, Short (1984) found significant improvement in both parent involvement and in appropriate child behavior.

6. *Cognitive and behavior therapy.* Our sixth principle refers to the enduring usefulness of cognitive and behavior theory for guiding both special education and research, theoretical systems eloquently reviewed by Gardner (1985). At the clinical level, the application of these two theoretical systems can be illustrated with the management of difficult behavior. Figure 1 outlines an iceberg to represent problems of aggression. The smaller portion of this entity shows above the waterline, or is visible in the form of specific behaviors like pushing, hitting, biting, or kicking. Below the waterline are possible explanations for the cause of particular aggressive behaviors. It could be frustration over communications deficits; therefore, hitting at the teacher rather than signaling for her attention. It

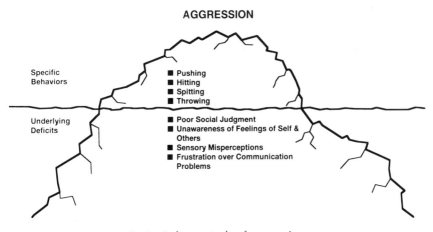

Fig. 1.   Iceberg metaphor for aggression.

could be a child's misperception of pain or inability to understand behavior rules. Through careful observation and assessment, the best explanatory cause is identified and used as the basis for intervention. If it is frustration over communication, we can teach a word, a sign, or a signal. If the aggressive hitting behavior decreases, our explanatory theory is supported. If, on the other hand, hitting continues, a different explanatory mechanism is involved.

At the level of empirical research, we have developed a communications curriculum (Watson, Lord, Schaffer, & Schopler, 1989). It includes data collection in four different semantics categories, especially important in the communication problems of autism.

7. *The generalist training model.* The seventh principle refers to intervention and training in the TEACCH system. That is, professionals concerned with autism are trained as generalists who are expected to know the entire range of problems raised by this disorder (Schopler, 1991). Traditionally in the United States, the field of mental health has emphasized specialization. Psychologists conducted evaluations, speech pathologists provided speech therapy, social workers specialized in family work, psychiatrists preferred psychotherapy, and so on. This is an understandable phenomenon considering the long training period of professionals in various disciplines. Unfortunately for families seeking help for their handicapped children, specialization structures professionals to be interested in or accountable for, primarily their own area of specialization. This increases the likelihood that parents receive inconsistent or contradictory opinions on diagnosis and treatment. Moreover, it makes it difficult for anyone to take professional responsibility for the entire child. The generalist model reduces these undesirable consequences of specialization. It enables staff to see the child from the parents' perspective and to work collaboratively with them. It increases staff responsibility, makes the job more interesting, and improves staff ability to use consultation from specialists more effectively.

From the perspective of training, we have developed an intensive multidiscipline training model. It incorporates didactic sessions on the eight topics we have found basic to the study and treatment of autism and related developmental disorders. These eight topics are presented in a didactic format during half of the training sessions and illustrated directly with a group of autistic children during the other half of the session. This training program was filmed by a Japanese documentary film group in 1986 and has been effectively applied in Belgium, France, Japan, and the United States (Asahi Shimbun, 1986).

## SUMMARY AND CONCLUSIONS

In this chapter I have tried to identify treatment principles and concepts that can apply to treatment programs across the spectrum of developmental disorders and mental retardation. The first part provides a summary description of North Carolina's university-based, statewide program for autism and related communication handicaps (TEACCH). Primary obstacles to the development of such a program were identified in the form of treatment theories and ideologies. When these are propelled to miracle-cure status by premature publicity and hype, relatively short-lived fads thrive while leading to unnecessary costs and needless disappointment. From our TEACCH experience, we find when programmatic priority is assigned to the nonspecific relationship informed by responsible empirical review of specific technology, specific techniques can be assigned according to individual needs. From these priorities, we have evolved seven treatment principles and concepts. These are amenable to both empirical research and evaluation of specific techniques. These have been shown useful in many different cultures and extended to other developmental problems.

## REFERENCES

Alpern, G. D. (1967). Measurement of "untestable" autistic children. *Journal of Abnormal Psychology, 72*, 478–496.

Asahi Shimbun (Producer). (1986). *Autism services with Division TEACCH.* Chapel Hill, NC: Health Sciences Consortium.

Axline, V. M. (1947). *Play therapy.* Boston: Houghton-Mifflin.

Bettison, S. (1991). Informal evaluation of Crossley's facilitated communication. *Journal of Autism and Developmental Disorders, 21*, 561–563.

Biklen, D. (1991). Communication unbound: Autism and praxis. *Harvard Educational Review, 60*, 291–314.

Bettelheim, B. (1967). *The empty fortress: Infantile autism and the birth of the self.* New York: Free Press.

Campbell, M. (1989). Pharmacotherapy in autism: An overview. In C. Gilberg (Ed.), *Diagnosis and treatment of autism* (pp. 203–218). New York: Plenum.

Cantwell, D. P., & Baker, L. (1984). Research concerning families of children with autism. In E. Schopler & G. Mesibov (Eds.), *The effects of autism on the family* (pp. 41–63). New York: Plenum.

Ciaranello, R. D. (1982). Hyperserotonemia in early infantile autism. *New England Journal of Medicine, 307*, 181–183.

Cummins, R. A., & Prior, M. P. (1992). Autism and facilitated communication: A reply to Biklen. *Harvard Educational Review, 62*, 228–241.

Eberlin, M., McConnachie, J., Ibel, S., & Volpe, L. (1993). Facilitated communication: A failure to replicate the phenomenon. *Journal of Autism and Developmental Disorders, 23*(3), 507–566.

Ekstein, R. (1954). The space child's time machine: A "reconstruction" in the psychotherapeutic treatment of a schizophrenic child. *American Journal of Orthopsychiatry, 24*, 492–506.

Frank, J. D. (1961). *Persuasion and healing.* Baltimore: Johns Hopkins University Press.

Gardner, H. (1985). *The mind's new science: A history of the cognitive revolution.* New York: Basic Books.

Geller, E., Ritvo, E. R., Freeman, B. J., & Yuwiller, A. (1982). Preliminary observations on effect of fenfluramine on blood serotonin and symptoms in three autistic children. *New England Journal of Medicine, 307*, 165–169.

Gualtieri, C. T., Evans, R. W., & Patterson, D. R. (1987). The medical treatment of autistic people: Problems and side effects. In E. Schopler & G. Mesibov (Eds.), *Neurobiological issues in autism* (pp. 373–388). New York: Plenum.

Kanner, L. (1943). Autistic disturbances of affective contact. *Nervous Child, 2,* 217–250.

Lansing, M., & Schopler, E. (1978). Individualized education: A public school model. In M. Rutter & E. Schopler (Eds.), *Autism: A reappraisal of concepts and treatment* (pp. 439–452). New York: Plenum.

Lipton, M. A., Werry, J. S., Gualtieri, C. T., & Schopler, E. (1982). Letter to the editor. Unpublished manuscript.

Lovaas, O. I. (1978). Parents as therapists. In M. Rutter & E. Schopler (Eds.), *Autism: A reappraisal of concepts and treatment* (pp. 369–378). New York: Plenum.

Lovaas, O. I. (1987). Behavioral treatment and normal educational and intellectual functioning in young autistic children. *Journal of Consulting and Clinical Psychology, 55,* 3–9.

Lovaas, O. I., Koegel, R. L., Simmons, J. Q., & Long, J. S. (1973). Some generalization follow-up measures on autistic children in behavior therapy. *Journal of Applied Behavior Analysis, 6,* 131–166.

Lovaas, O. I., Schaeffer, B., & Simmons, J. Q. (1965). Experimental studies in childhood schizophrenia: Building social behavior in autistic children by the use of electric shock. *Journal of Experimental Research in Personality, 1,* 99–109.

Marcus, L., Lansing, M., Andrews, C., & Schopler, E. (1978). Improvement of teaching effectiveness in parents of autistic children. *Journal of American Academy of Child Psychiatry, 17,* 625–639.

Mesibov, G. B. (1990). Normalization and its relevance today. *Journal of Autism and Developmental Disorder, 20,* 379–390.

Mesibov, G. B., Schopler, E., Schaffer, B., & Landrus, R. (1988). *Individualized assessment and treatment for autistic and developmentally disabled children. Vol. 4 Adolescent and adult psychoeducational profile (AAPEP).* Austin, TX: Pro-Ed.

Mesibov, G. B., Troxler, M., & Boswell, S. (1988). Assessment in the classroom. In E. Schopler & G. B. Mesibov (Eds.), *Diagnosis and assessment in autism* (pp. 261–270). New York: Plenum.

Nirje, B. (1969). The normalization principle and its human management implications. In R. Kugel & W. Wolfensberger (Eds.), *Changing patterns in residential services for the mentally retarded* (pp. 181–195). Washington, DC: U.S. Government Printing Office.

National Institutes of Health. (1990). Consensus development conference statement: Treatment of destructive behaviors in persons with developmental disabilities. *Journal of Autism and Developmental Disorders, 20,* 403–429.

Prior, M., & Cummins, R. (1992). Questions about facilitated communication and autism. *Journal of Autism and Developmental Disorders, 22,* 331–338.

Reichler, R. J., & Schopler, E. (1976). Developmental therapy: A program model for providing individual services in the community. In E. Schopler & R. J. Reichler (Eds.), *Psychopathology and child development: Research and treatment* (pp. 347–372). New York: Plenum.

Rimland, B. (1964). *Infantile autism.* New York: Appleton-Century-Crofts.

Rutter, M., & Schopler, E. (Eds.). (1978). *Autism: A reappraisal of concepts and treatment.* New York: Plenum.

Schopler, E. (1971). Parents of psychotic children as scapegoats. *Journal of Contemporary Psychotherapy, 4,* 17–22.

Schopler, E. (1987). Specific and nonspecific factors in the effectiveness of a treatment system. *American Psychologist, 42,* 376–383.

Schopler, E. (1993). Anatomy of a negative role model. In G. Brannigan & M. Merrens (Eds.), *The undaunted psychologist* (pp. 173–186). New York: McGraw-Hill.

Schopler, E. (1991). Training professionals and parents for teaching autistic children. In T. Ollendick,

J. Ratey, S. Mayfield, & E. Mikklesen (Codirectors), *Postgraduate advances in autism disorder: An independent-study course designed for individual continuing education* (pp. 1–9). Berryville, VA: Forum Medicam.

Schopler, E., Brehm, S. S., Kinsbourne, M., & Reichler, R. J. (1971). Effect of treatment structure on development in autistic children. *Archives of General Psychiatry, 24,* 415–421.

Schopler, E., & Hennike, M. J. (1990). Past and present trends in residential treatment. *Journal of Autism and Developmental Disorders, 20,* 291–298.

Schopler, E., Lansing, M., & Waters, L. (1983). *Individualized assessment and treatment for autistic and developmentally disabled children: Vol. 3. Teaching activities for autistic children.* Austin, TX: Pro-Ed.

Schopler, E., & Loftin, J. (1969). Thinking disorders in parents of psychotic children. *Journal of Abnormal Psychology, 74,* 281–287.

Schopler, E., & Mesibov, G. B. (1987). Introduction to neurobiological issues in autism. In E. Schopler & G. Mesibov (Eds.), *Neurobiological issues in autism* (pp. 3–11). New York: Plenum.

Schopler, E., & Mesibov, G. B. (1988). *Diagnosis and assessment in autism.* New York: Plenum.

Schopler, E., Mesibov, G., & Baker, A. (1982). Evaluation of treatment for autistic children and their parents. *Journal of the American Academy of Child Psychiatry, 21,* 262–267.

Schopler, E., Mesibov, G. B., De Vellis, R., & Short, A. (1981). Treatment outcome for autistic children and their families. In P. Mittler (Ed.), *Frontiers of knowledge in mental retardation. Vol. 1 Special educational and behavioral aspects* (pp. 293–301). Baltimore, MD: University Park.

Schopler, E., Mesibov, G., Shigley, H., & Bashford, A. (1984). Helping autistic children through their parents: The TEACCH model. In E. Schopler & G. B. Mesibov (Eds.), *The effects of autism on the family* (pp. 65–81). New York: Plenum.

Schopler, E., & Reichler, R. (1971). Parents as cotherapists in the treatment of psychotic children. *Journal of Autism and Childhood Schizophrenia, 1,* 87–102.

Schopler, E., & Reichler, R. J. (1972). How well do parents understand their own psychotic child? *Journal of Autism and Childhood Schizophrenia, 2,* 387–400.

Schopler, E., & Reichler, R. J. (1979). *Individualized assessment and treatment for autistic and developmentally disabled children. Vol. 1: Psychoeducational profile.* Austin, TX: Pro-Ed.

Schopler, E., Reichler, R. J., Bashford, A., Lansing, M., & Marcus, L. (1990). *Individualized assessment and treatment for autistic and developmentally disabled children. Vol. 1: Psychoeducational profile revised.* Austin, TX: Pro-Ed.

Schopler, E., Reichler, R. J., & Renner, B. R. (1988). *The Childhood Autism Rating Scale (CARS).* Los Angeles: Western Psychological Services.

Schopler, E., Short, A., & Mesibov, G. (1989). Relation of behavioral treatment to "normal functioning": Comment on Lovaas. *Journal of Consulting and Clinical Psychology, 57,* 162–164.

Short, A. B. (1984). Short-term treatment outcome using parents as cotherapists for their own autistic children. *Journal of Child Psychology and Psychiatry and Allied Disciplines, 25,* 443–458.

Strain, P. (1989, July). *Integrating persons with autism: Different perspectives.* Panel discussion at the Autism Society of America Conference, Seattle, WA.

Watson, L., Lord, C., Schaffer, B., & Schopler, E. (1989). *Teaching spontaneous communication to autistic and developmentally handicapped children.* Austin, TX: Pro-Ed.

Wolfensberger, W. (1972). *The principle of normalization in human services.* Toronto: National Institute on Mental Retardation.

# II

# Assessment Issues

# 5

# Self-Management of Problematic Social Behavior

## ROBERT L. KOEGEL, WILLIAM D. FREA, and ALAN V. SURRATT

### INTRODUCTION

The purpose of this chapter is to discuss self-management as a valuable aid in the treatment of problematic social behaviors in autism. Within this treatment, the child is taught to determine whether or not a target behavior has occurred, how to record the occurrence of the behavior, and how to recruit or obtain reinforcement. The use of self-management permits a large amount of behavior management without the continual presence of a treatment provider, thus increasing the amount of treatment provided as well as the number of settings where treatment takes place. Self-management is especially ideal for individuals whose primary treatment goals are in the area of pragmatic or social skills. In environments where it would be especially intrusive or stigmatizing to have a clinician present, self-management (in the absence of a clinician) may have significant advantages. Not only is it less stigmatizing without the presence of a therapist, but it also is more likely that opportunities for natural social exchanges will occur under such conditions. Self-regulation during such exchanges also has the potential for fine-tuning social skills as a result of peer modeling and feedback. Because children

ROBERT L. KOEGEL and WILLIAM D. FREA • Autism Research Center, University of California at Santa Barbara, Santa Barbara, California 93106-9490. ALAN V. SURRATT • Center on Human Development, University of Oregon, Eugene, Oregon 97403-1235.

*Behavioral Issues in Autism*, edited by Eric Schopler and Gary B. Mesibov. New York, Plenum Press, 1994.

with autism have many characteristics that make their behavior difficult for a single therapist to modify, incorporating self-management into a treatment package is especially advantageous. This is true to a large extent because of the need to observe and provide consequences for numerous behaviors across many settings. Further, although some of these behaviors occur infrequently, they are severely problematic when they do occur, thus requiring the therapist to maintain continuous vigilance over extended periods of time. For example, children with autism (1) exhibit low-probability excess behaviors that disrupt their environments; (2) fail to exhibit numerous appropriate behaviors that can enhance their development; and (3) exhibit certain behaviors that, even though they may occur rarely, have a major impact on nonhandicapped individuals judgments of autism. These characteristics result in the need for continuous and vigilant treatment intervention across significant portions of the day in order to produce socially meaningful treatment impacts. Self-management addresses this need by incorporating the child as an active contributor to his/her own treatment. The following characteristics of autism illustrate how self-management can be useful.

## CHARACTERISTICS OF AUTISM REQUIRING EXTENDED TREATMENT EFFORTS

### Disruptive Behavior

Certain low-frequency, but high-intensity behaviors disrupt the environment enough that even a rare occurrence of the behavior is problematic. Thus, a large amount of continuous vigilance is necessary in order to ensure that a treatment provider will be present when the behavior occurs. This is especially important because children with autism frequently exhibit disruptive behaviors that result in the interruption of their learning environments to the point where exclusion from the environment is considered for the child (cf. Koegel & Koegel, 1990). These behaviors range from tantrums to self-injurious behavior and aggression to disruptive or ostracizing self-stimulatory behaviors. That is, although the children's behavior may be uneventful for large periods of time, at seemingly unpredictable times they may engage in highly noticeable disruptive events with little provocation. For example, when presented with a minor demand, such as a request to sit in a chair or a request for a minor conversational interaction, a child may initiate severe screaming, kicking, or biting of self or others. At other times the child may be sitting quietly in a classroom, and then suddenly without obvious provocation begin to loudly chant in a repetitive stereotypic manner, disrupting the classroom atmosphere. Such behaviors, if they occurred in a nonhandicapped child might be characterized as reflecting an extreme lack of self-control and often lead to the conclusion that the person is unpredictable and may be at risk for being left unsupervised. As the examples discussed later in this chapter illustrate, self-management is ideally suited for such behaviors because it has the potential to solve the problems of providing continuous therapist vigilance, as well as the problem of needing to leave the children unsupervised.

## Unresponsivity to Social Stimuli

Although at times the children engage in severe excess behaviors such as those described above, at most other times children with autism are very unresponsive. They typically do not initiate interactions with others, and when others attempt to interact with them, the children usually try to avoid the interaction. Such characteristics result in an extremely low level of environmental interactions that can be detrimental to normal development (Burke & Cerniglia, 1990; Koegel & Felsenfeld, 1977; Koegel, Koegel, & O'Neill, 1989). Specifically, low levels of environmental interaction result in low levels of neural stimulation, which has been shown to be detrimental for both normal development and for recovery from neural dysfunction (Burke & Cerniglia, 1990). Also, low levels of environmental interaction result in minimal opportunities for environmental feedback, thus providing for minimal incidental learning (Hart & Risley, 1975). In short, there is a need to increase autistic children's responsiveness to a large variety of social and other environmental stimuli, across a very large number of different types of stimulus conditions. Further, if such responsivity is to be effective it must occur across extended periods of time. It is not likely to be enough for the child to interact socially in a clinic session for 30 minutes. Relatively large amounts of environmental stimulation spaced throughout the day appear to be necessary for normal development. Again, this results in a need for a therapy procedure that will have an impact throughout the day. The addition of self-management to a treatment package seems ideally suited for solving such problems (Koegel, Koegel, Hurley, & Frea, 1992).

## Pragmatic Behavior

Perhaps better than just about any other behavior, pragmatic behavior illustrates how severe the consequences can be of failing to self-manage behavior in the absence of a treatment provider. Children are often stigmatized by their peers due to even low-incidence behaviors that are viewed as odd or inappropriate in a social situation. The situations described below illustrate the complexity of treating pragmatic problems.

## Pragmatic Aspects of Communication

The pragmatic aspects of language are concerned with governing the use of language, and with the social aspects of language that rely on the speaker to deliver the message he or she is trying to communicate (Levison, 1983). Pragmatic aspects of language can be summarized by breaking them down into three broad categories (Prutting & Kirchner, 1987). (1) The control of the speech act, topic, turn taking, lexical selection, and stylistic variations. Examples of this are the ability to smoothly exchange the speaker and listener roles in a way that is appropriate in the specific context while varying the speech acts used in commenting, requesting, and questioning; the ability to select, introduce, maintain, and shift topics; the ability to take turns in a conversation when it breaks down; the ability to control pause time and interruption; the ability to give feedback; the ability to choose the appropriate words to convey the meaning desired; and the ability to adjust speaking style and tone (e.g., polite). (2) The paralinguistic aspects of speech require skills to control intelligibility and prosody. This requires the speaker to be able to monitor how well he or she is being understood. It also requires the person to control the loudness of the voice, the intonation and stress, and the fluency of the message (Duncan & Fiske, 1977; Scherer & Ekman, 1982). (3) The nonverbal aspects of speech require control of aspects of communication such as physical proximity, physical contact, body posture, gestures, facial expression, eye gaze, and hand movement. All of these skills are required to support the linguistic aspects of the message that is being given (Craig & Gallegher, 1982; Feldman, 1982; Hoffer & St. Clair, 1981; Von Raffel-Engel, 1980). Each of these areas require considerable monitoring and/or control by the speaker in order to communicate messages that are appropriate and meaningful to communicative partners.

## Pragmatic Deficits in Autism

Several of the above pragmatic areas appear repeatedly as deficits in descriptions of autism (Baltaxe, 1977; Loveland, Landry, Hughes, Hall, & McEvoy, 1988; Seibert & Oller, 1981). We will discuss particularly the absence of topic control, the absence of conversation initiation, the inappropriate use of facial expression and affect, inappropriate body posturing and gestures, and dysprosody. For example, children with autism often fail to shift appropriately from one topic to the next (Bernard-Optiz, 1982; Ricks & Wing, 1975). This is characterized by overly detailed explanations of favorite topics with a refusal to shift the topic regardless of cues given by the conversation partner. Children who exhibit this behavior often perseverate on a favorite topic or subject throughout an entire conversation and can maintain their fixation with a particular subject for years. In their experiences with many autistic persons, Ricks and Wing (1975, p. 208) found that "if the autistic person has a special interest, he is inclined to talk about this *ad nauseam* but without actually being able to discuss and explore any new angles on this subject. The same pieces of information tend to recur whenever the same subject is raised." They followed this explanation with an example of a child they came in contact with who loved to listen to and talk about music, but "his contribution invariably consisted of a list of all the records he owned and all the conductors he had heard."

By the very nature of the disorder, autism may inhibit children from pursuing social contact. Avoidance of social interaction also results in the child's reluctance to initiate conversation. Recently, our clinicians in Santa Barbara found that even when a child's responding to others is increased to nearly 100%, there is no increase in the autistic child's own initiations. A serious result of a child's refusal to initiate interactions may be a reluctance by the child's peers to continue to initiate interaction (Kohn, 1966). This serves to ensure the autistic child's isolation from social contact (Bartak, Rutter, & Cox, 1975; Rimland, 1964; Sorosky, Ornitz, Brown, & Ritvo, 1968; Wing, 1969).

Flat or inappropriate affect is also a common symptom of autism (Rimland, 1964). Inappropriate facial expression and affect can be seen in the failure to exhibit fear in dangerous situations, the display of laughter for no apparent reason, the failure to show interest or concern when someone is in pain, or profound irrational fears (Schreibman & Mills, 1983). It is common to find an autistic child who has a seemingly constant, placid expression, appearing to be totally emotionally detached.

Nonverbal aspects of language, such as hand movement or body posture, are also found to be inappropriate in many children with autism (McHale, Simeonson, Marcus, & Olley, 1980; Waterhouse & Fein, 1978). A pragmatic problem results when a person's gestures during conversation are inappropriate to the content of his or her speech. Erratic or exaggerated gestures are perceived as odd or distracting by the listener. Body posture also can be perceived as odd when, for example, the speaker is slumped over when telling someone about something exciting that happened, or just simply arching his or her back over an arm of a chair for no apparent reason. Similarly, autistic children seem to have a difficult time understanding and using visual language such as gestures. Though progress can often be made in teaching autistic children to understand gestures, progress is slow in teaching them to use gestures (Ricks & Wing, 1975; Wing, 1985).

Finally, children with autism often have dysprosic speech (Baltaxe, 1981, 1984; Baltaxe & Simmons, 1975; Rutter, 1970). Specific examples include expressionless speech (Kanner, 1943), rapid delivery and singsong intonation (Rutter, 1970), errors in stress assignment (Baltaxe, 1984), arrhythmic speech (Bagshaw, 1978), excessive high pitch without pitch change (Goldfarb, Braunstein, &

Lorge, 1956; Pronvost, Wakstein, & Wakstein, 1966), hoarseness, harshness, and hypernasality (Pronvost et al., 1966), vocal volume at too high or low a level, or varying intensity inappropriately (Fay, 1969; Goldfarb et al., 1956; Pronvost et al., 1966), and incorrect primary sentence stress (Baltaxe & Guthrie, 1987; Schreibman, Kohlenberg, & Britten, 1986). Self-management is ideally suited for the modification of such a large number of behaviors under a variety of complex stimulus conditions that may require prohibitive amounts of therapist time throughout the day (Koegel & Frea, 1993).

## Impact of Pragmatic Deficits

There are three important factors to be considered when viewing the impact of pragmatic deficits on children with autism. First, when pragmatic problems are viewed as the major problem in an autistic child, it is usually a case where the child has achieved great treatment gains, and only minor social skills problems are perceived as remaining. In this case, the minor problems, or the *pragmatic* problems are often overlooked by treatment providers in light of the progress the child has made. However, the child may still need to overcome serious obstacles. He or she may be attending a public school with nonhandicapped children who are not concerned with the treatment gains the child has made. They are, however, very interested in the bizarre behavior they see in any classmate. Thus, the child may be ostracized and excluded from peer interactions.

Our second point concerns the serious impact that even seemingly minor pragmatic problems might have on future development. Unfortunately in the real classroom this involves having the social skills to avoid peer rejections. It should be no surprise that peer acceptance is crucial for normal development. Children who are stigmatized tend to carry the role of the outcast into adulthood (Dodge, 1983). This affects all areas of their lives. Harry Stack Sullivan (1953) believed that the healthy, close relationship that the adult shares with his or her loved ones is dependent on the close bonds that were experienced in childhood and adolescence. Many still adhere strongly to this belief that friendships and peer acceptance are critical for healthy development. Other functions that friendships are believed to serve are consensual validation of interests, hopes, and fears; bolstering feelings of self-worth; providing affection and opportunities for intimate disclosure; promoting the growth of interpersonal sensitivity, serving as prototypes for later romantic, marital and parental relationships; providing instrument aid; providing opportunities for nurturing behavior; promoting a sense of reliable alliance; providing companionship (Sullivan, 1953; Furman & Buhrmester, 1985; Furman & Robbins, 1985); acting as a cultural institution for the transmission of social norms and knowledge; serving as a staging arena for behavior; serving as a context for the display of appropriate self-images (Fine, 1981); serving as a context for growth in social competence; providing emotional security and support; and acting as prototypes for later relations (Hartup & Sancillo, 1986; Strain, 1984).

By being on the fringes of the social aspects of their schools, high-functioning autistic children are at risk not only of suffering in the area of friendships, but also in the area of academics as well. Much of success in school depends on a healthy and happy relationship with peers (Quay & Jarrett, 1984; Michael, 1986). Support from peers, modeling friends, and learning from classmates are all valuable needs that are usually met for children, but may not be met for children with pragmatic deficits. Contrary to what many would like to believe, social integration does not result as a product of functional integration (Haring, 1990).

Our third point also deals with serious risks to the child's future. There is evidence suggesting that the stigmatizing effects that pragmatic deficits have may result in more serious behavior problems. Research on the communicative function of inappropriate behaviors support the hypothesis that social awkwardness and a sparse network of friends may cause the child to use more drastic means of communication or attention seeking (Carr & Durand, 1985; Dodge, 1983; Hunt, Alwell, & Goetz, 1988). Kenneth Dodge (1983) performed a short-term longitudinal study, where he found that the children who were rejected engaged in significantly more physical aggression than any of the other children. Earlier studies have found that physically aggressive and disruptive children consistently have significantly lower levels of academic achievement (Feldhusen, Thurston, & Benning, 1970a, 1970b).

*In summary,* the research described above suggests that autistic children may be at risk for continuing developmental problems unless intervention programs are designed in a manner taking into consideration a comprehensive variety of subtle aspects of communication. Thus, self-regulation of behavior throughout the day may be a prerequisite for normalized development. The discussion below illustrates this point.


## SELF-REGULATION OF BEHAVIOR

These types of problems (disruptive behavior, unresponsiveness to the environment, and inappropriate pragmatic skills) represent a myriad of behaviors that need to be modified under a very large number of stimulus conditions. It is neither practical nor desirable for a therapist to follow a child around for the amount of time or environments required for such widespread changes to occur. This is true especially because even rare instances of the behavior may have serious consequences, thus requiring the therapist to maintain continuous vigilance over long periods of time. One avenue, however, that provides a very practical and appropriate solution to this problem is a self-regulation approach to behavior change. During self-regulation of behavior, individuals initiate, monitor, evaluate, and reinforce their own behavior with minimal or no external influence (Litrownick, 1982; Kanfer & Hagerman, 1981). Additionally, the ability of individuals to direct their own behavior should be a vital element for the generalization and maintenance of newly acquired skills across a large numbers of settings and time (Lovett & Haring, 1989; O'Leary & Dubey, 1979; Sainato, Strain, Lefebvre, & Rapp, 1990).

As noted above, many people with developmental disabilities have difficulty in meeting societal expectations for personal independence (Grossman, 1983). The absence of self-regulatory behavior in this population may be a key factor contributing to their dysfunctions in learning and adaptive behavior (Whitman, 1990). Unfortunately, it has been a commonly held assumption that people with mental handicaps lack the cognitive abilities and social opportunities to learn self-management. However, studies are disproving this belief and showing self-regulatory strategies to be effective behavioral interventions for developmentally disabled populations (Fowler, 1984; Shapiro, 1981). This has even been the case with relatively young children (e.g., Sainato et al., 1990).

Self-regulation studies have used a variety of terminology and procedures relevant to the problems discussed in this chapter. For the purposes of this chapter, and somewhat consistent with other literature, the terms will be used as follows. *Self-regulation,* which is used interchangeably with *self-management,* is "the maintenance of behavior in the absence of any immediate environmental support or feedback" (Kanfer, 1971, p. 40). These are all-encompassing terms that include two main subcategories, self-monitoring and self-instruction. *Self-monitoring,* refers to attending to one's own behavior. It may incorporate the two separate functions of discriminating the occurrence of the behavior (self-evaluation) and recording that occurrence (self-recording) (Nelson, 1977). *Self-instruction* refers to "verbal statements to oneself which prompt, direct, or maintain behavior" (O'Leary & Dubey, 1979, p. 450). Recent studies also are displaying an increased emphasis on normalizing community placements by using *self-reinforcement* as a component of self-regulation. Although the large majority of studies report a need for some sort of reinforcement for self-management, the role of external reinforcers may be greatly minimized (cf. Koegel & Koegel, 1990). One way of achieving this is to teach the child to self-administer or self-recruit reinforcers from the natural environment. Interestingly, the use of self-reinforcement not only looks more natural, but it "may result in performance that exceeds that obtained when reinforcers are selected and delivered by external change agents" (Lagomarcino & Rusch, 1989, p. 297). Similarly, persons with severe handicaps have been taught to self-recruit feedback from their supervisors, with very positive results (Mank & Horner, 1987).

Although self-regulation does not appear to develop independently in many people with developmental disabilities, it appears to be possible for them to learn these skills (Koegel & Frea, 1993; Koegel, Koegel, Hurley, & Frea, 1992).

Unfortunately, the teaching of self-regulation skills to developmentally disabled children does not appear to be a common component in school curriculums (Sainato et al., 1990), even though the literature abounds with examples of research-based intervention strategies that incorporate self-regulation (e.g., Lagomarcino & Rusch, 1989; Moore, Agran, & Foder-Davis, 1989).

## Treatment Procedures

### Procedures for Self-Monitoring

In order to illustrate how one may utilize self-regulation in the treatment of autism, we will first describe the procedures one might use to teach self-monitoring. Following this description several case histories will be presented.

Self-monitoring training can be conceptualized as four broad steps: (1) pretraining; (2) training; (3) creating independence; and (4) generalization (cf. Koegel, Koegel, & Parks, 1991). The *pretraining* stage requires the clinician to first specifically define the behaviors that need to be treated. Ideally, a functional analysis also is conducted at this time in order to determine the function that the maladaptive behavior serves for the child. Once the target behavior and its function are defined, the therapist chooses a means for the child to measure the behavior. For example, if the child will be measuring the occurrences of a desirable behavior, a wrist counter such as those found in golfing supplies shops or discount stores may be used. Similarly, if the client needs to record the absence of a behavior, a wrist counter or a checklist with small boxes where the child may place a mark immediately following a set time interval may be employed. When the specified time intervals need to be particularly precise, or if the client does not know how to tell time, the end of the interval may be signaled using a watch with a repeat chronograph alarm function.

After a measurement device is selected, the therapist needs to identify functional reinforcers for the child. This may require some observation time if the child does not possess the verbal skills to express a desired reward. The rewards used at the beginning of treatment should be easy to deliver and capable of being enjoyed within a short period of time because intervals are often quite short in the initial stages. The final step in the pretraining stage is choosing an initial goal. At this early stage of training, the therapist typically needs to select a very small unit of behavior or unit of time that is easily attainable for the child in order to insure initial success. Later, the interval can be lengthened in order to attain independence for the child.

At this point self-monitoring *training* can begin. During this stage, the therapist has the recording device present as well as a variety of rewards for the child to choose. The therapist may start out modeling the inappropriate behavior and the appropriate behavior prior to the child's recording of the behavior. After the child has a good understanding of the target behavior, training on the recording of this behavior can begin. The reward should be visible to the child, but out of reach, during training. If a wrist counter is being used, the child should have it placed on his wrist and be told (or shown through modeling) how to press the button each time the target behavior is performed. The child is prompted to record the behavior after each occurrence. Whenever the child records without being prompted, immediate reinforcement and/or profuse praise is typically delivered. Because it is important to reinforce the act of accurately recording (rather than the target behavior itself), the monitoring of inappropriate behavior should also be reinforced. For example, if the child says, "I was yelling, so I don't get a point," the therapist might say, "That's right! Thanks for telling me; let's try again."

The third step in teaching self-monitoring, *creating independence,* is the ultimate goal of treatment. It focuses on increasing the time spent self-monitoring behavior, fading the student's reliance on prompts, and increasing the number of responses required for a reward. Increasing the self-management time is crucial regardless of the recording device used, whether it be increasing the time of the lesson each day or increasing the interval of the alarm until the child is at a level where he or she can function productively in the community for extended periods of time without needing to interact with the therapist. The number of responses necessary for a reward also can be gradually increased as the student learns to self-monitor behaviors. For example, the number of points on the wrist counter or the number of boxes that need to be checked can gradually be increased as the child's proficiency increases. The final step in creating independence is fading the presence of the treatment provider entirely. The method of fading the therapist depends on the specific needs of the student. One method is simply to step out of the room following an excuse or comment to the child. The time away can be gradually increased. Once the therapist is absent for extended periods of time, a method of validating the child's behavior in the absence of the therapist is developed. Fortunately, research shows that complete accuracy of self-monitoring behavior is not necessary in order for the procedure to work. Therefore, relatively simple methods of validation are possible. For example, when the therapist returns to the room where the child is recording, the therapist might ask a teacher or parent what the child was doing during the therapist's absence, and check the child's recording device. Only gross problems seem to be of concern. For example, only if the child does not press the wrist counter at all, or if the child presses it only as the therapist is about to enter the room, is remedial action required. Such problems are relatively infrequent. However, if they do occur, the therapist typically disallows any reinforcement for that time period.

The fourth and final stage of self-monitoring is training for *generalization* across settings. Once the behavior is occurring in the therapist's absence, it is fairly easy to teach it in other settings. This usually involves instructing the student that he or she can now earn points by engaging in the appropriate behavior in the new setting. Again, typically the child may need to be observed, with the therapist leaving for gradually increasing periods of time.

## Application of Self-Management to Stigmatizing Social Problems

The following case histories illustrate self-management interventions with a variety of children of different functioning levels.

### Carl: Self-Regulation of Responsivity to Peer Initiations

Carl was a 7-year old boy with autism. Although he was relatively high functioning and was in a regular second-grade classroom, he was having difficulty making friends, and he appeared very unhappy and unmotivated to go to school. School officials and family members were becoming concerned about the appropriateness of a regular classroom, even though he was functioning academically at a normal level. His clinician spent the first 2 weeks observing his behavior in the classroom and recording behaviors that seemed problematic. Her observations indicated that his most debilitating social deficit was his lack of responsivity to questions and other social initiations from peers and staff, making him appear severely abnormal and resulting in his having almost no friends. He was becoming almost completely socially isolated, with very little likelihood of the problem resolving itself. Self-management was selected as the intervention approach because it would be relatively unobtrusive and unlikely to interfere with natural social interactions.

The first step in treatment was to teach Carl to discriminate instances of responsiveness versus unresponsiveness to questions from his clinician. After each question, the clinician paused for about 3 seconds, and then asked Carl, "Did you answer?" After Carl was consistently able to respond appropriately ("Yes" or "No"), the next step in the program was begun. This second step involved familiarizing Carl with a wrist counter and teaching him to "press the button" each time he answered a question that the clinician asked. Carl liked the wrist counter because it "looked like a fancy watch," making the treatment relatively easy. Initially, he needed to be prompted to press the wrist counter each time he responded, but he quickly learned to respond without prompts. During this training Carl was told that he could earn a reinforcer of his choice (in this case, one fourth of a chocolate-chip cookie) after every three presses of his wrist counter. The next step in the program was to thin the schedule of reinforcement so that he was required to make 30 presses on the wrist counter in order to receive a chocolate-chip cookie. Generalization to his natural school setting was then programmed by asking his teacher and two of his classmates to prompt Carl to utilize the wrist counter at school. Carl's rate of responding to peer initiations rapidly increased. Other classmates appeared to become intrigued by Carl's "watch" and soon came over to interact as well. Carl's responses to their initiations seemed to foster other initiations as well, and Carl began to make new friends at school. Interestingly, as the program progressed Carl began to be less accurate in recording his responses. On some days he even forgot to wear his watch (although during the first few times he did this, he pressed a "pretend wrist counter"). Ultimately, he no longer wore the watch at all, although his rate of responsivity and social interactions with peers remained at a high level. Although the reasons for this are unclear, it appeared that the natural reinforcers of the peer interactions had taken over as the primary reinforcer for his responsiveness. His motivation for school increased, he appeared much happier, and it appeared that he had many more friends. At that point his clinician terminated her formal involvement with Carl, and it appears that his social responsivity is maintaining in the absence of further intervention.

## James: Self-Instruction for Reducing Stereotypy

James, a fourteen-year-old severely handicapped youth with autism, engaged in obtrusive stereotypic behavior that severely stigmatized him in the community. At 6 feet tall, he was very noticeable skipping down the sidewalk flailing his arms about his ears and above his head and producing loud unintelligible vocalizations. Behavioral observations indicated that such behaviors were incompatible with James's attention to other stimuli in his environment. As such, a self-instruction program to focus James's attention on other environmental stimuli seemed ideal. This program would permit continual intervention by producing an incompatible behavior and would not require the presence or continual vigilance of a clinician. The intervention proceeded as follows.

Following a discrimination training where the target behavior was modeled, James was provided with a wristwatch with a repeat alarm function. Every time the alarm sounded, James was prompted to say "I see a . . . ," and was provided with a token reinforcer each time he labeled an environmental stimulus. After several sessions, James would reliably label an environmental stimulus after each alarm without any prompting, and he was working to earn a considerable number of tokens prior to receiving a tangible reinforcer (a cup of ice cream). The alarm was then set to sound after every 15 seconds. At this point James began to look around during his community walks and to label stimuli (trees, fire trucks, buildings, etc.) each time the alarm sounded. The frequent alarms did not permit James enough time to stop observing his environment and to engage in stereotypic behavior. As a result, James was able to engage in brief community outings without exhibiting any stereotypic behavior at all. His periodic labeling of objects in his environment did not seem atypical to other individuals, and he began to appear as a person who was very interested in his environment and even began to interest other individuals in observing the events he was pointing out.

## Nicky: Self-Monitoring of Verbal Initiations

Nicky, a preschool child with autism, had been taught to self-monitor his responses to peer initiations and was doing quite well in that regard. However, he was still experiencing social problems at his preschool because he almost never initiated interactions himself. His clinician hypothesized that because Nicky already knew basic self-monitoring procedures, it might be relatively easy to merely add "initiating" as a target behavior. The treatment procedure went as follows. Nicky was given the self-monitoring wrist counter and told that he could now earn points (which could be exchanged for candy) if he went over and talked to other children. Initially, he was prompted to select a child and to press his wrist counter if he walked over to the child and said something. If on repeated initiations Nicky continued to perseverate on the same topic, he was prompted to "say something different" in order to earn points. Once this procedure was in effect, the schedule of reinforcement was thinned to one piece of candy for every 2 initiations recorded on the wrist counter, then to three, etc., until 10 initiations were accurately being recorded on the wrist counter and exchanged for reinforcers. Ultimately, the combination of initiating and responding to peers resulted in numerous brief conversational interactions taking place with the other children in his classroom, greatly increasing Nicky's level of social integration.

## SUMMARY

Overall, the above literature and case examples suggest that self-regulatory intervention strategies may have considerable application in the field of autism. Although the exact mechanism of such interventions is not completely understood, and the limits of applicability have not yet been defined, it nevertheless appears that the procedures are far enough developed at the present time to have significant applied value to a large number of children with autism. Continued research in this area is expected to produce significant advances in the autonomy, independence, and social integration of children with severe handicaps.

### ACKNOWLEDGMENTS

Funding for the development of this chapter was provided in part by the following research projects; "Research in Autism: Parent Intervention" (USPHS MH 28210 from the National Institute of Mental Health) and "A Rehabilitation Research and

Training Center on Community Referenced Technologies for Nonaversive Behavior Management" (NIDRR Cooperative Agreement #G0087C0234 from the U.S. Department of Education).

## REFERENCES

Bagshaw, N. B. (1978). *An acoustic analysis of fundamental frequency and temporal parameters of autistic children's speech.* Unpublished master's thesis. University of California, Santa Barbara.

Baltaxe, C. A. (1977). Pragmatic deficits in the language of autistic adolescents. *Journal of Pediatrics Psychology, 2,* 176–180.

Baltaxe, C. A. M. (1981). Acoustic characteristics of prosody in autism. In P. Mittler (Ed.), *New frontiers of knowledge in mental retardation* (1) (pp. 223–233). Baltimore: University Park.

Baltaxe, C. A. M. (1984). Use of contrastive stress in normal, aphasic, and autistic children. *Journal of Speech and Hearing Research, 27,* 97–105.

Baltaxe, C. A. M. & Guthrie, D. (1987). The use of primary sentence stress by normal, aphasic, and autistic children. *Journal of Autism and Developmental Disorders, 17,* 255–271.

Baltaxe, C. A. M., & Simmons, J. Q. (1975). Language in childhood psychosis: A review. *Journal of Speech and Hearing Disorders, 40,* 439–458.

Bartak, L., Rutter, M., & Cox, A. (1975). A comparative study of infantile autism and specific developmental receptive language disorder: 1. The children. *British Journal of Psychiatry, 126,* 127–145.

Bernard-Opitz, V. (1982). Pragmatic analysis of the communicative behavior of an autistic child. *Journal of Speech and Hearing Disorders, 47,* 99–109.

Burke, J. C., & Cerniglia, L. (1990). Stimulus complexity and autistic children's responsivity: Assessing and training a pivotal behavior. *Journal of Autism and Developmental Disorders, 20,* 233–253.

Carr, E. G., & Durand, V. M. (1985). Reducing behavior problems through functional communication training. *Journal of Applied Behavior Analysis, 18,* 111–126.

Craig, H., & Gallegher, T. (1982). Gaze proximity as turn regulators within three-party and two-party child conversations. *Journal of Speech and Hearing Research, 25,* 65–75.

Dodge, K. A. (1983). Behavioral antecedents of peer social status. *Child Development, 54,* 1386–1399.

Duncan, S., & Fiske, D. (1977). *Face to face interaction: Research, methods and theory.* Hillsdale, NJ: Lawrence Erlbaum.

Fay, W. H. (1969). On the basis of autistic echolalia. *Journal of Communication Disorders, 2,* 38–47.

Feldhusen, J. F., Thurston, J. R., & Benning, J. J. (1970a). Aggressive classroom behavior and school achievement. *Journal of Special Education, 4,* 431–439.

Feldhusen, J. F., Thurston, J. R., & Benning, J. J. (1970b). Longitudinal analysis of classroom behavior and school achievement. *Journal of Experimental Education, 38,* 4–10.

Feldman, R. (Ed.). (1982). *The development of nonverbal behavior in children.* New York: Springer-Verlag.

Fine, G. A. (1981). Friends, impression management, and preadolescent behavior. In S. R. Asher & J. M. Gottman (Eds.), *The development of children's friendships* (pp. 29–52). New York: Cambridge University Press.

Fowler, S. (1984). Introductory comments: The pragmatics of self-management for the developmentally disabled. *Analysis and Intervention of Developmental Disabilities, 4,* 85–89.

Furman, W., & Buhrmester, D. (1985). Children's perceptions of the personal relationships in their social networks. *Developmental Psychology, 21,* 1016–1024.

Furman, W., & Robbins, P. (1985). What's the point: Selection of treatment objectives. In B. Schneider, K. H. Rubin, & J. E. Ledingham (Eds.), *Children's peer relations: Issues in assessment and intervention* (pp. 41–54). New York: Springer-Verlag.

Goldfarb, W., Braunstein, P., & Lorge, I. (1956). A study of speech patterns in a group of schizophrenic children. *American Journal of Orthopsychiatry, 26,* 544–555.

Grossman, H. (1983). *Classification in mental retardation.* Washington, DC: American Association on Mental Deficiency.

Haring, T. G. (1990). Social relationships. In L. Meyer, C. A. Peck, & L. Brown (Eds.), *Critical issues in the lives of people with severe disabilities* (pp. 195–217). Baltimore: Brookes.

Hart, B., & Risley, T. R. (1975). Incidental teaching of language in the preschool. *Journal of Applied Behavior Analysis, 8,* 411–420.

Hartup, W. W., & Sancillio, M. F. (1986). Children's friendships. In E. Schopler & G. B. Mesibov (Eds.), *Social behavior in autism* (pp. 61–79). New York: Plenum.

Hoffer, B., & St. Clair, N. (Eds.). (1981). *Developmental kinesics: The emerging paradigm.* Baltimore: University Park.

Hunt, P., Alwell, M., & Goetz, L. (1988). Acquisition of conversation skills and the reduction of inappropriate social interaction behaviors. *Journal of the Association for Persons with Severe Handicaps, 13,* 20–27.

Kanfer, F. (1971). The maintenance of behavior by self-generated stimuli and reinforcement. In A. Jacobs & L. Sachs (Eds.), *The psychology of private events* (pp. 143–179). New York: Academic.

Kanfer, F., & Hagerman, S. (1981). The role of self-regulation. In L. Rehm (Ed.), *Behavior therapy for depression: Present status and future directions* (pp. 143–179). New York: Academic.

Kanner, L. (1943). Autistic disturbances of affective contact. *Nervous Child, 3,* 217–250.

Koegel, L. K., Koegel, R. L., Hurley, C., & Frea, W. D. (1992). Improving social skills and disruptive behavior in children with autism through self-management. *Journal of Applied Behavior Analysis, 25,* 341–354.

Koegel, L. K., Koegel, R. L., & Parks, D. R. (1991). *How to teach self-management to people with severe disabilities: A training manual.* Unpublished manuscript. University of California, Santa Barbara.

Koegel, R. L., & Felsenfeld, E. (1977). Sensory deprivation. In S. Gerber (Ed.), *Audiometry in infancy* (pp. 247–262). New York: Grune & Stratton.

Koegel, R. L., & Frea, W. D. (1993). Treatment of social behavior in autism through the modification of pivotal social skills. *Journal of Applied Behavior Analysis, 26,* 369–377.

Koegel, R. L., & Koegel, L. K. (1990). Extended reductions in stereotypic behavior of students with autism through a self-management treatment package. *Journal of Applied Behavior Analysis, 23,* 119–127.

Koegel, R. L., Koegel, L. K., & O'Neill, R. E. (1989). Generalization in the treatment of autism. In L. V. McReynolds & J. E. Spradin (Eds.), *Generalization strategies in the treatment of communication disorders* (pp. 116–131). Toronto: B. C. Decker.

Kohn, M. (1966). The child as a determinant of his peers' approach to him. *The Journal of Genetic Psychology, 109,* 91–100.

Lagomarcino, T., & Rusch, F. (1989). Utilizing self-management procedures to teach independent performance. *Education and Training in Mental Retardation, 24,* 297–305.

Levinson, S. (1983). *Pragmatics.* Cambridge: Cambridge University Press.

Litrownick, A. J. (1982). Special considerations in the self-management training of the developmentally disabled. In P. Karoly & F. Kanfer (Eds.), *Self-management and behavior change: From theory to practice* (pp. 315–352). New York: Pergamon.

Loveland, K. A., Landry, S. H., Hughes, S. O., Hall, S. K., & McEvoy, R. E. (1988). Speech acts and the pragmatic deficits of autism. *Journal of Speech and Hearing Research, 31,* 593–604.

Lovett, D., & Haring, K. (1989). The effects of self-management training on the daily living of adults with mental retardation. *Education and Training in Mental Retardation, 24,* 306–323.

Mank, D., & Horner, R. H. (1987). Self-recruited feedback: A cost-effective procedure for maintaining behavior. *Research in Developmental Disabilities, 8,* 91–112.

McHale, S. M., Simeonson, R. J., Marcus, L. M., & Olley, J. G. (1980). The social and symbolic quality of autistic children's communication. *Journal of Autism and Developmental Disorders, 10,* 299–310.

Michael, J. (1986). Repertoire-altering effects of remote contingencies. *Analysis of Verbal Behavior, 4,* 10–18.

Moore, S., Agran, M., & Foder-Davis, J. (1989). Using self-management strategies to increase the production rates of workers with severe handicaps. *Education and Training in Mental Retardation, 24,* 324–332.

Nelson, R. O. (1977). Methodological issues in assessment via self-monitoring. In J. D. Cone & R. P. Hawkins (Eds.), *Behavioral assessment: New directions in clinical psychology* (pp. 217–240). New York: Brunner-Mazel.

O'Leary, S., & Dubey, D. (1979). Applications of self-control by children: A review. *Journal of Applied Behavior Analysis, 12,* 449–465.

O'Neill, R. E. (1987). *Environmental interactions of normal children and children with autism.* Unpublished doctoral dissertation, University of California, Santa Barbara.

Pronvost, W., Wakstein, M., & Wakstein, D. (1966). A longitudinal study of the speech behavior and language comprehension of fourteen children diagnosed atypical or autistic. *Exceptional Child, 33,* 19–26.

Prutting, C. A., & Kirchner, D. M. (1987). A clinical appraisal of the pragmatic aspects of language. *Journal of Speech and Hearing Disorders, 52,* 105–119.

Quay, L. C., & Jarrett, O. S. (1984). Predictors of social acceptance in preschool children. *Developmental Psychology, 20,* 793–796.

Ricks, D. M., & Wing, L. (1975). Language, communication, and the use of symbols in normal and autistic children. *Journal of Autism and Childhood Schizophrenia, 5,* 191–222.

Rimland, B. (1964). *Infantile autism.* New York: Appleton-Century-Crofts.

Rutter, M. (1970). Autistic children: Infancy to adulthood. *Seminars in Psychiatry, 2,* 435–450.

Sainato, D. M., Strain, P. S., Lefebvre, D., & Rapp, N. (1990). Effects of self-evaluation on the independent work skills of preschool children with disabilities. *Exceptional Children, 56,* 540–549.

Scherer, K., & Ekman, P. (Eds.). (1982). *Handbook of methods in nonverbal behavior research.* Cambridge: Cambridge University Press.

Schreibman, L., Kohlenberg, B. S., & Britten, K. B. (1986). Differential responding to content and intonation components of a complex auditory stimulus by nonverbal and echolalic autistic children. *Analysis and Intervention in Developmental Disabilities, 6,* 109–125.

Schreibman, L., & Mills, J. I. (1983). Infantile autism. In T. J. Ollendick & M. Hersen (Eds.), *Handbook of child psychopathology* (pp. 105–129). New York: Plenum.

Seibert, T., & Oller, D. K. (1981). Linguistic pragmatics and language intervention strategies. *Journal of Autism and Developmental Disorders, 11,* 75–88.

Shapiro, E. (1981). Self-control procedures with the mentally retarded. In M. Hersen, R. Eisler, & P. Miller (Eds.), *Progress in behavior modification* (Vol. 12, pp. 265–297). New York: Academic.

Sorosky, A. D., Ornitz, E. M., Brown, M. B., & Ritvo, E. R. (1968). Systematic observations of autistic behavior. *Archives of General Psychiatry, 18,* 439–449.

Strain, P. S. (1984). Social behavior patterns of non-handicapped and handicapped-developmentally disabled friend pairs in preschools. *Analysis and Intervention in Developmental Disabilities, 4,* 15–28.

Sullivan, H. S. (1953). *The interpersonal theory of psychiatry.* New York: Norton.

Von Raffler-Engel, W. (Ed.). (1980). *Aspects of nonverbal communication.* Amsterdam: Swets & Zeitlinger.

Waterhouse, L., & Fein, D. (1978). Patterns of kinesic synchrony in autistic and schizophrenic children. In F. C. C. Peng & W. von Raffler-Engler (Eds.), *Language acquisition and developmental kinesics* (pp. 157–166). Hiroshima: Bunka Hyoron.

Whitman, T. (1990). Self-regulation and mental retardation. *American Journal on Mental Retardation, 4,* 347–362.

Wing, L. (1969). The handicaps of autistic children—A comparative study. *Journal of Child Psychology and Psychiatry, 10,* 1–40.

Wing, L. (1985). *Autistic children.* New York: Brunner-Mazel.

# 6

# Developmental Disorders and Broad Effects of the Environment on Learning and Treatment Effectiveness

JAMES A. MULICK and PATRICIA M. MEINHOLD

## INTRODUCTION

The idea of providing comprehensive yet individualized teaching and therapy for children with developmental disorders and other major handicaps is, at once, as attractive as it is difficult to achieve. The historic success of American mass education, its ability to contribute to a melding of diverse cultures, required an approach that did not emphasize the differences between students, but rather emphasized their common educational objectives. In the traditional approach, students were judged by their adaptability. The curriculum was designed to encourage acceptance of widely held social values and accepted cultural practices. Lack of student achievement, even lack of engagement with the educational process, quickly led teachers and others to judge that the *student* had failed. People with influence, like parents and community leaders, teachers and administrators, and even those students who were more readily engaged and successful, could exert strong pressure on students who were different to adapt to the style of

JAMES A. MULICK and PATRICIA M. MEINHOLD • Department of Pediatrics, The Ohio State University, and The Children's Hospital, Columbus, Ohio 43205.

*Behavioral Issues in Autism*, edited by Eric Schopler and Gary B. Mesibov. New York, Plenum Press, 1994.

education that was provided; or if still unsuccessful, to exit the educational system and then avoid other settings in which school achievement was a social prerequisite. This approach presupposes that failure leads to more failure and finally to exclusion.

Special education has emerged as a decidedly different educational enterprise in American culture. The implication of our present standards for special education is that the teaching approach used must be individualized, and failure, when it occurs, is a failure of the strategy or technology used, not the student. Individualized instruction and the use of specific treatments are superior to group methods, particularly if group methods fail to consider the impact of having a disability on a youngster's participation. We routinely teach braille reading to compensate for blindness; we teach sign language to compensate for deafness; we provide architectural modifications to improve school and community access to those with movement handicaps; and we use very specialized and individualized strategies to teach students with rare and complex disabilities.

This appreciation of individual differences and special needs exists side by side with the older view of mass education. We are often forced to reckon with the tension produced by conflict between these two cultures, that of achieving social (and educational) unity out of diversity, and that of achieving equality and fairness in the face of undeniable disadvantage. Each day, professionals, parents, and people with handicaps feel this tension personally and look for a resolution. Our partial solution (and solutions to conflicts between such powerful ideals are usually temporary and incomplete) is to seek to achieve the former, social and educational unity, through work on better understanding the individual meaning of the latter, of disadvantage, and to compensate for the impact of disability by using the tools of behavioral and biomedical science and technology to full advantage (Meinhold & Mulick, 1990b; Mulick & Kedesdy, 1988).

The purpose of this chapter is to illustrate the individual and ecological factors that determine treatment effectiveness in developmental disorders (especially autism and pervasive developmental disorders). The design of effective compensatory strategies rests on an understanding of the nature of individual factors affecting learning, and on the interactions between individual characteristics and the environments in which learning occurs. We will pay special attention to the effects of broad environmental factors (such as setting and context) on behavioral processes. These background conditions have been neglected in applied behavioral research until quite recently, partly as a result of researchers' preoccupation with the causes of disability and basic developmental or cognitive processes, and partly because they introduce considerable methodological complexity to the already complicated lives of researchers in this field. Finally, we will comment briefly on the implications of an ecological perspective for making policy decisions affecting the education and treatment of people with developmental disabilities.

## GENERAL PROCESS ASSUMPTIONS

Developmental disabilities affect important areas of intellectual and adaptive functioning, and are, by definition, long-term conditions requiring long-term compensatory assistance from others, and sometimes professional intervention. This is, in fact, a definition developed in the U.S. Congress to help determine eligibility for publicly funded services under the Developmentally Disabled Assistance and Bill of Rights Act (1975) and subsequent amendments. The concept has been adopted, with modifications, in other federal and state legislation in the United States, and has been embraced by professionals for some purposes. The developmental disability concept differs from the definitions of "handicapped children" in federal and state legislation based on PL 94-142, the Education for All Handicapped Children Act (1975), and its federal and state derivative and supplementary legislation. The Social Security Act defines disabilities manifested first during childhood in still different terms and uses professional assessments in slightly different ways to establish eligibility for funding. These and other disability laws (see Burgdorf, 1980; Turnbull, 1983) demonstrate wide recognition that some disabilities are things that set those affected by them apart from other people. Unfortunately, categories and terms developed for legislative and other social policy purposes are not very good for scientific classification and are even less useful in developing a scientific theory of normal and abnormal development. They are, therefore, not very good conceptual starting points for work on devising more effective compensatory and therapeutic interventions.

Scientific problem solving requires more stable definitions of terms than those subject to legislative and judicial revision. Hence, for all the popularity of newer or more socially acceptable terms, the research community clings to terms that assist in classification and description. For example, we still use mental retardation to refer to a condition of pervasive developmental delay and autism to refer to a cluster of abnormal characteristics that seem to covary in a subpopulation of disabled people.

Normal development is judged by (a) the attainment of major milestones and (b) learning new skills at an average rate. Retarded development is defined by marked delay or general failure of development and learning. The scientifically important question has been: How does such retardation come about? What prevents normal learning? Explanatory theories of mental retardation are generally based on the effects of (a) physical insults to the developing individual that alter physiological structures and functions affecting learning, (b) genetic and chromosome disorders leading to abnormal physical structures and functions of bodily systems affecting learning, (c) extreme environmental conditions, and (d) a combination of these types of influence (Baroff, 1986; Bijou & Dunitz-Johnson, 1981; Lipsitt, 1984; Matson & Mulick, 1983). The other developmental disabilities, most of which are closely associated with mental retardation, can be thought of as resulting from different admixtures of these abnormal developmental influences.

Autism, for example, is associated with characteristics such as (a) poor social relatedness, (b) both delayed and abnormal language and social development, (c) difficulty with concept formation and abstraction, (d) unusual motivational systems and preferences, (e) unusual patterns of learning about recurrent environmental cues, (f) auditory processing deficits, and (g) a preference for sameness and a seeming lack of spontaneity (Mesibov, Troxler, & Boswell, 1988). These characteristics, in turn, have been associated with impaired central nervous system (CNS) function, especially to those neurophysiological subsystems that, when damaged, result in social, communicative, and motivational abnormalities (e.g., Yeterian, 1987). Other frequent characteristics of people with some developmental disorders such as repetitive self-injury (e.g., Courchesne, 1989; Baumeister, Frye, & Schroeder, 1984; DeCatanzaro, 1978), impulsiveness (e.g., Thompson, Bjelajac, Huestis, Crinella, & Yu, 1989) and aggression (e.g., Mulick, Hammer, & Dura, 1991) have been explained by theories based, at least in part, on experimentally demonstrated neurophysiological or brain–behavior relationships.

The most important point to make here about these theories of etiology is that while physical insult and resulting abnormality of structure are implicated, the environment continues to have an explanatory role in two ways. First, the environment contributes to the severity and variability of these abnormal characteristics by providing the opportunity, or lack of opportunity, for their expression in abnormal behavior and learning. Second, the environment can provide compensatory experiences that make possible the adaptive learning that is accomplished by youngsters with these disorders and can at times make possible learning to overcome handicapping behavioral tendencies (Lovaas, 1987). The basic support for the role of the environment in moderating the expression of developmental disorders will be summarized in the next section.

## The Relevance of Context to Behavior and Learning

The environment is simply the entire set of events, settings, objects, and people that interacts with the behavior of individuals. The timing and sequence of environmental events and their contingent relationships with behavior comprise the subject matter of the behavior analysis of learning and development. Living beings are constantly interacting with the environment, but behavior analysts usually restrict their attention to only a few characteristics of the environment at a time. This is done for analytic convenience, not because there is a lack of evidence for the influence of many other variables.

## Antecedents

Environmental events can signal or cue behavior in a number of ways. Responding can be directly elicited (such as when food elicits salivation and gastric activity), but it can also be "cued" in other ways. The opportunity for a response to be reinforced (or punished) can be signaled by stimuli that have been present when that response has been reinforced or punished before. Discriminative stimuli are said to "set the occasion" for responding because they do not cause a response in the mechanical way that food elicits salivation, but instead make a particular class of responses more likely to occur for a period of time. A host of stimuli can come to affect responding in this way, including both external environmental events (transduced by receptors for distal stimuli such as the eyes, ears, and nose) and internal physical sensations. In fact, the sensations of bodily feedback produced by the actions of a learner probably "bridge the gap" in time between external discriminative events, behavior, and the consequences that comprise contingencies. "Awareness" of a contingency between a response and a consequence is not necessary for operant learning to occur, but awareness (i.e., following a rule or using cues other than those produced by the schedule itself, like watching a clock during a time-based schedule) may alter the effects of schedules of reinforcement under some conditions (Stoddard, Sidman, & Brady, 1988).

Another class of environmental events that act as antecedents for responding are more difficult to define and to describe in words, but the class has been called "setting factors." Setting factors represent a sort of inventory of potentially effective experiences from the view point of the learner. Thus they include the qualitative and quantitative potential of the environment and its relative enrichment or complexity. Setting factors can affect behavior by providing complex discriminative cues, and they can also determine the learner's momentary preferences (i.e., motivations). It has never been possible to provide a complete description of all setting factors affecting a given learner, but progress has been made in identifying the range of potential setting factors that teachers, parents, and therapists need to worry about if they wish to produce reliable learning. These factors can operate at the level of the individual learner, at the level of classroom or home settings and schedules, and even at the level of institutional or social policy.

## Consequences

In addition to providing the "cues that affect responding, the environment provides the consequences that are responsible for the strengthening, maintenance, and suppression of behavior through operant learning. An event is said to be a reinforcer if it increases an act's future likelihood when it follows that act very closely in time, or in cognitive terms, when the act seems to produce the reinforcer. Likewise, a punisher decreases the future likelihood of an act it follows closely in time, perhaps by increasing escape and avoidance behavior that competes for the time slot of the behavior that was punished, and perhaps by altering the motivational processes of the learner so that the effective range of reinforcement for ongoing behavior is perceived or "felt" differently by the learner. Altered reinforcer value in the face of punished responding might occur when, for example, after tuning in to all the television stations and finding the same live political event being broadcast on all the channels, a person decides to read a book.

It is important to point out that inhibition of behavior is probably an active form of learning, whether it is manifested by passive withholding of a target response or by active performance of an alternative behavior. The effects of punishment usually are enhanced by the availability of reinforcement for alternative behavior, and so are the suppressive effects of nonreward, at least for the short term. There remains a question as to whether temporarily reinforcing alternative behavior will, in the short term, substantially affect the probability of a response selected for punishment or extinction. There is experimental evidence to suggest that it may *not* under some conditions. Experiments from the animal laboratory on the temporary augmentation of the suppressive effects of extinction suggest that reinforcement of competing behavior might actually result in little advantage over extinction alone in terms of the total amount of nonreinforced responding required for response elimination (e.g., Leitenberg, Rawson, & Mulick, 1976; Rawson, Leitenberg, Mulick, & Lefebvre, 1977; Vyse, Rieg, & Smith, 1985). Likewise, experiments based on operant discrimination learning in subjects with mental retardation suggest that stimuli controlling nonreinforced responses (responses that are incompatible with reinforced responses controlled by other stimuli) are simply ignored and undergo no substantial change in their controlling relationship with the nonreinforced behavior during the period of time devoted to the alternative response–reinforcement relation (Huguenin & Touchette, 1980). In the natural environment, of course, neither nonreinforcement of the response to be reduced nor the permanent maintenance of alternative reinforcement (or punishment) contingencies can be guaranteed.

We seldom actually know the effective range of rewards and punishers operating for a given individual in the natural environment. Not only are we unable to directly measure the individual's momentary motivational state, but we also are unable to confirm directly those cues or events in the environment that are being experienced as positive or negative by the learner at any given time. Most learning demonstrations try to assure the effectiveness of reinforcers by seeing that access to them is denied to the learner except as a part of the contingency between the response to be acquired and the planned reinforcer. These motivational manipulations are sometimes referred to as "deprivation conditions" or "establishing operations" (Michael, 1982). In practice, despite attempting to stack the cards in favor of our choices, we always end up guessing that our selected reinforcer (or punisher) will be effective in the context of competing motivational influences. This is in contrast to the situation in the laboratory, where competing influences can be minimized and there can be more confidence about what cues and reinforcers are operating.

## Interactionist Perspective

Individuals are always interacting with a very complex environment. Identifying and analyzing the effective features of the environment is further complicated by the fact that an individual's behavior itself generates stimuli that can affect further responding *and* influence the behavior of others. Behavior is thought to flow sequentially in time as a result of the discriminative stimulus functions of sensory experiences provided by the environment and by the actions of the learner "bridging the gap" in time between behavior and reinforcement. Contingencies operate via the timing of their occurrence. Schedules of reinforcement are excellent examples of the seamless flow of behavior produced by cues leading to acts producing reinforcement.

An operant analysis of the effects of the environment on learning and development suggests that even the simple mother–infant dyad, the basis for much learning prerequisite for normal development, is very complex indeed. Mother–infant interaction is the context for the early development of socialization and language, diurnal entrainment of activity cycles, the elaboration of many early motor and perceptual-motor sequences, and for the acquisition of numerous other behavioral patterns. The outcome of a dyadic interaction depends on the behavior of each participant (e.g., is the infant sleepy or hungry or in pain; and is the mother anxious, or painfully in need of allowing her milk to flow, or hoping to feel her baby return the love she feels?). Each participant's behavior is dependent on the state of deprivation that precedes the encounter and on the host of discriminative and motivational factors provided by the environment (e.g., the presence of other people with their own motivations, the familiarity of the setting, whether it is night or day, the room temperature, noise level, and other setting factors).

Individuals are embedded in layers of environmental influence—levels of influence on behavior that we can begin to understand from an interactionist or ecobehavioral perspective (Schroeder, 1990). We will examine how these levels of influence are relevant to the unique learning and treatment needs of people with disabilities. The organization of the remainder of the chapter will follow a sequence of increasing complexity. We will begin with factors affecting the individual directly and move to progressively more distant environmental influences. In each type of example, we will try to demonstrate the interaction of influences at one level of analysis with factors at other levels, in keeping with our interactionist perspective.

## INDIVIDUAL FACTORS

By individual factors, we are referring to internal events and conditions that alter learning and performance in broader environmental contexts. Many members of this class of variable are biological ones. They include momentary effects of homeostatic feedback mechanisms, illnesses and handicapping conditions, and biomedical interventions. We will discuss two of these variables—physical illness and psychoactive drugs.

### Illness and Health

Illness should be differentiated functionally from a handicap in terms of its effect on individual behavior. By illness we refer to a medical condition that is progressive, with changes in its effects on bodily systems as it progresses. Illnesses affect operant learning in many ways. They can alter the effectiveness of cues when they affect sensation (e.g., otitis media and conductive hearing loss) and perception (e.g., delirium). They can alter the range of possible behavioral alternatives by affecting motor movements directly (e.g., swelling or stiffness) or through the general fatigue they might engender. Finally, they can alter the value of reinforcers by affecting sensory feedback from behavior (e.g., pain), and homeostatic regulating mechanisms and CNS motivational systems (e.g., salt hunger during adrenal failure, excessive thirst in diabetes). Illnesses can even become cues and reinforcers for the individual. For example, when you feel a headache you might take an analgesic, and when you have a headache you might be able to avoid an unpleasant obligation. They can represent punishers as well, like gastrointestinal illness producing avoidance of a new food that was consumed just before feeling sick.

Our group at The Ohio State University has had an opportunity to work for several years with a large, stable population of multihandicapped children and adults (described in Meinhold & Mulick, 1990a, pp. 112–118). This population has a high rate of physical illness owing to their frail conditions and complications of their handicapping conditions. Furthermore, their lack of functional communication makes it difficult for medical personnel to detect some acute illnesses during routine physical examinations. We discovered that behavior change associated with disease-related sensory consequences (i.e., apparent discomfort and aggression or changes in the frequency of self-injury) or abrupt changes in preferred reinforcers could be the most obvious indication of an acute illness in this group (Gunsett, Mulick, Fernald, & Martin, 1989).

Reaction to illness is highly individual. Not all infants with ear infections engage in head banging, but some apparently do, and ear infections may be a frequent antecedent of first-time head banging (DeLissovoy, 1963). Our clinical experience reinforces this correlation but suggests that resolution of the acute illness does not consistently change the rate of head banging. Presumably, social or even sensory reinforcers take over the maintenance of head banging after the illness is over. Similarly, aggression may be related to an acute illness, either because it is elicited by the resulting discomfort, or because others treat the individual differently when the illness is present and establish conditions appropriate for either escape-related aggression or positively reinforced aggression (Mulick, Hammer, & Dura, 1991).

Handicapping conditions alter learning, too, but the condition is not progressive, and so the effects are slightly different. These effects are more like static setting conditions. In autism, for example, altered auditory processing may change the effectiveness of certain cues and make certain auditory stimuli effective as reinforcers and others effective as punishers (e.g., noise, speech) in ways that would be less likely to be seen in people not classified as autistic. Stimulus overselectivity during the acquisition of a discrimination is another example of learning, in this case learning to rely on narrow elements of the complex natural environment as cues (Huguenin & Touchette, 1980), that seems more likely to evolve in people with autism (e.g., Kolko, Anderson, & Campbell, 1980). Unlike acute illness, these contextual factors will probably remain effective in an individual long enough so that compensatory strategies, not temporary adaptation and medical treatment, will be needed.

## Drugs as Stimuli

Psychotropic medication has revolutionized the care of people with mental illness in the last 60 years. Among the most dramatic effects are those seen in the treatment of schizophrenia, where neuroleptic medication can greatly reduce some of the characteristic and most troubling symptoms such as auditory hallucinations and distorted perception and thinking. Psychostimulants are effective with youngsters who have difficulty attending selectively to the environment and aid in the reduction of increased generalized activity. Some affective disorders respond well to several types of antidepressant medications. The list of accomplishments in modern psychopharmacology is very long and very impressive. The value of psychopharmacology, however, has been less impressive in mental retardation and developmental disabilities.

The effects of neuroleptic medication (major tranquilizers) on stereotypies have been studied for a long time. Even after discounting methodologically flawed studies, real reductions in stereotyped movements among some developmentally disabled subpopulations are probably to be expected with this class of drug (e.g., pervasive developmental disorder, see Campbell, 1985). But response to neuroleptic treatment of stereotypies (and the response to withdrawal of neuroleptic treatment) may be idiosyncratic and setting specific (Aman & White, 1988; Hollis & St. Omer, 1972; Marholin, Touchette, & Stewart, 1979). Further, the reduction in rate of stereotypic motor behavior, at least when produced by chlorpromazine, may extend to all classes of motor behavior (Hollis & St. Omer, 1972) and may not actually result in the increase in adaptive behavior that one would expect from the decreased preoccupation with stereotypy (Aman, White, & Field, 1984). The benefit in reducing stereotypy, at least in terms of the hoped-for expansion of response repertoires in people with mental retardation and developmental disabilities, is far from clear for the entire class of neuroleptics. Drug-efficacy studies should be conducted in such a way that objective behavioral measures show the effects, if any, on target symptoms and collateral behavior. Studies should especially note how alterations in behavioral symptoms interact with other adaptive and maladaptive activities in natural settings. Global ratings alone, the usual measure in drug studies, even when supplemented with concurrent laboratory measures of behavior, can't detect the response-response (i.e., changes in rates or duration of response as a function of changes in other responses) and behavior-setting (i.e., differential response as a function of ongoing behavior, alternative opportunities, available reinforcers, etc.) interactions, which are needed to refine our understanding of the real risks and benefits of drug treatment.

Psychoactive drugs can modify the effects of environmental stimuli, in much the same way as that suggested for acute illnesses. Other interesting aspects of such drugs are their potential to function as environmental stimuli (Ho, Richards, & Chute, 1978; Thompson & Pickens, 1971). Any drugs with high voluntary self-administration potential, such as some analgesics, sedatives, muscle relaxers, psychostimulants, and minor tranquilizers, by definition, function as positive reinforcers. Drug addiction is an example of such behavior. There is reason to believe these drugs would function as reinforcers when administered by another person as well. Some drugs, such as dextroamphetamine and ethanol, can function as discriminative stimuli and fairly reliably produce state-dependent learning. Other medications may even function as punishers through the induction of unpleasant side effects.

It is plausible, therefore, to advise parents and physicians to consider the stimulus properties of drugs and their timing of administration when using them. The reinforcing and associative properties of some drugs might, if used contingent on the occurrence (or the increase in frequency) of behavior problems, make matters worse over the long term, in much the same way that contingent social attention has been shown to increase (or reinforce) problem behavior in some children. Our clinical observation of mentally retarded patients given PRN orders for minor tranquilizers and analgesics supports this view, but in the absence of controlled studies on the subject, the putative reinforcing effects of drugs cannot be separated from the effects of the social attention attendant on administering them (a positive reinforcement effect) or from the effects of removing discomfort (or anxiety) contingent on problem behavior (a negative reinforcement effect).

The following example illustrates the clinical application of a drug's stimulus properties. After consulting with the physician and parent about the disturbed pattern of sleep in a youngster with severe multiple handicaps, it seemed that increasing evening doses of a benzodiazepine drug, prescribed to help induce relaxation and sleep, were failing to induce sleep as expected. We suggested trying noncontingent administration of a fixed (lower) dose of the drug about 20 minutes following a planned series of evening activities terminated by low-intensity parent–child interaction in the child's bedroom. Within about 2 weeks, a dramatic reversal had occurred, and the child was falling asleep before drug administration. Presumably, the correlation of relaxation and low activity with the drug's effects promoted behavior compatible with falling asleep. Practical guidelines for the clinical application of both the main therapeutic effect and the stimulus properties of psychotropic drugs will require new research. The most useful line of research to pursue would be to examine commonly prescribed drugs in a variety of practical and naturalistic situations such as classrooms, homes, and recreational settings.

One theory of self-injurious behavior (SIB) involves the opioid–peptide system in the brain (see Bernstein, Hughes, Mitchell, & Thompson, 1987; Cataldo & Harris, 1982). The involvement of the brain's own production of opiatelike polypeptides (for which there are opioid receptor cells in the CNS and other parts of the body that account for the commonly observed effects of both the plant-derived and endogenous substances) would suggest that SIB is maintained, in part, by either (a) the reinforcing effect of the release during physical trauma of these naturally occurring morphinelike substances, or (b) their analgesic property, through blunting the direct punishing effect of SIB and thereby allowing other environmental reinforcers to maintain the SIB. Neither theory has been unequivocally supported as yet (nor have other mechanisms of action in which opioid peptides may play a part in SIB), but the possibility of treating SIB by administering drugs that selectively block opiate receptor cells is under active experimental investigation (e.g., Barrett, Feinstein, & Hole, 1989; Lienemann & Walker, 1989). Time will tell whether this approach will result in more effective pharmacological and behavioral treatments for SIB.

Finally, drug administration can serve as a cue for a change in the behavior of caregivers and teachers. Behavioral reactivity to the presence of medication has been reported frequently, and such expectancy effects are usually controlled by the use of placebo and blind-observer control procedures in valid drug studies. Observer reactivity, and ways to control for it, has been reviewed extensively in literature devoted to research methodology (e.g., Connors, 1985). This leads however, to the discussion of other setting variables that affect normal and abnormal behavior.

## SETTING FACTORS

Beginning with studies conducted during the mid-1970s at the University of North Carolina at Chapel Hill and Murdoch Center, we have been involved in research of our own and with that of associates in which the emphasis has been on the effectiveness of therapeutic interventions *as a function of the general environmental context* (see Vyse & Mulick, 1988; Vyse & Mulick, 1990; Meinhold & Mulick, 1990a). The North Carolina SIB Project (see Schroeder, Kanoy, Mulick, Rojahn, Thios, Stephens, & Hawk, 1982) research, for example, demonstrated that overcorrection for pica in adults with profound mental retardation was more effective in an environment offering more opportunities for engagement with other people and stimulating objects (Mulick, Barbour, Schroeder, & Rojahn, 1980). Other studies demonstrated that particular types of clothing could alter the adaptive behavior and maladaptive severe SIB and self-restraint of subjects in programmed environments and, as a result, affect the accessibility of their behavior to positive reinforcement (Rojahn, Mulick, McCoy, & Schroeder, 1978; Rojahn, Schroeder, & Mulick, 1980). Our group extended the earlier findings of Berkson and Davenport (1962), Berkson and Mason (1964) and Guess and Rutherford (1967), that object manipulation and toy play could decrease the rate of topographically incompatible stereotyped behavior, to the case of repetitive SIB (Mulick, Hoyt, Rojahn, & Schroeder, 1978; Schroeder et al., 1982). We documented the dramatic effects of group composition and client sensory deficit on a variety of adaptive and maladaptive behavior classes shown in people with mental retardation and SIB (Schroeder et al., 1982). Others, working with some of the clients in our program, documented the fact that time-out effectiveness was dependent on the function of SIB in the individual's repertoire and the type of setting used for time-in (Solnick, Rincover, & Peterson, 1977). We noted the correlation of SIB with deficient communication skills (Schroeder, Schroeder, Smith, & Dalldorf, 1978) and experimented with the use of alternative and nonspeech communication skill training and multicomponent adaptive behavior curriculums to help displace SIB and other maladaptive behavior. By the middle of the 1970s, it was apparent that no behavior problem or therapeutic approach could be understood completely without consideration of its relationship to other substitutable and covarying responses of the client, the client's membership in a social group, and the characteristics of the physical environment (Schroeber, Mulick, & Rojahn, 1980).

## Incentive and Motivation

Carr (1977) was among the first to speculate at length about the possible motives affecting the expression of SIB and stereotyped behavior. Since that time, it has become clear to many researchers and probably most parents that motives for abnormal and disturbing behavior are difficult to pin down, even if you know what you're looking for. The motives change over time, especially in those with more severe retardation, and many different motivations may affect the expression of a single maladaptive behavior.

Iwata and his colleagues at the John F. Kennedy Institute in Baltimore described a useful clinical measure of behavior in which the abnormal activity is observed in several distinct environmental contexts in order to make inferences about the behavior's relationship to maintaining variables (Iwata, Dorsey, Slifer, Bauman, & Richman, 1982). The process of making these systematic observations across conditions was called a functional analysis, but there is no single way to do a functional analysis. Touchette, MacDonald, and Langer (1985) described another, more naturalistic, method to understand behavior in terms of its possible maintaining variables, called the scatter plot. Ecobehavioral analysis, using simultaneous multiple-response measures across multiple individuals in the same environment (e.g., Vyse & Mulick, 1988; Tarnowski, Rasnake, Linscheid, & Mulick, 1989), is a still more naturalistic and labor-intensive way to help make the same kinds of inferences. The techniques described in Schroeder et al. (1982) using a matched partial correlation technique to analyze multiple response data in groups, are at the extreme end of the continuum of labor intensiveness in ecobehavioral research. Which approach is best among these and others available? It really depends how much resolution and validity you feel you need to be able to draw useful conclusions. Clinical work and classroom teaching are fairly low-resolution activities, where it is often easier (at least in the absence of contrary regulatory or administrative constraints) to abandon a failed approach than to be sure you have the correct and complete answer before you make any move at all.

We have been using the clinical laboratory approach to study some of the same problems since about 1985 at The Ohio State University and The Children's Hospital in Columbus. It has proved most useful with people who have very limited response repertoires, like infants and those with profound retardation and mobility limitations. After Carr (1977), possible motivations for abnormal behavior in toddlers are (a) escape from instructional or performance demands, (b) positive reinforcement, (c) negative social reinforcement, and (d) self-stimulation. Accordingly, we have observed toddlers interacting with their parents in a relatively demanding social situation (a play session during which the parent directs the child's activities and attention), in a low-demand situation (a play session during which the parent follows the child's interests), and in a situation where the child is alone for a period of time. We add a condition we refer to as the "parent-report" condition, in which the setting simulates conditions the parent describes as likely to result in the problem behavior. We videotape the conditions in succession for about 5-minutes each (depending on the number of conditions and the age of the child) and use rest periods of variable duration to help reduce carryover effects. The data are analyzed by taking counts and durations of behavior by condition from the videotape.[1]

The behavior of one 30-month-old boy who was referred for self-injury and excessive screaming will be used to demonstrate the approach. He was felt to fit the classification of Pervasive Developmental Disorder. His Bayley Mental Developmental Index was 66 with downward scatter due to failures on many language items to a much lower level than his test average. His Vineland Adaptive Behavior Scale suggested better nonverbal than communication-related functioning with standard scores of 66 in the Communication Domain, 76 in the Daily Living Skills Domain, 61 in the Socialization Domain, and 93 in the Motor Domain. The history indicated babbling at about 1.5 years and then decreasing vocal production except for screaming. His behavior at home was described as including spinning himself and objects, staring at electric fans, arranging objects in patterns and then rearranging them, and frequently exhibiting extreme food preferences for a week or two at a time. He was, however, inseparable from and very clingy to his mother, and made good eye contact when he seemed to want something. Rocking and head banging began at about 24 months. There was a history of recurrent otitis media, but his ears were clear and hearing was assessed normal at the time of the evaluation (see Figure 1).

The usual functional analysis shows how the target behavior occurs as a function of the planned conditions. This child's SIB was body slamming against the floor or walls. Figure 1 indicates that disruptive screaming and SIB occur only during the "parent-report" condition, in this case: mother present reading a book but ignoring the child. The SIB in this toddler was not related to the demand condition, consistent with the parental report. Instead, the behavior seemed to be related to the well-known conception of a temper tantrum, disruptive behavior carried out to gain parental attention and therefore under positive reinforcement control.

Our procedure allows us to measure other behavior. This permits a more detailed analysis and can be used to validate the conditions and interpretations suggested by the gross functional analysis. Figure 2 shows the SIB, "body slams," plotted against parent verbal directives. It can be seen that there is no correlation between the two. Figure 3 shows a correlation between the SIB and the disruptive screaming, raising the possibility of a response class and the possibility that reducing one would also reduce the other. This phenomenon has been reported for some types of disruptive behaviors. For example, Friman and Hove (1987) noted that the elimination of stereotyped thumb sucking in two boys who also had more

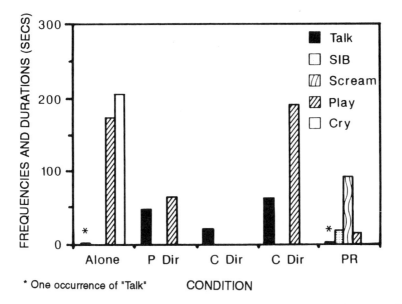

Fig. 1. Adaptive and Maladaptive behavior by condition. Frequency of social vocalizations (Talk), self-injurious body-slams (SIB) and disruptive screaming (Scream), and duration in seconds of object engagement (Play) and crying (Cry) under each experimental condition. (Alone = parent leaves the room; P Dir = parent-directed play; C Dir = Child-directed play; PR = parent report [parent reading]).

than 20-square centimeter bald spots each from hair pulling (the hair pulling normally cooccurred with the thumb sucking), resulted in elimination of hair pulling, too. Knell and Moore (1988) reported the same result, elimination of hair pulling when thumb sucking was eliminated, in a normal 39-month-old boy. In our case, Figure 4 shows the crying that did occur (which could be reliably differentiated from the disruptive screaming by our observers) did not covary with screaming and occurred during different conditions. This provides some indirect evidence for the response class hypothesis, and at least differentiates the screaming from normal protest crying that is typical when a child's mother exits the room. Figure 5 shows the duration of adaptive toy play, and indicates that while the SIB we observed did occur when play was low, SIB did not occur when the toy play was completely absent in the child-directed play condition. In this condition, the mother just goes along, elaborating and participating in whatever the child selects to do.

Finally, Figure 6 shows various types of parent talk plotted as a function of our hypothesized motivational conditions. The first grouping shows that what we called Parent-Directed Play (P Dir) has the most talk, mostly directives, filler, and

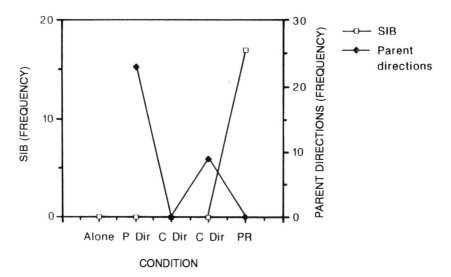

Fig. 2. Parent directions and self-injury by condition. Relative frequencies of self-injurious body-slams (SIB) and parent directions under each experimental condition. (Alone = parent leaves the room; P Dir = parent-directed play; C Dir = child-directed play; PR = parent report [parent reading]).

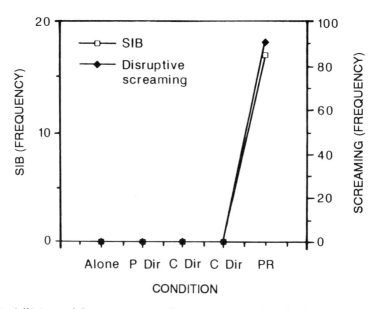

Fig. 3. Self-injury and disruptive screaming by condition. The relationship between frequency of self-injurious body-slams (SIB) and disruptive screaming (Scream) under each experimental condition. (Alone = parent leaves the room; P Dir = parent-directed play; C Dir = child-directed play; PR = parent report [parent reading]).

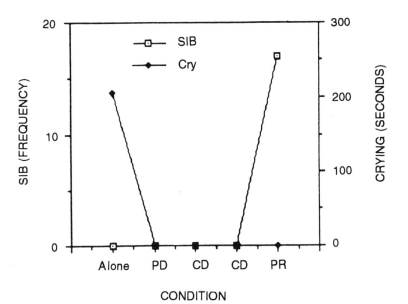

Fig. 4. Self-injury and crying by condition. The relationship between frequency of self-injurious body-slams (SIB) and duration of crying in seconds under each experimental condition. (Alone = parent leaves the room; P Dir = parent-directed play; C Dir = child-directed play; PR = parent report [parent reading]).

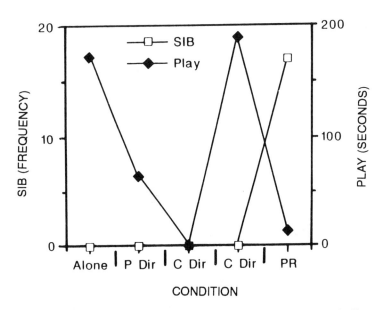

Fig. 5. Self-injury and play by condition. The relationship between frequency of self-injurious body-slams (SIB) and duration of object engagement in seconds (Play) under each experimental condition. (Alone = parent leaves the room; P Dir = parent-directed play; C Dir = child-directed play; PR = parent report [parent reading]).

a little praise. The low-demand condition (Child-Directed Play) resulted in no talk by the mother; she just played along with her child, who was nonverbal and initiated no speech. There were some directive comments and a few reprimands (not of the target behavior, which did not occur) during the second child-directed play condition. Finally, this mother was a good follower of our instruction to ignore the SIB during the "parent-report" condition, and no parent talk occurred. This functional analysis suggested that the SIB for this child was coercive or tantrumlike, reinforced by parental attention. It suggests a treatment similar to those reported for other coercive behaviors. There was little evidence that increasing toy play or simple social interaction skills would have eliminated the SIB, which did not occur when the mother had been engaged with the child or when she was completely absent from the room. The suggested treatment, time-out, has been successful.

## Alternative Actions

By the early 1970s, it was clear that behavior considered problematic was typical of barren, unstimulating environments. A simple response competition

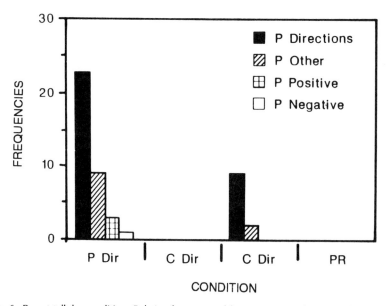

Fig. 6. Parent talk by condition. Relative frequency of four categories of parent talk under each experimental condition. (P Directions = parent directs child's actions; P Other = Other comments such as labeling the child's activities; P Positive = Positive comments to the child such as praise; P Negative = reprimands).

model of choice and time allocation had suggested this would be true. Most workers tried to stack the cards as much as possible to promote adaptive behavior of mentally retarded people through providing as many behavioral alternatives and reinforcers as possible, and this alone produced modest reductions in problem behavior (Horner, 1980; Schroeder, Rojahn, & Mulick, 1978).

The response to environmental opportunities is not assured, however, if the person lacks behavior required to take advantage of the opportunities for adaptive behavior. Sometimes the alternative behavior must be taught. Mulick et al. (1978) showed that the alternative adaptive behavior effectively competes with SIB and stereotypy if it is *topographically incompatible* and inherently engaging for the individual. Unfortunately, opportunities to learn alternatives are sometimes less appealing to the individual than are some high-rate stereotypies. Mace, Browder, and Lin (1987) showed that stereotypies can even be functionally related to teaching sessions and act as escape responses. They reduced stereotypy by (a) decreasing task difficulty and increasing reinforcement and (b) using paced instructions so that the stereotypy no longer successfully escaped from the demands. Of course, a concurrent choice analysis of these data would suggest the same outcome and treatment, that is, individuals generally maximize reinforcement unless constrained from doing so. Thus, stereotypies may be chosen simply because their reinforcement value is greater than the alternatives'. This implies that alternative opportunities alone, even familiar ones, will be insufficient treatment without also adjusting the relative reinforcement values.

For example, Dura, Mulick, Hammer, and Meyers (1990) investigated environmental illumination levels and the acquisition of joystick control over computer-generated sensory reinforcers in profoundly mentally retarded children with multiple physical handicaps. These children functioned at level similar to that of very young infants. Many such children acquire responses reinforced by sensory events displayed on a CRT (the computer's video screen) quite readily with a few physical or verbal prompts. These particular youngsters, however, had failed to respond to conventional prompting. They seemed to be more interested in the social interaction than the CRT. Reducing the ambient illumination, so that the TV screen provided the most visible source of visual stimulation in the room, served to establish the response reliably in some of these difficult-to-engage youngsters and decreased the need for distracting social prompts.

Sometimes stereotypies are so high rate that virtually all behavioral variability is eliminated. This usually occurs only in people with profound mental retardation and multiple physical and neurological impairments. One such individual we had an opportunity to evaluate fit this category. She was a 22-year-old non-ambulatory female with a diagnosis of profound mental retardation, autism, seizure disorder, and cerebral palsy (etiology unknown). Her hand mouthing was so constant that she required occasional medical restraint to allow healing of the breakdown of her skin on the hand. She held on to virtually no objects when given the chance, even during meals, but obviously had the necessary manual dexterity to do so. Physical prompting usually resulted in more vigorous hand mouthing if possible, and active attempts to escape physical proximity if prompting was continued.

Using a rationale developed by the second author, we evaluated a simple response-prevention technique during brief sessions, at first of 5 minutes and, after a discontinuation for a few weeks due to medical orders to restrain all opportunity for mouthing while her skin healed, for 2 minutes. This is shown in Figure 7. We compared two conditions, blocking hand mouthing (lower) with no blocking (upper).[2] Session order was randomized each day. The same objects were made available on her lap board in each condition. Much to our surprise, we observed

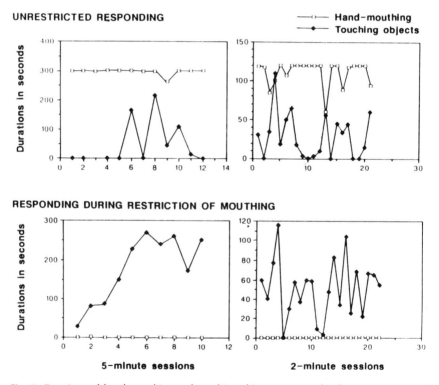

Fig. 7. Durations of hand mouthing and touching objects (in seconds) during 5-minute and 2-minute observation sessions. Unrestricted sessions (top panels) and restriction of mouthing sessions (bottom panels) were both conducted in a randomly assigned order on each observation day (they are separated here for ease of interpretation).

the acquisition of manual object exploration as a reinforcer. The blocking procedure, just manually stopping her hand from reaching her mouth, produced touching objects and holding objects during blocking sessions *in the absence of any
experimental contingency between object touching and mouthing.* However, the
object manipulation also began occurring during the sixth nonblocking session
when she was under no constraints whatsoever. Apparently, some disruption of the
mouthing preoccupation was required to allow the reinforcer sampling to occur
that was prerequisite to the choice of alternative behavior.

## Social Ecology

Most education and treatment is provided in group settings as a matter of
cost-effectiveness. The treatment received, however, is sometimes inadequate or
counterproductive. Schroeder et al. (1982) showed that the presence and absence
of a single newcomer or disruptive client dramatically altered the rates of many
adaptive and maladaptive behaviors of others in group settings serving people with
mental retardation and behavioral disturbances. It was as if the entire habitual set
of social and individual interactions in the setting had been thrown out of balance
by such intrusions. This is what we mean by a social ecology. Literally, changes
in one part of such complex social environments produce dramatic changes in
other parts of the social environments. The reality of these potential effects is the
context in which teaching and treatment procedures, as well as new social relationships, are imposed on people with handicaps by planners and programmers.

Vyse and Mulick (1988) made observations in a classroom serving mostly
ambulatory youngsters with mental retardation and other developmental disorders.
A multicategory data system was used to time sample the behavior of students and
teachers, with the unit of analysis the teaching "day." The analysis revealed
significant correlations between categories of student behavior, both within individuals and between individuals, and the behavior of teachers. In the example
shown in Figure 8, Ann shows more aggression on days when teacher attention
was high, days when she was also likely to receive higher rates of positive social
attention from adults, be more socially interactive, and be less likely to engage in
planned work or play activities. She also received less inattention (proximity
without interaction) on days when she was more aggressive, and more inattention
and less positive teacher attention on days when she was more likely to engage in
planned work or play. The fact that she appeared to have been reprimanded more
on days with high levels of other maladaptive behaviors was not significantly
correlated with the other significant behavioral relationships. These relationships
can be interpreted as revealing inadvertent social reinforcement of aggression and

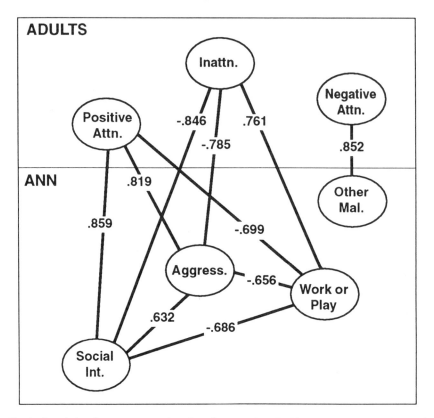

Fig. 8. Correlations between categories of teacher attention (Positive Attention, Inattention, and Negative attention), and categories of student behavior (Aggression, Other Maladaptive Behaviors, Social Interaction, and Work or Play) and correlations between pairs of student behaviors (reproduced by permission, from Vyse & Mulick, 1988).

off-task behavior. The situation, however, is even more complicated than the figure suggests. Not depicted are the significant behavioral correlations between the teachers' and her classmates' behavior on the same days. The overall pattern of relationships probably would have changed if the teachers had tried to alter their pattern of interaction with Ann, and there might have been effects on all the other people in this classroom social ecology. These idiosyncratic but reliable behavioral patterns, the habitual distribution of cues and consequences over time, may be responsible for the great durability of maladaptive behavior patterns in stable social groups and for the failure of social behavior change in one setting to generalize reliably to another setting.

## CUSTOMS, RULES, AND REGULATIONS

These individual and social–ecological interrelationships do not exist accidentally. They exist as a function of other social and institutional structures. All people behave within constraints partly imposed by cultural and administrative rules and government regulations. The cultural and social contexts of individual behaviors has been discussed in the anthropological literature aptly and entertainingly by Harris (1979, 1985), and similar thinking is being applied to problems in clinical psychology and behavior therapy (e.g., Biglan, Glasgow, & Singer, 1990). No one has applied such an analysis to problems in mental retardation and developmental disabilities yet, but the need to do so is becoming readily apparent.

## Normalization

Ideological reasoning alone, perhaps best symbolized by the normalization construct in this field, does not generate reliably effective rules for the construction of therapeutic environments for people with handicaps. Mulick and Kedesdy (1988) demonstrated how normalization concepts tend to be contradicted by some things we have learned from the functional analysis of SIB. Normal-appearing environments by themselves, even environments characterized by social advantage, do not assure normal behavioral outcomes. Handicaps sometimes require extraordinary environmental modifications, including modifications of quite normal rules for social conduct. We do not suggest that segregation and devaluation of people with handicaps is indicated by a scientific analysis, just that rules derived from an abstract and idealized sociopolitical analysis may not be useful in developing effective individualized treatment approaches. Treatment for a behavioral abnormality is not necessarily accomplished through a normal human relationship; therapeutic relationships sometimes require extraordinary persistence, objectivity, analysis, effort, and so forth.

For example, a strong version of normalization holds that normal means are themselves normalizing. Wolfensberger and Glenn (1975) once argued that normalization goals have been partially fulfilled once normative processes have been instituted, regardless of other outcomes. Normal environments do, of course, provide opportunities for learning that are not available in segregated, restricted, crowded, unpleasant institutional environments. But that contrast does not include individualization and careful analysis. It sidesteps completely the actual level of specificity needed. Thus, transfer of adults from an institution to a community residence can be, and has been, reported to be associated with not only increases in adaptive behavior, but also increases in maladaptive behavior (e.g., Fine, Tangeman, & Woodward, 1990). Normal environments make some things easier and some things remarkably harder.

## Rules, Regulations, and Rewards

The final point to be made is that real environments are affected by the reward systems in place for all their inhabitants. Human service and professional workers in this field carry out their activities according to the rules promulgated by their employers, and employers often make rules in response to cultural standards and government regulations. Many of these rules affect the time allocated to various activities by caregivers and professionals, the time available affects both how and what is done by workers, and we have already seen that interpersonal behavior affects the learning opportunities and reinforcers available for the recipients of services. The same external forces operate within the family, in terms of cultural practices and the formal rules and laws enforced by the government.

Rules and regulations can be seen to affect many events that are influential at the level of individual behavior. We will summarize one example from a recent analysis of a private ICF/MR for nonambulatory people with profound mental retardation we examined from a contextualist and ecobehavioral point of view (Meinhold & Mulick, 1990a). The state involved used a per diem reimbursement system based on level of need, in which *more* money was provided for *less* resident independence. We could only speculate that this kind of reimbursement system might encourage greater disability, not less, among residents. But there was more. We found the contingencies of financial reimbursement for services were tied to a format in which any logged discrepancy between planned and delivered habilitation services (in quantitative terms like time spent or number of actions performed) resulted in retroactive loss of funding for the services delivered over the preceding month. Overproviding services was thus severely discouraged even as paperwork accuracy was encouraged. This is an instructive response-competition model. Further, incidental teaching and response-contingent interventions were nearly impossible to define under this system in such a way that funding for them could even be requested. They were, in fact, underused approaches at the facility we examined. We had to conclude that the force of the regulatory contingencies could have, in turn, produced counterhabilitative contingencies of reinforcement for the residents who lived in such a system. This conclusion is supported by considering the implications of contingencies imposed on staff by the relative effort required for habilitative programming, time pressures, resident medical needs, and the lack of countervailing reinforcers for supervisors to encourage habilitative efforts.

## CONCLUSION: THE CASE FOR ENVIRONMENTAL IMPACT STATEMENTS

What are the implications of these examples, besides the obvious one that the functional environment is exceedingly complex? There are a few implications worth commenting on in closing. They pertain to the way we solve clinical learning and behavior problems, the organization of service environments, and the policies governing developmental disability services. They can be summed up rather neatly, however (but see Meinhold & Mulick, 1990b, for a more complete discussion of *decision analysis*): **Before agreeing to the next new idea anyone in this field (no matter how authoritative a source he/she may seem to be) offers as a solution to a problem, require him/her to provide an environmental impact statement.**

This is in no way facetious. Treatment proposals should be based *at least* on a discussion of relevant functional relationships for the client, a statement of expected benefit, and a discussion of possible side effects. Treatment and educational initiatives can and should be responsive to the individual needs of the people they are designed to help. We have described the breadth of individual–environment interactions that are known to influence learning and development. Many of these can be analyzed (or at least estimated) as direct effects or side effects of any treatment or policy proposal. Cost considerations should be acknowledged because they are real, and they will exert their influence anyway (Paisey, Whitney, & Moore, 1989). Ethical and legal considerations should be included in an impact statement, particularly insofar as they are relevant to the specific treatment proposal.

Changes in program structure, which usually have effects on individual behavior at several levels of social organization, would require a somewhat more complicated analysis. For example, the ecobehavioral analysis reported in Vyse and Mulick (1988) was initiated in response to a proposed change in a state regulation governing how many students could be placed in a class with a single teacher and aide. The results suggest that altering teacher–student ratios should be done with caution in view of the significant role played by teacher to student behavioral interaction in maintaining appropriate behavior and student learning. A decision to change a student's classroom placement is another example of a program-level decision that can be expected to have effects on the behavior of the youngster in question and other students as well (Schroeder et al., 1982). Finally, proposed changes in curriculum or teaching methodology (e.g., moving to computer-based instruction for some skills) should be evaluated on a pilot basis for students with many different types of developmental disabilities before major investments or systemwide commitments are made.

Proposed changes in federal and state regulations, especially those involving program funding or reimbursement rates, should have the most extensive environmental impact statements of all. They will affect the most people. At present, such changes are usually justified either ideologically or on the basis of a limited direct cost-benefit analysis. There is, however, good reason to believe that regulatory effects reach the individual level of interaction more reliably than was realized before, and in some surprising ways. These broad effects should be acknowledged by would-be social architects, and they should be required to submit for public comment a thorough analysis of the probable range of effects of proposed regulatory changes. Such an analysis should begin with effects on administrative decisions and activities that would be likely to be affected (e.g., personnel actions and staffing levels, professional services, program expansion or contraction, etc.), include the plausible effects on staff on or caregiver activity schedules, and project the probable effects of the changes on staff to client (or student) and client to client interaction. Experience with developing these *regulatory ecobehavioral impact* statements will improve their accuracy, and public access to the information will contribute to a more effective and responsive regulatory system.

ACKNOWLEDGMENTS

The authors are grateful to many staff and administrators of the Heinzerling Memorial Foundation for cooperating with a segment of the clinical research described in this manuscript. The first author was supported in part by U.S. Department of Health and Human Services MCH Special Project MCJ 009053 during preparation of this manuscript. This work was completed while the second author was a postdoctoral Fellow in Pediatric Psychology in the Department of Pediatrics at The Ohio State University. She is now at the Department of Psychology, Western Michigan University, Kalamazoo, MI.

## NOTES

1. Interobserver reliability was assessed for 40% of observation sessions based on simple percentage agreement between two trained observers. All percentages exceeded 80% (range = 81%–100%; average = 93%).
2. Interobserver reliability between two trained observers was assessed during 49% of observation sessions. Interclass (generalizability) coefficients (Berk, 1979) were .9997 for hand-mouthing and .9973 for touching objects.

## REFERENCES

Aman, M. G. (1987). Overview of pharmacotherapy: Current status and future directions. *Journal of Mental Deficiency Research, 31,* 121–130.

Aman, M. G., & White, C. J. (1988). Thioridazine dose effects with reference to stereotypic behavior in mentally retarded residents. *Journal of Autism and Developmental Disorders, 18,* 355–366.

Aman, M. G., White, A. J., & Field, C. J. (1984). Chlorpromazine effects on stereotypic and conditioned behavior: A pilot study. *Journal of Mental Deficiency Research, 28,* 253–260.

Baroff, G. S. (1986). *Mental retardation: Nature, cause and management* (2d ed.). New York: Hemisphere.

Barrett, R. P., Feinstein, C., & Hole, W. T. (1989). Effects of naloxone and naltrexone on self-injury:

A double-bind, placebo controlled analysis. *American Journal on Mental Retardation, 93*, 644–651.

Baumeister, A. A., Frye, G. D., & Schroeder, S. R. (1984). Neurochemical correlates of self-injurious behavior. J. A. Mulick & B. L. Mallory (Eds.), *Transitions in mental retardation, Volume 1: Advocacy, technology, and science* (pp. 207–227). Norwood, NJ: Ablex.

Berk, R. A. (1979). Generalizability of behavioral observations: A classification of interobserver agreement and interobserver reliability. *American Journal of Mental Deficiency, 83*, 460–472.

Berkson, G., & Davenport, R. K. (1962). Stereotyped movements in mental defectives. *American Journal of Mental Deficiency, 66*, 849–852.

Berkson, G., & Mason, W. A. (1964). Stereotyped movements in mental defectives: IV. The effects of toys and the character of the acts. *American Journal of Mental Deficiency, 88*, 511–524.

Bernstein, G. A., Hughes, J. R., Mitchell, J. E., & Thompson, T. (1987). Effects of narcotic antagonists on self-injurious behavior: A single case study. *Journal of the American Academy of Child and Adolescent Psychiatry, 26*, 886–889.

Biglan, A., Glasgow, R. E., & Singer, G. (1990). The need for a science of larger social units: A contextual approach. *Behavior Therapy, 21*, 195–215.

Bijou, S. W., & Dunitz-Johnson, E. (1981). Interbehavioral analysis of developmental retardation. *The Psychological Record, 31*, 305–329.

Burgdorf, R. (1980). *The legal rights of handicapped persons.* Baltimore: Brookes.

Cataldo, M. F., & Harris, J. (1982). The biological basis for self-injury in the mentally retarded. *Analysis and Intervention in Developmental Disabilities, 2*, 21–39.

Campbell, M. (1985). Schizophrenic disorders and pervasive developmental disorders/infantile autism. In J. M. Wiener (Ed.), *Diagnosis and psychopharmacology of childhood and adolescent disorders* (pp. 113–150). New York: Wiley.

Carr, E. G. (1977). The motivation of self-injurious behavior: A review of some hypotheses. *Psychological Bulletin, 84*, 800–816.

Christian, W. P. (1987). Executive management of human service programs for clients who are developmentally disabled. In J. A. Mulick & R. F. Antonak (Eds.), *Transitions in mental retardation, Volume 2: Issues in therapeutic intervention* (pp. 235–253). Norwood, NJ: Ablex.

Conners, C. K. (1985). Methodological assessment issues in pediatric psychopharmacology. In J. M. Wiener (Ed.), *Diagnosis and psychopharmacology of childhood and adolescent disorders* (pp. 69–110). New York: Wiley.

Courchesne, E. (1989). Neuroanatomical systems involved in infantile autism: The implications of cerebellar abnormalities. In G. Dawson (Ed.), *Autism: Nature, diagnosis, and treatment* (pp. 119–143). New York: Guilford.

DeCatanzaro, D. A. (1978). Self-injurious behavior: A biological analysis. *Motivation and Emotion, 2*, 45–65.

DeLissovoy, V. (1963). Headbanging in early childhood: A suggested cause. *Journal of Genetic Psychology, 102*, 109–114.

Developmentally Disabled Assistance and Bill of Rights Act. (1975). 42 U.S.C. Secs. 6001–6081.

Dura, J. R., Mulick, J. A., Hammer, D., & Myers, E. G. (1990). Establishing independent microcomputer use in people with multiple handicaps, profound mental retardation, and a history of learning failure. *Computers in Human Behavior, 6*, 177–183.

Education for All Handicapped Children Act. (1975), 20 U.S.C. Secs. 1401 et seq. (P.L. 94-142).

Fine, M. A., Tangeman, P. J., & Woodward, J. (1990). Changes in adaptive behavior of older adults with mental retardation following deinstitutionalization. *American Journal on Mental Retardation, 94*, 661–668.

Friman, P. C., & Hove, G. (1987). Apparent covariation between child habit disorders: Effects of successful treatment for thumb sucking on untargeted chronic hair pulling. *Journal of Applied Behavior Analysis, 20*, 421–425.

Gunsett, R. P., Mulick, J. A., Fernald, W. B., & Martin, J. L. (1989). Brief report: Indications for medical screening prior to behavioral programming for severely and profoundly mentally retarded clients. *Journal of Autism and Developmental Disorders, 19,* 167–172.

Guess, D., & Rutherford, G. (1967). Experimental attempts to reduce stereotypy among blind retardates. *American Journal of Mental Deficiency, 71,* 984–986.

Harris, M. (1979). *Cultural materialism: The struggle for a science of culture.* New York: Basic Books.

Harris, M. (1985). *The sacred cow and the abominable pig: Riddles of food and culture.* New York: Simon & Schuster.

Ho, B. T., Richards, D. W., & Chute, D. L. (1978). *Drug discrimination and state dependent learning.* New York: Academic.

Hollis, J. H., & St. Omer, V. V. (1972). Direct measurement of psychopharmacologic response: Effects of chlorpromazine on motor behavior of retarded children. *American Journal of Mental Deficiency, 76,* 397–407.

Horner, R. D. (1980). The effects of an environmental "enrichment" program on the behavior of institutionalized profoundly retarded children. *Journal of Applied Behavior Analysis, 13,* 473–491.

Huguenin, N. H., & Touchette, P. E. (1980). Visual attention in retarded adults: Combining stimuli which control incompatible behavior. *Journal of the Experimental Analysis of Behavior, 33,* 77–86.

Iwata, B. A., Dorsey, M. F., Slifer, K. J., Bauman, K. E., & Richman, G. S. (1982). Toward a functional analysis of self-injury. *Analysis and Intervention in Developmental Disabilities, 2,* 3–20.

Kolko, D. J., Anderson, L., & Campbell, M. (1980). Sensory preferences and overselective responding in autistic children. *Journal of Autism and Developmental Disorders, 10,* 259–271.

Knell, S. M., & Moore, D. J. (1988). Childhood trichotillomania treated indirectly by punishing thumb sucking. *Journal of Behavior Therapy and Experimental Psychiatry, 19,* 305–310.

Leitenberg, H., Rawson, R. A., & Mulick, J. A. (1975). Extinction and reinforcement of alternative behavior. *Journal of Comparative and Physiological Psychology, 88,* 640–652.

Lienemann, J., & Walker, F. (1989). Naltrexone for treatment of self-injury. *American Journal of Psychiatry, 146,* 1639–1640.

Lipsitt, L. P. (1984). Mental retardation: A view from the infant learning laboratory. In J. A. Mulick & B. L. Mallory (Eds.), *Transitions in mental retardation, Volume 1: Advocacy, technology, and science* (pp. 249–260). Norwood, NJ: Ablex.

Lovaas, O. I. (1987). Behavioral treatment and normal education and intellectual functioning in young autistic children. *Journal of Consulting and Clinical Psychology, 55,* 3–9.

Mace, F. C., Browder, D. M., & Lin, Y. (1987). Analysis of demand conditions associated with stereotypy. *Journal of Behavior Therapy and Experimental Psychiatry, 18,* 25–31.

Marholin, D., Touchette, P. E., & Stewart, R. M. (1979). Withdrawal of chronic chlorpromazine medication: An experimental analysis. *Journal of Applied Behavior Analysis, 12,* 159–171.

Matson, J. L., & Mulick, J. A. (Eds.). (1983). *Handbook of mental retardation.* New York: Pergamon.

Meinhold, P. M., & Mulick, J. A. (1990a). Counter-habilitative contingencies in residential institutions. In S. R. Schroeder (Ed.), *Ecobehavioral analysis and developmental disabilities: The twenty-first century* (pp. 105–121). New York: Springer-Verlag.

Meinhold, P. M., & Mulick, J. A. (1990b). Risks, choices and behavioral treatment. *Behavioral Residential Treatment, 5,* 29–44.

Mesibov, G. B., Troxler, M., & Boswell, S. (1988). Assessment in the classroom. In E. Schopler & G. B. Mesibov (Eds.), *Diagnosis and assessment in autism* (pp. 261–270). New York: Plenum.

Michael, J. (1982). Distinguishing between the discriminative and motivational functions of behavior. *Journal of the Experimental Analysis of Behavior, 37,* 149–155.

Mulick, J. A., Barbour, R., Schroeder, S. R., & Rojahn, J. (1980). Over-correction of pica in two profoundly retarded adults: Analysis of setting effects, stimulus and response generalization. *Applied Research in Mental Retardation, 1,* 241–252.

Mulick, J. A., Hammer, D., & Dura, J. R. (1991). Assessment and management of antisocial and hyperactive behavior. In J. L. Matson & J. A. Mulick (Eds.), *Handbook of mental retardation* (2nd ed., pp. 397–412). New York: Pergamon.

Mulick, J. A., Hoyt, P., Rojahn, J., & Schroeder, S. R. (1978). Reduction of a "nervous habit" in a profoundly retarded youth by increasing independent toy play. *Journal of Behavior Therapy and Experimental Psychiatry, 9,* 25–30.

Mulick, J. A., & Kedesdy, J. H. (1988). Self-injurious behavior, its treatment, and normalization. *Mental Retardation, 26,* 223–229.

Paisey, T. J. H., Whitney, R. B., & Moore, J. (1989). Person–treatment interactions across nonaversive response-deceleration procedures for self-injury: A case study of effects and side effects. *Behavioral Residential Treatment, 4,* 69–88.

Pueschel, S. M., & Mulick, J. A. (1990). *Prevention of developmental disabilities.* Baltimore: Paul H. Brookes.

Rawson, R. A., Leitenberg, H., Mulick, J. A., & Lefebvre, M. (1977). Recovery of extinction responding in rats following discontinuation of reinforcement of alternative behavior: A test of two explanations. *Animal Learning and Behavior, 5,* 451–457.

Rojahn, J., Mulick, J. A., McCoy, D., & Schroeder, S. R. (1978). Setting effects, adaptive clothing, and the modification of head-banging and self-restraint in two profoundly retarded adults. *Behavioral Analysis and Modification, 2,* 185–196.

Rojahn, J., Schroeder, S. R., & Mulick, J. A. (1980). Ecological assessment of self-protective devices in three profoundly retarded adults. *Journal of Autism and Developmental Disorders, 10,* 59–66.

Schroeder, S. R. (Ed.). (1990). *Ecobehavioral analysis and developmental disabilities: The twenty-first century.* New York: Springer-Verlag.

Schroeder, S. R., Kanoy, J. R., Mulick, J. A., Rojahn, J., Thios, S. J., Stephens, M., & Hawk, B. (1982). Environmental antecedents which affect management and maintenance of programs for self-injurious behavior. J. C. Hollis & C. E. Myers (Eds.), *Life-threatening behavior.* Washington, dC: AAMD (Monograph No. 5).

Schroeder, S. R., Mulick, J. A., & Rojahn, J. (1980). The definition, taxonomy, epidemiology, and ecology of self-injurious behavior. *Journal of Autism and Developmental Disorders, 10,* 417–432.

Schroeder, S. R., Rojahn, J., & Mulick, J. A. (1978). Ecobehavioral organization of developmental day care for the chronically self-injurious. *Journal of Pediatric Psychology, 3,* 81–88.

Schroeder, S. R., Schroeder, C. S., Smith, B., & Dalldorf, J. (1978). Prevalence of self-injurious behaviors in a large state facility for the retarded: A three year follow-up study. *Journal of Autism and Childhood Schizophrenia, 8,* 261–269.

Solnick, J. V., Rincover, A., & Peterson, C. R. (1977). Some determinants of the reinforcing and punishing effects of time out. *Journal of Applied Behavior Analysis, 10,* 415–424.

Stoddard, L. T., Sidman, M., & Brady, J. V. (1988). Fixed-interval and fixed ratio reinforcement schedules with human subjects. *The Analysis of Verbal Behavior, 6,* 33–44.

Tarnowski, K. J., Rasnake, L. K., Linscheid, T. R., & Mulick, J. A. (1989). Ecobehavioral characteristics of a pediatric burn injury unit. *Journal of Applied Behavioral Analysis, 22,* 101–109.

Thompson, R., Bjelajac, V. M., Huestis, P. W., Crinella, F. M., & Yu, J. (1989). Inhibitory deficits in rats rendered "mentally retarded" by early brain damage. *Psychobiology, 17,* 61–76.

Thompson, T., & Pickens, R. (1971). *Stimulus properties of drugs.* New York: Appleton-Century-Crofts.

Touchette, P. E., MacDonald, R. F., & Langer, S. N. (1985). A scatter plot for identifying stimulus control of problem behavior. *Journal of Applied Behavior Analysis, 18,* 343–351.

Turnbull, H. R. (1983). Parents, disabled children, and defederalization: Life on the razor's edge of public selfishness. In J. A. Mulick & S. M. Pueschel (Eds.), *Parent-professional partnerships in developmental disability services* (pp. 207–232). Cambridge, MA: Academic Guild.

Vyse, S. A., & Mulick, J. A. (1988). Ecobehavioral assessment of a special education classroom: Teacher-student behavioral covariation. *Journal of the Multihandicapped Person, 1,* 201–216.

Vyse, S. A., & Mulick, J. A. (1990). Ecobehavioral assessment: Future directions in the planning and evaluation of behavioral intervention. In S. R. Schroeder (Ed.), *Ecobehavioral analysis and developmental disabilities: The twenty-first century* (pp. 228–244). New York: Springer-Verlag.

Vyse, S. A., Rieg, T. S., & Smith, N. F. (1985). Reinforcement-based response elimination: The effects of response-reinforcement interval and response specificity. *The Psychological Record, 35,* 365–376.

Wolfensberger, W., & Glenn, L. (1975). *PASS: A method for the quantitative evaluation of human services.* Toronto: National Institute on Mental Retardation.

Yeterian, E. H. (1987). Childhood autism as a forebrain disorder: Review of a neural model and selected brain imaging and drug therapy studies. In J. A. Mulick & R. F. Antonak (Eds.), *Transitions in Mental Retardation, Volume 2: Issues in therapeutic intervention* (pp. 235–253). Norwood, NJ: Ablex.

# III

# Treatment Issues

# 7

# Assessment and Treatment of Self-Injurious Behavior

BRIAN A. IWATA, JENNIFER B. ZARCONE, TIMOTHY R. VOLLMER, and RICHARD G. SMITH

The immediate trauma and chronic risks associated with self-injurious behavior (SIB) make it perhaps the most dramatic behavior disorder among individuals diagnosed with autism and related developmental disabilities. The disorder actually consists of a diverse array of responses having multiple origins, and the only common feature shared by all SIB is that it "produces physical injury to the individual's own body" (Tate & Baroff, 1966). In this chapter, we describe the demography and etiology of SIB, and review current approaches to assessment and treatment.

## DEFINITION, RISK, AND PREVALENCE

An initial diagnosis of SIB usually is not difficult because the behavior either is observed directly or is associated with noticeable injuries, often in the form of abrasions, contusions, or lacerations. SIB is further differentiated from accidental injury or that caused by aggression because the trauma is recurrent and self-inflicted. Numerous forms of topographies or SIB have been documented in the

BRIAN A. IWATA and RICHARD G. SMITH • Department of Psychology, The University of Florida, Gainesville, Florida 32611. JENNIFER R. ZARCONE • Department of Behavioral Psychology, The Kennedy Institute, 707 North Broadway, Baltimore, Maryland 21205. TIMOTHY R. VOLLMER • Department of Psychology, Louisiana State University, Baton Rouge, Louisiana 70803.

*Behavioral Issues in Autism*, edited by Eric Schopler and Gary B. Mesibov. New York, Plenum Press, 1994.

literature, including aerophagia (air swallowing), biting, eye gouging, head banging and head hitting, hitting or slapping other body parts, inserting fingers or
objects in body cavities, mouthing hands or objects, pica (ingesting inedible
substances), rumination (repeatedly regurgitating and reswallowing food),
scratching, trichotillomania (hair pulling), and vomiting (Maurice & Trudel,
1982). The injuries produced by these behaviors can be quite varied depending on
response topography and intensity: amputation of body parts (usually fingers)
from biting, body disfigurement (as in cauliflower ear) from hitting, bone fracture
from hitting and banging, enucleation of the eye from gouging, hair and surface
tissue loss from hair pulling or scratching, hematoma and internal organ damage
from hitting, poisoning, intestinal rupture from pica, retinal detachment or con-
cussion from head banging, and wound infection as a secondary problem.

In addition to the medical risks associated with SIB, social and educational
risks often result when individuals are excluded from activities and programs for
which they would otherwise qualify. Furthermore, SIB is a frequently cited reason
for institutionalization and for failure to find suitable community placement for
individuals already institutionalized (Russo, Carr, & Lovaas, 1980).

The epidemiology of SIB has not been studied thoroughly, and current
estimates of prevalence are based on relatively small samples. DeLissovoy (1961)
found the incidence of noninjurious head banging in normal infants to be 15.2%.
The behavior appeared at about 8 months of age, usually occurred at bed times,
and was gone by about 25 months. Prevalence among individuals with mental
retardation and autism ranges from 6.5% (Borthwick, Meyers, & Eyman, 1981) to
28% (Fovel, Lash, Barron, & Roberts, 1989) and is distinguished from that found
in nonhandicapped populations due to its relative severity and chronicity. Degree
of retardation (Griffin, Williams, Stark, Altmeyer, & Mason, 1984) and restrictive
residential placement (Borthwick et al., 1981) both have been associated with a
higher prevalence of SIB. Head hitting and head banging are the most commonly
seen forms of SIB, accounting for more than 50% of all observed cases (Griffin
et al., 1984; Maurice & Trudel, 1982). Mortality rates associated with SIB are
unknown but estimated to be small because protective measures are taken with
individuals having a history of severe injury.

## ETIOLOGY AND MAINTAINING VARIABLES

SIB is a complex disorder with multiple determinants. There is evidence that
some SIB may be induced through biological mechanisms (e.g., see Cataldo &
Harris, 1982), but reviews of the literature (e.g., Bachman, 1972; Carr, 1977)
indicate that most SIB is learned (operant) behavior. Therefore, only brief discussion of biological factors associated with SIB will be provided here, with
greater emphasis placed on the role of learning mechanisms.

## Biological Factors

### Genetic and Congenital Disorders

SIB has been associated with several specific syndromes and medical problems, most notably the Lesch-Nyhan (Lesch & Nyhan, 1964; Nyhan, 1976) and Cornelia deLange (Johnson, Ekman, Friesen, Nyhan, & Shear, 1976) syndromes, chronic otitis media or ear infection (DeLissovoy, 1963), and frontal lobe seizure (Gedye, 1989). The extremely high prevalence of SIB (above 90%) in the Lesch-Nyhan syndrome provides compelling evidence for a biological basis. However, although the cause of Lesch-Nyhan syndrome is well known, no specific mechanism for SIB has been identified, and medical forms of treatment have had no effect on either the biological or the behavioral aspects of the disorder. The relationship between SIB and other medical problems, such as otitis media, may actually be due to learning rather than biological causation (see Environmental and Behavioral Factors).

### Mechanical and Biochemical Factors

Studies with laboratory animals have shown that stereotypies and sometimes SIB can be induced through a variety of surgical and chemical preparations, including lesion to the brain (Jones & Barraclough, 1978) and injection or ingestion of alcohol (Charmove & Harlow, 1970) or caffeine (Peters, 1967). Although there is no direct evidence that these factors account for the development of SIB in humans, results of basic research suggest that SIB in some individuals may be one of a number of nonspecific motor disturbances resulting from neurological trauma.

### Endogenous Opioid Theory

Research on the neurobiology of pain regulation has led to the discovery of an endogenous opioid system, which includes specific opioid peptides, receptor sites, and mechanisms of action (Snyder, 1977, 1984). Extremely high levels of physiological stress stimulate release of endogenous opioids (e.g., endorphins), which increase tolerance to pain-producing stimuli. Additional research has demonstrated the reinforcing effects of endorphins in an operant, self-administration paradigm with laboratory animals (Belluzzi & Stein, 1977). These potential pain-reducing and reinforcing aspects of endogenous opioids suggest two hypotheses for the development and maintenance of SIB. First, if the occurrence of SIB increases the "pain threshold," the behavior may be just as susceptible as noninjurious responses to the effects of environmental consequences (see Environmental and Behavioral Factors). Second, it is possible that SIB in some individuals may be maintained through the release of endorphins, analogous to narcotic self-administration. Both of these explanations involve rather complex pharmacological and behavioral interactions, and supporting evidence is extremely mixed at the present time (for additional discussion, see King, McCracken, & Poland, 1991, and DeMet & Sandman, 1991). Nevertheless, the endogenous opioid hypotheses have led to the evaluation of a class of drugs that may have specific suppressive effects on SIB. These drugs—the opiate antagonists—will be described briefly in the section on pharmacologic approaches to treatment.

## Environmental and Behavioral Factors

The most successful treatments for SIB have been those derived from principles of operant conditioning (Favell, Azrin, Baumeister et al., 1982). The fact that SIB can thus be "unlearned" provides retrospective support for the view that much of SIB is operant behavior. Early accounts of the development of SIB stressed the role of positive reinforcement inadvertently delivered as adult attention and comfort to children following episodes of SIB (Lovaas & Simmons, 1969). Subsequent research has revealed that SIB may be strengthened through positive or negative reinforcement, which may be delivered either socially (by another individual) or automatically (directly produced by the behavior).

### Social-Positive Reinforcement

Lovaas and Simmons (1969) provided striking evidence that attention from caring adults, when delivered contingent on the occurrence of SIB, may serve as positive reinforcement. Such consequences often are unavoidable and are even dictated based on universal standards of humane care. Although attention and comfort interrupt SIB temporarily, they may increase its overall rate if the individual receives relatively little attention in the absence of SIB or for the occurrence of other behaviors (Smolev, 1971).

### Automatic-Positive Reinforcement

Some behaviors directly provide stimulation that serves as positive reinforcement. These responses often have been referred to as "stereotypic," or "self-stimulatory" behaviors due to their seemingly nonfunctional appearance and continued occurrence independent of the social environment. A functional description of these behaviors suggests that they are maintained by directly produced or "automatic" consequences (Skinner, 1969). Theoretical accounts of the source of automatic reinforcement, ranging from perceptual stimulation (Lovaas, Newsom, & Hickman, 1987) to endogenous opioids (Cataldo & Harris, 1982), have been difficult to verify empirically.

## Social-Negative Reinforcement

Events that are removed or prevented contingent on the occurrence of behavior may strengthen behavior through the process of negative reinforcement. Escape from or avoidance of "undesirable" events may take a number of forms, some of which are relatively innocuous (e.g., noncompliance). Unfortunately, many developmentally disabled individuals have not acquired socially appropriate escape behaviors and use other means to terminate aversive situations, including tantrums and other forms of disruption, destructive behavior, aggression, and SIB (see Iwata, 1987, for a more extensive discussion of how severe behavior disorders may be inadvertently shaped using negative reinforcement).

## Automatic-Negative Reinforcement

Some responses directly (i.e., automatically) terminate or at least attenuate ongoing stimulation. Scratching the skin temporarily alleviates the "itch" associated with an insect bite, rubbing the temples "soothes" a headache, and tapping the jaw provides "distraction" from a toothache. These behaviors may persist when more adaptive means of terminating "aversive states" associated with physical discomfort are not available. Thus, face hitting may occur whenever there is localized pain to the head or face, and it may later continue due to the additional irritation it produces. This type of automatic-negative reinforcement may account for observed correlations between specific medical conditions and SIB noted previously. For example, one form of SIB—head banging—has been associated with ear infections in children (DeLissovoy, 1963). Although ear infections do not produce head banging per se, their presence may create an aversive situation that is attenuated by striking or banging the head.

## PRETREATMENT CONSIDERATIONS

Few parents or professionals express concern when an individual with severe developmental delay requires hundreds of training sessions in order to acquire a new skill as long as there is some indication that progress is being made. This approach to treatment based on gradual improvement over time does not apply to behavior disorders; it is assumed that problems like SIB can be eliminated immediately. But given that SIB often has a long and complex learning history, including the presence of other behavior problems as well as significant behavior deficits, it is unlikely that SIB can be eliminated quickly or permanently. Thus, an emerging approach to treatment emphasizes risk management in the short run combined with a series of behavioral assessment procedures leading to the development of long-term interventions that gradually reduce the frequency of problem behavior. This section describes steps to be taken prior to the actual implementation of treatment.

## Medical Screening and Risk Management

Because of the obvious risks associated with SIB and the possibility that some SIB may be occasioned by preexisting medical problems, a thorough examination should be conducted as the first step in a comprehensive approach to treatment.

### Preexisting Medical Disorders

It has been noted previously that some recurrent medical conditions, such as ear infections, dental problems, or allergies may produce a painful or discomforting situation that is attenuated through SIB. Cyclical episodes of highly specific SIB may suggest the presence of such conditions (e.g., ear punching, localized scratching, etc.), which should be ruled out or identified and treated.

### Internal Injuries Caused by SIB

Some topographies of SIB are known to produce primarily internal damage that is not immediately apparent to the observer. Examples include forceful contact against the head (head banging, head hitting, face punching) that can produce skull fractures and retinal damage, pica leading to hemorrhage or perforation of internal organs, and chronic vomiting or rumination that can cause a variety of nutritional problems such as malnourishment and dehydration. Identification of injuries caused by these forms of SIB, if not already documented in an individual's medical history, may require the use of radiologic procedures.

## Surface Tissue Damage

The most common injuries caused by SIB are skin lacerations and contusions. These outcomes are readily observable as well as sensitive to changes in the frequency and intensity of SIB. Thus, in cases where SIB does not cause internal damage, measurement of surface injuries provides a good estimate of current risk prior to treatment and an outcome indicator following the completion of treatment. Several methods have been used to document the extent of such injuries, including informal notation, identification of injury locations on a body (e.g., burn) chart, and quantification of injuries based on number, type, location, and severity (Iwata, Pace, Kissel, Nau, & Farber, 1990).

## Protection from Risk

Because no therapy will eliminate SIB immediately, interim steps must be taken to protect an individual from further injury prior to and during the course of treatment. A variety of restraint devices and protective appliances have been developed for such purposes (e.g., Richmond, Schroeder, & Bickel, 1984; Spain, Hart, & Corbett, 1984). Although many state guidelines regard mechanical forms of restraint as more intrusive than physical restraint (i.e., holding), data from a number of studies (e.g., Hill & Spreat, 1987) indicate that mechanical restraint is associated with a lower prevalence of injuries to both staff and clients and is therefore a safer procedure to use.

## Assessment of Adaptive Behavior and Identification of Reinforcers

### Key Adaptive Behaviors

Although the development of socially appropriate forms of behavior may not directly reduce the frequency of SIB, it will at least provide the individual with alternative means for obtaining reinforcement. In theory, any "new" adaptive response could compete with SIB from the standpoint of time allocation, but three classes of behaviors are particularly relevant due to the functions they serve. Their role in the treatment of SIB will be described in a later section of this chapter; they are noted here because deficits in any of the three should be identified prior to treatment. First, independent interaction with the physical environment (also called solitary leisure skills, toy play, etc.) provides an opportunity for reinforcement and learning new skills that does not require the constant intervention or even the presence of a teacher or therapist (Singh & Millinchamp, 1987). Second, communication skills that serve the functions of "I want" and "I don't want" allow the individual to obtain needed items when they are not immediately available, to get help, or to terminate ongoing aversive events (Cipani, 1990). Finally, compliance with instructions allows the individual to both tolerate and benefit from training (Mace et al., 1988).

## Identification of Reinforcers for Increasing Adaptive Behavior

Consideration of motivational factors is perhaps the most overlooked aspect of client training. Little attention is paid to finding new reinforcers; instead, easily available forms of stimulation (e.g., attention and food) are used repeatedly to the point of satiation. Individuals with severe behavioral deficits often have had limited access to potentially reinforcing events; therefore, an important aspect of increasing motivation will require frequent exposure to a wide range of sensory experiences and activities. Several methods have been developed to formally incorporate reinforcement assessment procedures into ongoing treatment programs (Fisher et al., 1992; Green, Reid, Carnipe, & Gardner, 1991; Pace, Ivancic, Edwards, Iwata, & Page, 1985) and to arrange training sessions so as to maximize reinforcer effectiveness (Egel, 1981; Vollmer & Iwata, 1991).

## Functional Analysis of Variables Maintaining SIB

Over the past 10 years, an increasing amount of research has focused on the development of methods for identifying the source(s) of reinforcement for problems such as SIB. This area of research has come to be known as the "functional analysis" of behavior disorders (see Mace, Lalli, & Pinter Lalli, 1991, and Iwata, Vollmer, & Zarcone, 1990, for recent reviews), and it has direct implications for the selection of treatment procedures. By revealing the contingencies that maintain a behavior disorder, functional analyses allow one to identify (a) the antecedent conditions that are likely to occasion the behavior, (b) the source of reinforcement (e.g., social positive) that, unless eliminated, will lead to recurrences of the behavior in the future, (c) the procedural form of extinction (e.g., attention withdrawal in the case of social-positive reinforcement) that should be incorporated into the treatment program, (d) the competing contingencies, reinforcers, and responses that will form the basis of treatment (behavioral replacement), and (e) the reinforcement-based approaches to treatment that are unlikely to be effective.

Although there is significant variation among procedures used to identify the motivational features of SIB, all have in common an attempt to identify the antecedent events or contexts that occasion behavior and the consequent events likely to serve as reinforcers. Three general approaches to conducting functional analyses have been reported in the literature. They differ in terms of the type of data collected and the degree to which environmental events are manipulated versus merely observed.

## Anecdotal or Indirect Methods

A number of interview formats, checklists, and rating scales have been developed to solicit information about situations in which behavior problems are more or less likely to occur. These procedures range from somewhat open-ended questionnaires (e.g., Gambrill, 1977) to more structured formats designed to identify relevant antecedent and consequent events (e.g., Sulzer-Azaroff & Mayer, 1977). The most recent attempt to refine anecdotal approaches to assessment for SIB was described by Durand and Crimmins (1988), who designed a 16-item checklist called the Motivation Assessment Scale (MAS). Each item consists of a question about the circumstances under which SIB may or may not occur, and answers are provided by way of a Likert-type scale ranging from 0 ("never") to 6 ("always"). The responses (numeric selections) can be summed or averaged to yield a total for each of four possible functions for SIB: positive reinforcement through attention, positive reinforcement through access to materials, negative reinforcement through escape, or "sensory" (i.e., automatic) reinforcement. Durand and Crimmins evaluated several characteristics of the MAS and concluded that the instrument was both a reliable and valid method for identifying variables maintaining SIB. Subsequent attempts to establish the reliability of the MAS, using both correlational and percentage agreement statistics, have not replicated the Durand and Crimmins results (Newton & Sturmey, 1991; Zarcone, Rodgers, Iwata, Rourke, & Dorsey, 1991). For example, Zarcone et al. reported mean interobserver agreement as less than 20% for a sample of 55 self-injurious individuals, each of whom was scored on the MAS by two teachers or therapists. Thus, the simplicity and efficiency of methods such as the MAS, which are major advantages of anecdotal approaches to assessment, appear to be outweighed by their reliance on subjective opinion or faulty memory. These types of instruments might be used as preliminary information-gathering devices but should not be considered adequate for the purpose of behavioral assessment.

## Descriptive (Correlational) Analysis

More objective than interview approaches, descriptive analyses involve direct observation of behavior (e.g., SIB) and the physical and social situations in which it occurs (Bijou, Peterson, & Ault, 1968). Inferences about maintaining variables are based on observed correlations between SIB and the occurrence of specific events. Touchette, MacDonald, and Langer (1985) described a simple approach to descriptive analysis called the "Scatter Plot," in which observers record instances of the target behavior within 30-minute intervals to determine if there is any distributional pattern of behavior across time of day. If so, the individual's activity schedule could be altered in an attempt to reduce inappropriate behavior. An example of the type of data sheet used for scatter plot recording is provided in Figure 1. Although this approach represents a clear improvement over anecdotal methods, it provides little or no information on specific sequences of behavior. A second approach to descriptive analysis does allow for sequential recording but contains little or no provision for quantification of data across time. This type of procedure commonly makes use of an "A-B-C" (antecedent-behavior-consequence) chart (Sulzer-Azaroff & Mayer, 1977), on which the teacher or caretaker notes time and setting and writes brief descriptions of events occurring immediately prior to and following instances of the target behavior (see Figure 2). An extension of the open-ended ABC analysis was developed recently by Pyles and Bailey (1990). Their data forms include for a given individual a list of prespecified events, which an observer merely checks as behavioral sequences occur. A third type of descriptive analysis is based on the work of Bijou et al. (1968), which emphasizes the use of objective behavioral definitions, time-based data collection procedures using brief time intervals (e.g., 10 seconds), and the assessment of observer reliability. Data gathered in this manner can be summarized as conditional probabilities based on observed frequencies of behavior and a variety of antecedent or consequent events. Although used extensively as a general observation procedure, interval and time sampling methods have certain limitations because they do not allow very good control over the environmental contexts in which behavior occurs. Data may not reveal functional relationships between behavior and highly intermittent sources of reinforcement. In addition, the typical contexts for behavior may contain multiple elements (i.e., interactional sequences), any one of which could account for behavioral maintenance (e.g., as in escape from tasks accompanied by teacher attention contingent on inappropriate behavior).

## Functional (Experimental) Analysis

In order to verify the effects of suspected variables or to clarify ambiguous descriptive data, assessment conditions may be arranged to allow systematic introduction and removal of these variables, while observing their effects on behavior. Two general models for conducting functional analyses of behavior disorders have evolved. The first model examines the effects of a single variable whose influence on behavior is suspected based on previous information (e.g.,

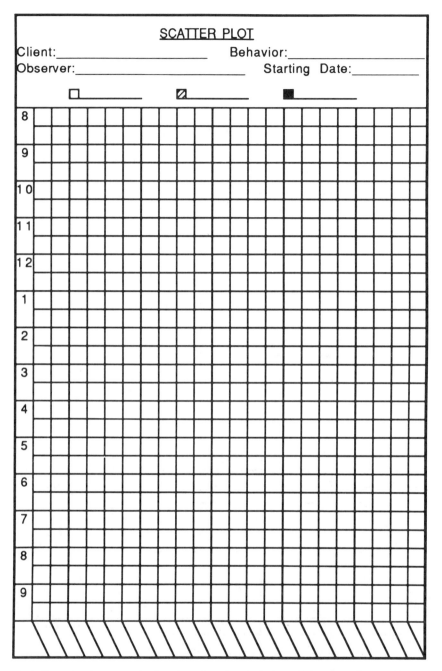

Fig. 1. Example of a scatter plot data sheet for estimating behavioral frequency (low, medium, or high) indicated by the fill pattern within half-hour intervals throughout the day.

| A-B-C CLIENT RECORD |||||||
|------|----------|-----------|----------|-------------|--------------|
| Client:_____ ||| Behavior:_____ |||
| Observer:_____ ||| Date:_____ |||
| Time | Location | Frequency | Activity | Antecedents | Consequences |
|  |  |  |  |  |  |
|  |  |  |  |  |  |
|  |  |  |  |  |  |
|  |  |  |  |  |  |
|  |  |  |  |  |  |
|  |  |  |  |  |  |
|  |  |  |  |  |  |
|  |  |  |  |  |  |
|  |  |  |  |  |  |
|  |  |  |  |  |  |
|  |  |  |  |  |  |
|  |  |  |  |  |  |
|  |  |  |  |  |  |
|  |  |  |  |  |  |
|  |  |  |  |  |  |
|  |  |  |  |  |  |
|  |  |  |  |  |  |
|  |  |  |  |  |  |
|  |  |  |  |  |  |
|  |  |  |  |  |  |
|  |  |  |  |  |  |
|  |  |  |  |  |  |
|  |  |  |  |  |  |
|  |  |  |  |  |  |
|  |  |  |  |  |  |
|  |  |  |  |  |  |
|  |  |  |  |  |  |
|  |  |  |  |  |  |
|  |  |  |  |  |  |
|  |  |  |  |  |  |
|  |  |  |  |  |  |

Fig. 2. Example of an Antecedent–Behavior–Consequence data sheet for identifying environmental correlates of a target behavior.

anecdotal report or naturalistic observation). Lovaas and Simmons (1969) identified adult attention as a positive reinforcer for SIB, and Carr, Newsom, and Binkoff (1980) used similar procedures to demonstrate that escape from tasks could serve as a negative reinforcer for aggressive behavior. The second model allows for the examination of more than one maintaining variable using either reversal (Carr & Durand, 1985) or multielement (Iwata, Dorsey, Slifer, Bauman, & Richman, 1982) designs. Both models involve exposing an individual to at least one "test" condition in which the variable of interest is present (e.g., contingent attention for SIB), and another "control" condition in which the variable is absent (e.g., no attention, noncontingent attention, DRO, etc.). Table 1 outlines the basic "test" and "control" conditions appropriate to the four learned functions of SIB. It is important to note that the "automatic" functions are difficult to identify because the reinforcing event produced by the behavior might not be amenable to control or even to direct observation. The test for automatic-negative reinforcement, for example, is usually impossible due to our lack of control over events that occasion such behavior (e.g., headaches). Nevertheless, results obtained from functional analyses usually will reveal orderly relationships between specific

Table 1. Test and Control Conditions for
Identifying the Maintaining Variables for SIB

---

*Social-positive reinforcement* (attention-maintained SIB)
    Test condition
        Deprivation from specific reinforcement (e.g., attention, materials, etc.)
        Contingent reinforcement
    Control condition
        Noncontingent reinforcement

*Automatic-positive reinforcement* (self-stimulatory SIB)
    Test condition
        General deprivation or lack of stimulation
    Control condition
        Noncontingent stimulation

*Social-negative reinforcement* (escape from tasks or other social situations)
    Test condition
        Work requirements (aversive stimulation)
        Contingent reinforcement (escape)
    Control condition
        No aversive stimulation

*Automatic-negative reinforcement* (attenuation of pain or discomfort)
    Test condition
        Biological condition
    Control condition
        No biological condition

---

environmental events and SIB. Once these events have been identified, treatments procedures can be developed to directly eliminate or reverse the process by which SIB has been strengthened.

## The Problem of Self-Restraint

Defined as self-initiated confinement incompatible with SIB or preference for such confinement, self-restraint is comprised of several related topographies: (a) apparent self-restraint, usually by placing arms inside articles of clothing or wrapping them in sheets or towels; (b) other forms of behaviors that seemingly prevent the occurrence of SIB (e.g., holding on to objects); and (c) observed preference for being placed in mechanical restraint. Although the variables that produce and maintain self-restraint are of interest in their own right (see Smith, Iwata, Vollmer, & Pace, 1992, for an analysis of these variables), the practical significance of self-restraint is that it interferes with performance of learned skills as well as acquisition of new behaviors. In extreme cases of chronic self-restraint, problems almost as serious as SIB may result, including muscular atrophy, arrested motor development, limited range of motion, and loss of function. Prevalence estimates have varied widely so that the extent of the problem is unknown. Bruhl, Fielding, Joyce, Peters, and Wiesler (1982) noted that over half of their clients in an intensive treatment program had exhibited self-restraint at one time, whereas calculations based on other data (Fovel et al., 1989) suggest that self-restraint may occur in as few as 10% of the self-injurious population generally. Fovel et al. did note that the occurrence of self-restraint was highly predictive of SIB (19 out of 20 self-restrainers had a history of SIB).

Because self-restraint interferes with SIB and a number of other behaviors, it also interferes with attempts to conduct functional analyses of SIB. For example, some individuals have been observed to engage in almost continuous self-restraint when allowed to do so, and to engage in almost continuous SIB when self-restraint is not allowed (Smith et al., 1992). For these reasons, SIB and self-restraint often have been treated in combination using one of two general approaches. The first consists of attempts to reduce the frequency of one behavior (e.g., SIB) while maintaining a low frequency of the other behavior (e.g., self-restraint). Favell, McGimsey, and Jones (1978) provided a particularly interesting example of this approach. Working with individuals who exhibited a preference for mechanical restraints, the investigators arranged a contingency in which access to restraints was available following increasingly longer time intervals during which the subjects exhibited no SIB. Thus, restraints were used as reinforcers for the absence of SIB, qualifying the procedure as an example of differential reinforcement of other behavior (reinforcement procedures are described in greater detail in the next section of this chapter).

A second approach to treatment has involved the gradual modification of restraint topography using shaping or fading procedures. Rojahn, Mulick, and Schroeder (1980) used this approach to replace one form of self-restraint (arms wrapped in shirt) with a more "appropriate" topography (hands in pockets) by requiring the subject to wear a jacket. Pace, Iwata, Edwards, and McCosh (1986) were able to fade restraints almost completely for two individuals who self-restrained, wore restraints, and exhibited SIB. For one individual, full-arm splints were gradually shortened and then finally replaced with tennis wristbands. For the second individual, self-restraint (hands in pants) was first transferred to another restraint (inflatable arm splints) and then later faded by reducing the air pressure in the splints. In both cases, intensive treatment was aimed at strengthening alternative behavior (play with toys and compliance with training tasks) as restraints were faded.

## LEARNING-BASED APPROACHES TO TREATMENT

Behavior-reduction procedures based on operant learning principles have proliferated over the years to the point where it is often difficult to identify the critical component(s) of treatment given only a descriptive label. In actuality, most if not all learning therapies designed to reduce the frequency of behavior achieve their effects in one of four ways. First, some interventions modify antecedent conditions so as to alter the susceptibility of behavior to reinforcement. Second, other interventions eliminate reinforcement for the behavior through extinction. Third, still other interventions are based on differential reinforcement for the absence of the target behavior (DRO) or for the occurrence of an alternative behavior (DRA). Finally, one group of procedures directly reduces behavior through the delivery of punishment (or through a related principle—response cost). These general classes of intervention do not specify any particular therapeutic operation, which perhaps explains how a relatively small set of principles could yield such a large number of "unique" treatments described in the literature. A more serious problem arises when our emphasis on procedural novelty (i.e., technique) obscures the underlying basis for treatment. For example, "planned ignoring" may be a benign and therefore preferred method of time-out, but because it amounts to cessation of attention, planned ignoring will only be effective as treatment (extinction) for behavior maintained by social-positive reinforcement. A shift in emphasis to "behavioral function" allows one to select or design treatment components based on their ability to alter the conditions currently maintaining the behavior problem. In this section, we outline variations in treatment procedure based on the modification of antecedent conditions, extinction, and reinforcement applied to the different functions of SIB. Approaches to treatment based on punishment are addressed at the end of this section.

## Modification of Antecedent Conditions: Establishing Operations

Until recently, the influence of antecedent events on behavior has been described primarily from a stimulus control perspective. An example will illustrate the limitations of such an approach. For an individual whose SIB is maintained by attention, several antecedent conditions one might alter would include the therapist, setting, and ongoing activity. Yet these changes are rarely made without *also* changing the reinforcement contingency for the behavior (i.e., no longer reinforcing SIB and instead reinforcing an alternative response). Thus, the effects of most antecedent changes are confounded with and determined by consequent changes; that is, consequences determine changes in stimulus control. If SIB continues to be reinforced by the new therapist in the new setting during the new activity, one would expect little in the way of therapeutic outcome.

There are, however, conditions under which antecedent modifications can change behavior without regard to consequences. Important to an understanding of these conditions is the concept of "establishing operation" or EO (Michael, 1982), which is defined as any operation that temporarily alters the effectiveness of a given stimulus to serve as a reinforcer for a given behavior. For behavior maintained by positive reinforcement, the EO often is some form of deprivation (e.g., from food or water); for escape and avoidance behavior, the EO usually is aversive stimulation (e.g., intense light, noise). The effects of EOs are diminished when responding produces reinforcement, as in attention-getting behavior that terminates when attention is delivered or as in aggression that produces escape, but EOs also can be attenuated prior to responding merely by providing noncontingent access to the reinforcer. For example, Vollmer and Iwata (1991) recently demonstrated how operant performance maintained by commonly used reinforcers— food, social interaction, and music—could be increased or decreased by limiting or providing access to these events prior to experimental sessions. In the same way, when the reinforcer maintaining SIB can be identified, noncontingent reinforcement (NCR) would be expected to decrease the behavior.

Using NCR as the basis for antecedent change, specific procedures can be formulated for different sources of reinforcement. For SIB maintained by social-positive reinforcement (e.g., attention), NCR would consist of a richer schedule of noncontingent attention. While studying the effects of a variety of attention manipulations on SIB, Anderson, Dancis, and Alpert (1978) and Lovaas and Simmons (1969) included the noncontingent delivery of attention as one control procedure and observed decreases in SIB. Vollmer, Iwata, Zarcone, Smith, and Mazaleski (1993) recently extended this line of research by examining the therapeutic effects of NCR. Working with three individuals whose SIB was attention maintained, Vollmer et al. initially delivered noncontingent attention on an almost continuous schedule (every 10 seconds) and observed marked reductions in SIB. SIB remained low as the schedule was gradually thinned until it reached 5 minutes, which was determined to be a practical schedule for implementation. Similar procedures have been used to decrease SIB that was presumably maintained by the direct (automatic) reinforcers it produced. For example, noncontingent vibration produced decreases in head banging (Bailey & Meyerson, 1970), noncontingent delivery of food decreased rumination (Rast, Johnston, Drum, & Conrin, 1981), and access to toys reduced stereotypic SIB (Favell, McGimsey, & Schell, 1982).

Because the establishing operation for escape behavior often involves presentation of an aversive task, NCR for such behavior would entail noncontingent task removal or modification, which can be accomplished in several ways. Carr, Newsom, and Binkoff (1976) "embedded" demands within entertaining stories, which apparently reduced the aversiveness of the demands; Weeks and Gaylord-Ross (1981) reduced task complexity by substituting "easy" tasks in place of "difficult" ones; and Pace, Iwata, Cowdery, Andree, and McIntyre (1993) initially reduced task frequency by placing fewer demands on their subjects. Because additional interventions were included in each of these studies, the effects of demand modification per se are unknown, and further research is needed to clarify these results. SIB maintained by pain attenuation (automatic negative reinforcement) provides perhaps the most obvious example supporting the use of NCR that, in the case of this behavioral function, involves removing the discomfort associated with the disorder. This approach to treatment has been described anecdotally on occasion (as in "We took care of her dental problems, and the behavior problem also went away"), but a relationship between these events has not been demonstrated in any studies published to date.

Because interventions based solely on the alteration of establishing operations do not necessarily abolish the reinforcement contingency responsible for maintaining the behavior problem, there exists the possibility that antecedent changes could reduce behavior and maintain it at a low level *in spite of the fact* that it still is reinforced; if so, antecedent interventions would be particularly useful in situations where extinction is not feasible (see below). On the other hand, it is also possible that the effects of antecedent change procedures may be compromised to the extent that reinforcement, in fact, does continue.

## Discontinuation of Reinforcement: Extinction

The principle of extinction—behavioral reduction through withholding of reinforcement—is conceptually simple but difficult to implement with SIB for two reasons. First, the correct use of extinction requires that the behavior be allowed to continue, thereby placing the individual at greater risk. This problem can be alleviated somewhat by establishing the risk of the behavior prior to treatment and supplementing extinction with the use of protective equipment if necessary. A second and more general difficulty with extinction is that translation from principle to procedure often has not taken into account the source of reinforcement for the behavior. "Discontinuation of reinforcement" typically has involved cessation of ongoing events, and this procedural variation is so common that some textbooks define extinction solely through reference to "ignoring," time-out, and other examples of stimulus termination (e.g., LaVigna & Donnellan, 1986). Yet, research has shown that procedural time-out can serve different functions, not all of which are behavior reducing (Plummer, Baer, & LeBlanc, 1977; Solnick, Rincover, & Peterson, 1977), and the same is true more generally of procedural approaches to defining extinction. The procedures that define extinction in a given situation are determined by the specific nature of reinforcement to be "discontinued."

Extinction for behavior maintained by attention and other forms of social-positive reinforcement has been firmly established in the literature as the "withholding of previously given positive reinforcement following emission of the target behavior" (Harris & Ersner-Hershfield, 1978, p. 1355). The "withholding" often takes the form of not reacting to the behavior, which has been translated roughly into "ignoring" as a specific procedural description and time-out as a more general form of limited access to reinforcement. Although extinction has been reported to be a successful treatment for a wide range of behavior problems, including aggression (Mace, Page, Ivancic, & O'Brien, 1986) and SIB (Harmatz & Rasmussen, 1969), extinction as a sole means of intervention has rarely been used and is not considered to be highly effective. This conclusion, however, is based on an unknown proportion of treatment studies in which the "ignoring" variant of extinction was applied to behavior not maintained by social-positive reinforcement.

Extinction procedures for SIB maintained by automatic-positive reinforcement are more difficult to develop due to the fact that the specific reinforcers directly produced by the behavior usually cannot be seen. Nevertheless, when it is possible to identify a behavior's automatic reinforcers, extinction might be implemented by arranging conditions so that the consequences are attenuated. This form of extinction has been called "sensory extinction" and has been applied to stereotypic mannerisms (Rincover, Cook, Peoples, & Packard, 1979) as well as SIB (Dorsey, Iwata, Reid, & Davis, 1982; Rincover & Devany, 1982). Procedurally, sensory extinction has involved mechanical intervention that disrupts the stimulation produced by a behavior but that does not interfere with the behavior per se. Examples include padding walls or furniture, or having individuals wear padded equipment.

Results of a functional analysis are particularly important when considering the use of extinction with escape behavior. To the extent that the "ignoring" variant of extinction involves cessation of interaction, it will serve as negative reinforcement for escape behavior and exacerbate the problem. Extinction of escape is achieved through prevention of escape. Procedurally, this requires presentation of escape-provoking stimuli (e.g., work tasks and related instructions) and not removing these activities contingent on the occurrence of SIB. Two studies describing the use of extinction for escape-maintained SIB were reported by Iwata, Pace, Kalsher, Cowdery, & Cataldo (1990) and Steege, Wacker, Berg, Cigrand, & Cooper (1989). Data from a subsequent study (Pace et al., 1993) suggested that the behavior-reducing effects of escape extinction were accelerated when the treatment was combined with an antecedent modification (reduction of demand frequency).

The final case for which extinction might be examined consists of SIB maintained by its pain-attenuating consequences. Aside from the fact that it would be very difficult to arrange a situation in which behavior does not terminate ongoing stimulation (e.g., as in scratching that does not relieve an itch), there is little justification for this type of extinction because it leaves the individual in a state of discomfort with no effective means of dealing with the problem. Furthermore, the elimination of such behavior through extinction may reduce caregivers' ability to determine that the individual is, in fact, in need of physical intervention or medical attention.

## Differential Reinforcement

Although treatment procedures based on antecedent changes and extinction can be highly effective in reducing SIB, they do not explicitly strengthen alternative behaviors that are either less dangerous or more socially acceptable. Behavioral replacement of this type is achieved through differential reinforcement of other behavior (DRO) and differential reinforcement of alternative behavior (DRA), and several variations of both procedures have been reported in the literature (see Vollmer & Iwata, 1992, for a recent review). Because DRO involves delivering reinforcement for the nonoccurrence of behavior during some interval of time, the procedure is somewhat similar to extinction in that appropriate behavior is not directly shaped. In fact, results of a recent study indicate that the behavior-reducing effects of DRO are primarily a function of the extinction component and not the reinforcement component of the contingency (Mazaleski, Iwata, Vollmer, Zarcone, & Smith, 1993). Therefore, emphasis here is placed on DRA procedures.

Day, Rea, Schussler, Larsen, and Johnson (1988) described an interesting application of DRA as treatment for SIB maintained by access to toys. Treatment consisted of making these items unobtainable following SIB. Additionally, when subjects did not engage in SIB, they were required to make specific vocal and gestural responses in order to obtain toys. The intervention thus combined an extinction procedure with differential reinforcement for appropriate "requesting" behavior. Similar types of consequences (toys and other reinforcing objects) may be used to reduce "self-stimulatory" SIB. Here, however, the newly selected objects should be available noncontingently so that the stimulation can compete successfully with that immediately available from the SIB. Favell, McGimsey, and

Schell (1982) described a more response-specific form of DRA based on the presumed reinforcer produced by the SIB: Toys providing visual stimulation were given to an individual who engaged in eye poking, and popcorn was given to an individual who engaged in pica.

Differential reinforcement as treatment for escape behavior has taken several different forms. First, more potent positive reinforcement than that currently available can be used to strengthen the alternative behavior. Mace and Belfiore (1990) used this approach to increase compliance with instructions and reduce escape. They first identified instructions for which there was a high probability of compliance. When these were presented in a 3:1 ratio with instructions for which compliance was low, escape behavior decreased and compliance increased. A second approach involves negative reinforcement (i.e., a break from the task, avoidance of prompts, etc.) instead of positive reinforcement made contingent on compliance (Iwata et al., 1990). A third example of DRA involves reinforcement of alternative escape behaviors. Steege et al. (1990) used such an approach while treating two individuals who exhibited SIB in training situations. Contingent on pressing a microswitch (activating a tape recorder that played the words "Stop"), brief (10-second) breaks from training were provided.

DRA procedures applied to pain-attenuating behavior would involve establishing new responses that reduce discomfort either indirectly (as in requesting aid from another) or directly (as in self-medication). Initially, individuals might be taught an alternative behavior indicating a painful condition; this alternative behavior could be strengthened using either positive reinforcement (e.g., praise, materials, etc.) or negative reinforcement (alleviation of the discomfort). Individuals who are capable of learning more complex behaviors might later be taught to directly alleviate discomforting conditions through self-medication. Although simple in concept, these behaviors are probably difficult to establish for two reasons. First, the ideal context for teaching the alternative response is one in which the source of discomfort (e.g., headache) is present, but these occasions do not occur frequently. Second, reinforcement (pain attenuation) is probably immediate following SIB but perhaps significantly delayed following the alternative response (signaling another, which eventually produces medication).

## Punishment

Behavior reduction via punishment includes a wide variety of procedures ranging from innocuous forms of verbal reprimand (or even facial gestures) to stimulation that most would describe as painful if not highly uncomfortable. For this reason, consideration of punishment as a single class of procedures for the purpose of regulation is almost impossible. From the standpoint of learning principles, on the other hand, all punishment procedures achieve their effects in the same manner. Punishment (contingent stimulus delivery) reduces behavior by overriding whatever source of reinforcement is maintaining the behavior. Thus, of the four general classes of behavior-reduction procedures (modification of antecedent events, extinction, differential reinforcement, and punishment), punishment is the only group whose effectiveness does not require identification of the maintaining variables for the behavior disorder. This fact suggests that, given the arbitrary use of reinforcement-based versus punishment procedures as treatment, one would expect a higher degree of success with punishment, a finding that has been supported repeatedly in the literature (e.g., Axelrod & Apsche, 1983; Matson & DiLorenzo, 1984).

The most effective stimulus used as punishment for SIB has been brief and relatively mild cutaneous shock applied to the arm or leg (see Carr & Lovaas, 1983, for a review and Linscheid, Iwata, Ricketts, Williams, & Griffin, 1990, for a recent example). Other forms of punishment used with SIB have included facial screening (Lutzker & Wesch, 1983; Watson, Singh, & Winton, 1986); overcorrection (Foxx & Bechtel, 1983; Halpern & Andrasik, 1986); time-out (Brantner & Doherty, 1983; Rolider & Van Houten, 1985); water mist applied to the face (Dorsey, Iwata, Ong, & McSween, 1980); and extraneous sounds, smells, and tastes (Bailey, 1983). Interventions in this class should be reserved for SIB that has been determined to be of high risk or that has been resistant to other forms of treatment. As with extinction, punishment does not result in the learning of appropriate behaviors as replacement for SIB; therefore, concurrent use of reinforcement procedures is important. Finally, punishment must be used only in compliance with applicable federal, state, and institutional regulations.

## OTHER TREATMENT APPROACHES

Although learning therapies comprise the largest and most successful class of treatments for SIB, numerous other approaches have been tried with varying degrees of success. Most prevalent among these are pharmacologic interventions, which are reviewed elsewhere in this volume (for another recent review, see Thompson, Hackenberg, & Schaal, 1991). One class of drugs, the opiate antagonists, is described briefly here because of its special relevance to the treatment of SIB. Two other approaches to treatment, sensory-integration therapy and gentle teaching, are included in this section because they have been proposed as alternatives to some of the behavioral interventions described in this chapter.

### Pharmacologic Intervention: The Opiate Antagonists

Commonly used as treatment for heroin overdose, opiate antagonists selectively block the effects of opiate drugs at the receptor site in the brain. As a result, they also increase sensitivity to pain-producing stimuli. These two characteristics of opiate antagonists suggest two interesting theories of action when applied as treatment for SIB: (a) extinction of SIB maintained by positive reinforcement in the form of endorphin release (see previous discussion of biological factors), or (b) enhanced "automatic" punishment of SIB through drug-induced lowering of the pain-perception threshold. Davidson, Kleene, Carroll, and Rockowitz (1983) published the first report on the use of naloxone with one self-injurious individual, for whom SIB was reduced by 50% initially but recovered to baseline levels by the fifth day of treatment. Most recent research (e.g., Sandman, Barron, & Colman, 1990) has focused on the use of naltrexone, a drug that is both longer acting and more easily administered than naloxone. Although much of the research to date has not been well controlled and findings have been mixed, suppression of SIB with the opiate antagonists has been superior to that found with other drugs (see Herman, 1991, for review).

## Sensory-Integration Therapy

Based on the neurodevelopmental work of Ayers (1972, 1974), Lemke (1974) proposed that SIB may be a symptom of general central nervous system damage, and suggested the use of multiple forms of sensory stimulation and exercise, collectively called sensory-integrative (S-I) therapy, as treatment. The goal of intervention was to reduce SIB by improving sensorimotor coordination. Three subsequent reports (Bright, Bittick, & Fleeman, 1981; Dura, Mulick, & Hammer, 1988; Wells & Smith, 1983) described the successful treatment of SIB using S-I therapy, but the studies contained a number of methodological problems, including inadequate measurement, the absence of baseline data, and, most important, the delivery of physical stimulation that was confounded with social stimulation. Mason and Iwata (1990), in evaluating S-I therapy as treatment for three individuals with SIB, included a number of control procedures in their study. Their results indicated that sensory-stimulation exercises based on S-I therapy had little effect on SIB when social stimulation was not part of the treatment. Thus, although S-I therapy may have a number of beneficial effects, specific reduction of SIB does not appear to be one of them.

## Gentle Teaching

Described as a humanistic treatment whose "central strategy is to resignify diadic interactions through unconditional value-giving and its frequent elicitation, while giving warm assistance and protection when necessary" (McGee & Gonzalez, 1990), gentle teaching stands in marked contrast to behavioral therapies based on contingencies of reinforcement or punishment. By emphasizing the development of warm human relationships, it is assumed that gentle teaching will result in "bonding," a generalized social attachment between caregiver and client. Through the process of bonding, the client learns the value of positive social interaction, participates more readily in instructional activities, and ceases engaging in oppositional behavior. Outcome data showing reductions in aggression, property destruction, and SIB have been presented by McGee and colleagues (McGee & Gonzalez, 1990; McGee, Menolascino, Hobbs, & Menousek, 1987). However, numerous attempts to replicate these findings under well-controlled conditions have failed to show similar therapeutic effects (see Barrera & Teodoro, 1990, and Jones, Singh, & Kendall, 1991, as illustrative studies, and Jones & McCaughy, 1992, for a recent review).

A major difficulty has been the lack of objective specification of treatment components comprising gentle teaching. In perhaps the most complete list of procedures presented to date, McGee and Gonzalez (1990) itemized 10 supportive techniques used throughout treatment: (a) errorless teaching, (b) task analysis and modification, (c) prompting, (d) coparticipation in tasks, (e) the use of tasks as vehicles to focus on positive interactions, (f) identification and reduction of precursors to problem behaviors, (g) reduced frequency of instructions, (h) choice making, (i) fading assistance, and (j) personalized verbal interactions. Little or no additional description was provided for these techniques; nevertheless, the terms used suggest a heavy emphasis on antecedent task simplification (a,b,c,d,g), noncontingent positive reinforcement in the form of attention and access to desired things (e,h,j), and noncontingent negative reinforcement through removal of "unwanted" items (f). Although our classification of these components may not be widely endorsed, it at least begins to operationalize the ingredients of gentle teaching according to known principles of learning. With additional specification, one might be able to determine which if any of these components actually is present in the treatment package, and whether their inclusion or exclusion has any effect on outcome.

## SUMMARY

Self-injurious behavior (SIB) is a serious and chronic disorder associated with multiple risks. Although data suggest that some SIB may be related to organic factors, in most cases the behavior appears to be a learned response, maintained by either social or automatic sources of reinforcement. A systematic approach to treatment involves the following steps: risk assessment and management, identification of replacement behaviors as well as reinforcers for strengthening these behaviors, and the use of functional analysis methodology to identify the variables currently maintaining SIB. Behavioral approaches to treatment attempt to reduce SIB through several means: removal of the antecedent conditions (e.g., deprivation, aversive stimulation) that occasion SIB, elimination of reinforcement. for SIB through extinction, or differential reinforcement. Another class of interventions, punishment, attempts to override the current source of reinforcement for SIB.

## REFERENCES

Anderson, L., Dancis, J., & Alpert, M. (1978). Behavioral contingencies and self-mutilation in Lesch-Nyhan disease. *Journal of Consulting and Clinical Psychology, 46,* 529–536.

Axelrod, S., & Apsche, J. (1983). *The effects of punishment on human behavior.* New York: Academic.

Ayers, A. J. (1972). *Sensory integration and learning disorders.* Los Angeles: Western Psychological Services.

Ayers, A. J. (1974). *The development of sensory integrative theory and practice.* Dubuque, IA: Kendall/Hunt.

Bachman, J. A. (1972). Self-injurious behavior: A behavioral analysis. *Journal of Abnormal Psychology, 80,* 211–224.

Bailey, J., & Meyerson, L. (1970). Effect of vibratory stimulation on a retardate's self-injurious behavior. *Psychological Aspects of Disability, 17,* 133–137.

Bailey, S. L. (1983). Extraneous aversives. In S. Axelrod & J. Apsche (Eds.), *The effects of punishment on human behavior* (pp. 247–284). New York: Academic.

Barrera, F. J., & Teodoro, G. M. (1990). Flash bonding or cold fusion? A case analysis of gentle teaching. In A. C. Repp & N. N. Singh (Eds.), *Perspectives on the use of nonaversive and aversive interventions for persons with developmental disabilities* (pp. 199–214). Sycamore, IL: Sycamore Publishing.

Belluzzi, J. D., & Stein, L. (1977). Enkephalin may mediate euphoria and drive-reduction reward. *Nature, 266,* 556–558.

Bijou, S. W., Peterson, R. F., & Ault, M. H. (1968). A method to integrate descriptive and experimental field studies at the level of data and empirical concepts. *Journal of Applied Behavior Analysis, 1,* 175–191.

Borthwick, S. A., Meyers, C. E., & Eyman, R. K. (1981). Comparative adaptive and maladaptive behavior of mentally retarded clients of five residential settings in three western states. In R. H. Bruininks, C. E. Meyers, B. B. Sigford, & K. C. Lakin (Eds.), *Deinstitutionalization and community adjustment of mentally retarded people* (pp. 351–359). Washington, DC: American Association on Mental Deficiency.

Brantner, J. P., & Doherty, M. A. (1983). A review of timeout: A conceptual and methodological analysis. In S. Axelrod & J. Apsche (Eds.), *The effects of punishment on human behavior* (pp. 87–132). New York: Academic.

Bright, T., Bittick, K., & Fleeman, B. (1981). Reduction of self-injurious behavior using sensory integrative techniques. *American Journal of Occupational Therapy, 35,* 167–172.

Bruhl, H. H., Fielding, L. H., Joyce, M., Peters, W., & Wiesler, N. (1982). Thirty-month demonstration project for the treatment of self-injurious behavior in severely retarded individuals. In J. H. Hollis & C. E. Meyers (Eds.), *Life threatening behavior* (pp. 191–275). Washington, DC: American Association on Mental Deficiency.

Carr, E. G. (1977). The motivation of self-injurious behavior: A review of some hypotheses. *Psychological Bulletin, 84,* 800–816.

Carr, E. G., & Durand, V. M. (1985). Reducing behavior problems through functional communication training. *Journal of Applied Behavior Analysis, 18,* 111–126.

Carr, E. G., & Lovaas, O. I. (1983). Contingent electric shock as a treatment for severe behavior problems. In S. Axelrod & J. Apsche (Eds.), *The effects of punishment on human behavior* (pp. 221–245). New York: Academic.

Carr, E. G., Newsom, C. D., & Binkoff, J. A. (1976). Stimulus control of self-destructive behavior in a psychotic child. *Journal of Abnormal Child Psychology, 4,* 139–153.

Carr, E. G., Newsom, C., & Binkoff, J. (1980). Escape as a factor in the aggressive behavior of two retarded children. *Journal of Applied Behavior Analysis, 13,* 101–117.

Cataldo, M. F., & Harris, J. (1982). A biological basis for self-injury in the mentally retarded. *Analysis and Intervention in Developmental Disabilities, 2,* 21–39.

Charmove, A. S., & Harlow, H. F. (1970). Exaggeration of self-aggression following alcohol ingestion in rhesus monkeys. *Journal of Abnormal Psychology, 75,* 207–209.

Cipani, E. (1990). "Excuse me: I'll have . . . " Teaching appropriate attention-getting behavior to young children with severe handicaps. *Mental Retardation, 28,* 29–33.

Davidson, P. W., Kleene, B. M., Carroll, M., & Rockowitz, R. J. (1983). Effects of naloxone on self-injurious behavior: A case study. *Applied Research in Mental Retardation, 4,* 1–4.

Day, R. M., Rea, J. A., Schussler, N. G., Larsen, S. E., & Johnson, W. L. (1988). A functionally based approach to the treatment of self-injurious behavior. *Behavior Modification, 12,* 565–589.

DeLissovoy, V. (1961). Head banging in early childhood: A study of incidence. *Journal of Pediatrics, 58,* 803–805.

DeLissovoy, V. (1963). Head banging in early childhood: A suggested cause. *Journal of Genetic Psychology, 102,* 109–114.

DeMet, E. M., & Sandman, C. A. (1991). Models of the opiate system in self-injurious behavior: A reply. *American Journal of Mental Retardation, 95,* 694–696.

Dorsey, M. F., Iwata, B. A., Ong, P., & McSween, T. (1980). Treatment of self-injurious behavior using a water mist: Initial response suppression and generalization. *Journal of Applied Behavior Analysis, 13,* 343–353.

Dorsey, M. F., Iwata, B. A., Reid, D. H., & Davis, P. A. (1982). Protective equipment: Continuous and contingent application in the treatment of self-injurious behavior. *Journal of Applied Behavior Analysis, 15,* 217–230.

Dura, J. R., Mulick, J. A., & Hammer, D. (1988). Rapid clinical evaluation of sensory integrative therapy for self-injurious behavior. *Mental Retardation, 26,* 83–87.

Durand, V. M., & Crimmins, D. B. (1988). Identifying the variables maintaining self-injurious behavior. *Journal of Autism and Developmental Disorders, 18,* 99–117.

Egel, A. L. (1981). Reinforcer variation: Implications for motivating developmentally disabled children. *Journal of Applied Behavior Analysis, 14,* 345–350.

Favell, J. E., Azrin, N. H., Baumeister, A. A., Carr, E. G., Dorsey, M. F., Forehand, R., Foxx, R. M., Lovaas, O. I., Rincover, A., Risely, T. R., Romanczyk, R. G., Russo, D. C., Schroeder, S. R., & Solnick, J. V. (1982). The treatment of self-injurious behavior. *Behavior Therapy, 13,* 529–554.

Favell, J. E., McGimsey, J. F., & Jones, M. L. (1978). The use of physical restraint in the treatment of self-injury and as a positive reinforcement. *Journal of Applied Behavior Analysis, 11,* 225–242.

Favell, J. E., McGimsey, J. F., & Schell, R. M. (1982). Treatment of self-injury by providing alternate sensory activities. *Analysis and Intervention in Developmental Disabilities, 2,* 83–104.

Fisher, W., Piazza, C. C., Bowman, L. G., Hagopian, L. P., Owens, J. C., & Slevin, I. (1992). A comparison of two approaches for identifying reinforcers for persons with severe and profound disabilities. *Journal of Applied Behavior Analysis, 25,* 491–498.

Fovel, J. T., Lash, P. S., Barron, D. A., Jr., & Roberts, M. S. (1989). A survey of self-restraint, self-injury, and other maladaptive behaviors in an institutionalized retarded population. *Research in Developmental Disabilities, 10,* 377–382.

Foxx, R. M., & Bechtel, D. R. (1983). Overcorrection: A review and analysis. In S. Axelrod & J.

Apsche (Eds.), *The effects of punishment on human behavior* (pp. 133–220). New York: Academic.

Gambrill, E. D. (1977). *Behavior modification: Handbook of assessment, intervention, and evaluation.* San Francisco: Jossey-Bass.

Gedye, A. (1989). Extreme self-injury attributed to frontal lobe seizures. *American Journal on Mental Retardation, 94,* 20–26.

Green, C. W., Reid, D. H., Carnipe, V. S., & Gardner, S. M. (1991). A comprehensive evaluation of reinforcer identification processes for persons with profound multiple handicaps. *Journal of Applied Behavior Analysis, 24,* 537–552.

Griffin, J. C., Williams, D. E., Stark, M. T., Altmeyer, B. K., & Mason, M. (1984). Self-injurious behavior: A state-wide prevalence survey, assessment of severe cases, and follow-up of aversive programs. In J. C. Griffin, D. E. Williams, M. T. Stark, B. K. Altmeyer, & H. K. Griffin (Eds.), *Advances in the treatment of self-injurious behavior* (pp. 1–25). Austin: Texas Planning Council for Developmental Disabilities.

Halpern, L. F., & Andrasik, F. (1986). The immediate and long-term effectiveness of overcorrection in treating self-injurious behavior in a mentally retarded adult. *Applied Research in Mental Retardation, 7,* 59–65.

Harmatz, M. G., & Rasmussen, W. A. (1969). A behavior modification approach to head banging. *Mental Hygiene, 53,* 590–593.

Harris, S. L., & Ersner-Hershfield, R. (1978). Behavioral suppression of seriously disruptive behavior in psychotic and retarded patients: A review of punishment and its alternatives. *Psychological Bulletin, 85,* 1352–1375.

Herman, B. H. (1991). Effects of opioid receptor antagonists in the treatment of autism and self-injurious behavior. In J. Ratey (Ed.), *Mental retardation: Developing pharmacotherapies* (pp. 107–137). Washington, DC: American Psychiatric Press.

Hill, J., & Spreat, S. (1987). Staff injury rates associated with the implementation of contingent restraint. *Mental Retardation, 25,* 141–145.

Iwata, B. A. (1987). Negative reinforcement in applied behavior analysis: An emerging technology. *Journal of Applied Behavior Analysis, 20,* 361–387.

Iwata, B. A., Dorsey, M. F., Slifer, K. J., Bauman, K. E., & Richman, G. S. (1982). Toward a functional analysis of self-injury. *Analysis and Intervention in Developmental Disabilities, 2,* 3–20.

Iwata, B. A., Pace, G. M., Kalsher, M. J., Cowdery, G. E., & Cataldo, M. F. (1990). Experimental analysis and extinction of self-injurious escape behavior. *Journal of Applied Behavior Analysis, 23,* 11–27.

Iwata, B. A., Pace, G. M., Kissel, R. C., Nau, P. A., & Farber, J. M. (1990). The Self-Injury Trauma (SIT) Scale: A method for quantifying surface tissue damage caused by self-injurious behavior. *Journal of Applied Behavior Analysis, 23,* 99–110.

Iwata, B. A., Vollmer, T. R., & Zarcone, J. R. (1990). The experimental (functional) analysis of behavior disorders: Methodology, applications, and limitations. In A. C. Repp & N. N. Singh (Eds.), *Perspectives in nonaversive and aversive interventions with developmentally disabled persons* (pp. 301–330). Sycamore, IL: Sycamore Publishing.

Johnson, H. G., Ekman, P., Friesen, W., Nyhan, W. L., & Shear, C. (1976). A behavioral phenotype in the deLange syndrome. *Pediatric Research, 10,* 843–850.

Jones, I. H., & Barraclough, B. M. (1978). Auto-mutilation in animals and its relevance to self-injury in man. *Acta Psychiatrica Scandinavica, 58,* 40–47.

Jones, L. J., Singh, N. N., & Kendall, K. A. (1991). Comparative effects of gentle teaching and visual screening on self-injurious behavior. *Journal of Mental Deficiency Research, 38,* 37–47.

Jones, R. S. P., & McCaughy, R. E. (1992). Gentle teaching and applied behavior analysis: A critical review. *Journal of Applied Behavior Analysis, 25,* 853–867.

King, B. H., McCracken, J. T., & Poland, R. E. (1991). Deficiency in the opioid hypotheses of self-injurious behavior. *American Journal of Mental Retardation, 95,* 692–694.

La Vigna, G. W., & Donnellan, A. M. (1986). *Alternatives to punishment: Solving behavior problems with nonaversive strategies.* New York: Irvington.

Lemke, H. (1974). Self-abusive behavior in the mentally retarded. *American Journal of Occupational Therapy, 28,* 94–97.

Lesch, M., & Nyhan, W. L. (1964). A familial disorder of uric acid metabolism and central nervous system function. *American Journal of Medicine, 36,* 561–570.

Linscheid, T. R., Iwata, B. A., Ricketts, R. W., Williams, D. E., & Griffin, J. C. (1990). Clinical evaluation of the Self-Injurious Behavior Inhibiting System (SIBIS). *Journal of Applied Behavior Analysis, 23,* 53–78.

Lovaas, O. I., Newsom, C. D., & Hickman, C. (1987). Self-stimulatory behavior and perceptual reinforcement. *Journal of Applied Behavior Analysis, 20,* 45–68.

Lovaas, O. I., & Simmons, J. Q. (1969). Manipulation of self-destruction in three retarded children. *Journal of Applied Behavior Analysis, 2,* 143–157.

Lutzker, J. R., & Wesch, D. (1983). Facial screening: History and critical review. *Australia and New Zealand Journal of Developmental Disabilities, 9,* 209–223.

Mace, F. C., & Belfiore, P. (1990). Behavioral momentum in the treatment of escape-motivated stereotypy. *Journal of Applied Behavior Analysis, 2,* 507–514.

Mace, F. C., Hock, M. L., Lalli, J. S., West, B. J., Belfiore, P., Pinter, E., & Brown, D. K. (1988). Behavioral momentum in the treatment of noncompliance. *Journal of Applied Behavior Analysis, 21,* 123–141.

Mace, F. C., Lalli, J. S., & Pinter Lalli, E. (1991). Functional analysis and treatment of aberrant behavior. *Research in Developmental Disabilities, 12,* 155–180.

Mace, F. C., Page, T. J., Ivancic, M. T., & O'Brien, S. (1986). Analysis of environmental determinants of aggression and disruption in mentally retarded children. *Applied Research in Mental Retardation, 7,* 203–221.

Mason, S. A., & Iwata, B. A. (1990). Artifactual effects of sensory-integrative therapy on self-injurious behavior. *Journal of Applied Behavior Analysis, 23,* 362–370.

Matson, J. L., & DiLorenzo, T. M. (1984). *Punishment and Its Alternatives: New perspectives for behavior modification.* New York: Springer-Verlag.

Maurice, P., & Trudel, G. (1982). Self-injurious behavior: Prevalence and relationships to environmental events. In J. H. Hollis & C. E. Meyers (Eds.), *Life-threatening behavior: Analysis and intervention* (pp. 81–103). Washington: American Association on Mental Deficiency.

Mazaleski, J. L., Iwata, B. A., Vollmer, T. R., Zarcone, J. R., & Smith, R. G. (1993). Analysis of the reinforcement and extinction components in DRO contingencies with self-injury. *Journal of Applied Behavior Analysis, 26,* 143–156.

McGee, J. J., & Gonzalez, L. (1990). Gentle teaching and the practice of human interdependence: A preliminary group study of 15 persons with severe behavioral disorders and their caregivers. In A. C. Repp & N. N. Singh (Eds.), *Perspectives on the use of nonaversive and aversive interventions for persons with developmental disabilities* (pp. 237–254). Sycamore, IL: Sycamore Publishing.

McGee, J. J., Menolascino, F. J., Hobbs, D. C., & Menousek, P. E. (1987). *Gentle teaching: A non-aversive approach to helping persons with mental retardation.* New York: Human Sciences Press.

Michael, J. L. (1982). Distinguishing between discriminative and motivational functions of stimuli. *Journal of the Experimental Analysis of Behavior, 37,* 149–155.

Newton, J. T., & Sturmey, P. (1991). The Motivation Assessment Scale: Inter-rater reliability and internal consistency in a British sample. *Journal of Mental Deficiency Research, 35,* 472–474.

Nyhan, W. L. (1976). Behavior in the Lesch-Nyhan Syndrome. *Journal of Autism and Childhood Schizophrenia, 6,* 235–252.

Pace, G. M., Ivancic, M. T., Edwards, G. L., Iwata, B. A., & Page, T. J. (1985). Assessment of stimulus preference and reinforcer value with profoundly retarded individuals. *Journal of Applied Behavior Analysis, 18,* 249–255.

Pace, G. M., Iwata, B. A., Cowdery, G. E., Andree, P. J., & McIntyre, T. (1993). Stimulus (instructional) fading during extinction of self-injurious escape behavior. *Journal of Applied Behavior Analysis, 26,* 205–212.

Pace, G. M., Iwata, B. A., Edwards, G. L., & McCosh, K. C. (1986). Stimulus fading and transfer in the treatment of self-restraint and self-injurious behavior. *Journal of Applied Behavior Analysis, 19,* 381–389.

Peters, J. M. (1967). Caffeine induced hemorragic automutilation. *Archives Internationales de Pharmacodynomie et de Therapy, 169,* 139–146.

Plummer, S., Baer, D. M., & LeBlanc, J. M. (1977). Functional considerations in the use of time out and an effective alternative. *Journal of Applied Behavior Analysis, 10,* 689–705.

Pyles, D. A. M., & Bailey, J. S. (1990). Diagnosing severe behavior problems. In A. C. Repp & N. N. Singh (Eds.), *Perspectives on the use of nonaversive and aversive interventions for persons with developmental disabilities* (pp. 381–401). Sycamore, IL: Sycamore Publishing.

Rast, J., Johnston, J. M., Drum, C., & Conrin, J. (1981). The relation of food quantity to rumination behavior. *Journal of Applied Behavior Analysis, 14,* 121–130.

Richmond, G., Schroeder, S. R., & Bickel, W. (1984). Tertiary prevention of attrition related to self-injurious behavior. In K. D. Gadow (Ed.), *Advances in learning and behavioral disabilities* (Vol. 5, pp. 97–116). Greenwich, CT: JAI.

Rincover, A., Cook, R., Peoples, A., & Packard, D. (1979). Sensory extinction and sensory reinforcement principles for programming multiple adaptive behavior change. *Journal of Applied Behavior Analysis, 12,* 221–233.

Rincover, A., & Devany, J. (1982). The application of sensory extinction procedures to self-injury. *Analysis and Intervention in Developmental Disabilities, 2,* 67–81.

Rojahn, J., Mulick, J. A., & Schroeder, S. R. (1980). Ecological assessment of self-protective devices in three profoundly retarded adults. *Journal of Autism and Developmental Disorders, 10,* 59–66.

Rolider, A., & Van Houten, R. (1985). Movement suppression time-out for undesirable behavior in psychotic and severely developmentally delayed children. *Journal of Applied Behavior Analysis, 18,* 275–288.

Russo, D. C., Carr, E. G., & Lovaas, O. I. (1980). Self-injury in the pediatric population. In J. Ferguson & C. B. Taylor (Eds.), *Comprehensive handbook of behavioral medicine* (pp. 23–41). Holliswood, NY: Spectrum.

Sandman, C. A., Barron, J. L., & Colman, H. (1990). An orally administered opiate blocker, naltrexone, attenuates self-injurious behavior. *American Journal of Mental Retardation, 95,* 93–102.

Singh, N. N., & Millinchamp, C. J. (1987). Independent and social play among profoundly mentally retarded adults: Training, maintenance, generalization, and long-term follow-up. *Journal of Applied Behavior Analysis, 20,* 23–34.

Skinner, B. F. (1969). *Contingencies of reinforcement: A theoretical analysis.* New York: Appleton-Century-Crofts.

Smith, R. G., Iwata, B. A., Vollmer, T. R., & Pace, G. M. (1992). On the relationship between self-restraint and self-injurious behavior. *Journal of Applied Behavior Analysis, 23,* 433–445.

Smolev, S. R. (1971). Use of operant techniques for the modification of self-injurious behavior. *American Journal of Mental Deficiency, 76,* 295–305.

Snyder, S. H. (1977). Opiate receptors in the brain. *New England Journal of Medicine, 296,* 266–271.

Snyder, S. H. (1984). Drug and neurotransmitter receptors in the brain. *Science, 224,* 22–31.

Solnick, J. V., Rincover, A., & Peterson, C. R. (1977). Some determinants of the reinforcing and punishing effects of time out. *Journal of Applied Behavior Analysis, 10,* 415–424.

Spain, B., Hart, S. A., & Corbett, J. (1984, November). The use of appliances in the treatment of severe self-injurious behavior. *Occupational Therapy,* 353–357.

Steege, M. V., Wacker, D. P., Berg, W. K., Cigrand, K. K., & Cooper, L. J. (1989). The use of behavioral assessment to prescribe and evaluate treatments for severely handicapped children. *Journal of Applied Behavior Analysis, 22,* 22–33.

Steege, M. W., Wacker, D. P., Cigrand, K. C., Berg, W. K., Novak, C. G., Reimers, T. M., Sasso, G. M., & DeRaad, A. (1990). Use of negative reinforcement in the treatment of self-injurious behavior. *Journal of Applied Behavior Analysis, 23,* 459–467.

Sulzer-Azaroff, B., & Mayer, G. R. (1977). *Applying behavior-analysis procedures with children and youth.* New York: Holt, Rinehart & Winston.

Tate, B. G., & Baroff, G. S. (1966). Aversive control of self-injurious behavior in a psychotic boy. *Behaviour Research and Therapy, 4,* 281–287.

Thompson, T., Hackenberg, T., & Schaal, D. (1991). Pharmacologic treatments for behavior problems in developmental disabilities. In U.S. Department of Health and Human Services, *Treatment of destructive behaviors in persons with developmental disabilities* (NIH Publication No. 91-2410, pp. 343–445). Bethesda, MD: National Institute of Health.

Touchette, P. E., MacDonald, R. F., & Langer, S. N. (1985). A scatter plot for identifying stimulus control of problem behavior. *Journal of Applied Behavior Analysis, 18,* 343–351.

Vollmer, T. R., & Iwata, B. A. (1991). Establishing operations and reinforcement effects. *Journal of Applied Behavior Analysis, 24,* 279–291.

Vollmer, T. R., & Iwata, B. A. (1992). Differential reinforcement as treatment for behavior disorders: Procedural and functional variations. *Research in Developmental Disabilities, 13,* 393–417.

Vollmer, T. R., Iwata, B. A., Zarcone, J. R., Smith, R. G., & Mazaleski, J. L. (1993). The role of attention in the treatment of attention-maintained self-injurious behavior: Noncontingent reinforcement (NCR) and differential reinforcement of other behavior (DRO). *Journal of Applied Behavior Analysis, 26,* 9–21.

Watson, J., Singh, N. N., & Winton, A. S. W. (1986). Suppressive effects of visual and facial screening on self-injurious finger-sucking. *American Journal of Mental Deficiency, 90,* 526–534.

Weeks, M., & Gaylord-Ross, R. (1981). Task difficulty and aberrant behavior in severely handicapped students. *Journal of Applied Behavior Analysis, 14,* 449–463.

Wells, M., & Smith, D. W. (1983). Reduction of self-injurious behavior of mentally retarded persons using sensory integrative techniques. *American Journal of Mental Deficiency, 87,* 664–666.

Zarcone, J. R., Rodgers, T. A., Iwata, B. A., Rourke, D. A., & Dorsey, M. F. (1991). Reliability analysis of the Motivation Assessment Scale: A failure to replicate. *Research in Developmental Disabilities, 12,* 349–360.

# 8

# Treatment of Family Problems in Autism

## SANDRA L. HARRIS

## INTRODUCTION

There is little dispute among professionals that autism is a biologically based disorder, probably of multiple etiologies (e.g., Schopler & Mesibov, 1987). Although biological in origin, it also appears to be the case that how a family responds to a child's autism can, in some cases, influence the child's educational gains and manifestation of behavior problems. A chaotic, disorganized family, or a clinically depressed parent, will have difficulty creating the kind of consistency to which these youngsters best respond. Thus, family problems may influence the development of the child with autism. Conversely, the child's disability can have a major impact on family functioning. These two factors may intertwine, with family dysfunction heightening the child's needs, and the child's behavior problems intensifying family difficulties.

To understand the special demands imposed on families of children and adolescents with autism it is helpful to remember that all parenting is sometimes stressful. Even "good" kids go through bad times, and difficult children who experiment with drugs, are depressed, or defy parental authority in ways that are destructive of themselves or others, contribute to a family atmosphere that can be painful for all involved.

Will there be a reader of this chapter who has not encountered some of life's intensely painful moments? Children get in serious trouble. Parents die. Husbands or wives loose jobs. Couples divorce. Those are normative events that we all

---

SANDRA L. HARRIS • Graduate School of Applied and Professional Psychology, Rutgers, The State University of New Jersey, Busch Campus, Piscataway, New Jersey 08855-0819.

*Behavioral Issues in Autism*, edited by Eric Schopler and Gary B. Mesibov. New York, Plenum Press, 1994.

confront. There is no way to evade suffering a share of life's injuries, but some of us cope better than others with these disappointments and losses. That is true for families who have a child with autism, just as it is true for others. It is therefore important to understand not only the specific sources of stress that these special needs families experience, but also how they cope with these demands, the factors that determine which families will respond more or less effectively to the stresses in their lives, and how their coping may impact on the child's developmental progress.

The present chapter examines briefly the current literature on the impact of a child's autism upon the family, some of the variables that may enhance or undermine family functioning in the face of stress, and ways to help families learn to cope with these special demands. The chapter considers the functioning of the essentially healthy family called upon to respond to extraordinary demands, as well as the family already at risk for dysfunction for whom the presence of a child with special needs may lead to maladaptive behavior on the part of one or more family members, and how family functioning may influence the child's behavior.

## THE IMPACT OF THE CHILD'S AUTISM ON THE FAMILY

The stress of raising a child with autism varies across the family's life cycle and varies with the extent of the child's disability. In addition, the specific effects of these stressful events differ according to the roles of the family members. In spite of this variability, and the complexity such variation injects into the measurement process, the literature does support the notion that these families, as a group, face demands that are beyond the ordinary.

### Mothers and Fathers

Mothers report greater distress in parenting a child with autism than do fathers (e.g., Bristol, Gallagher, & Schopler, 1988; Wolf, Noh, Fisman, & Speechley, 1989). Mothers of children with autism suffer restrictions on their personal time and freedom, may endure a loss of self-esteem because they view themselves as having "failed" in their parenting role, and report feelings of depression, anger, fatigue and tension (DeMyer, 1979; Holroyd, 1974; Wolf et al., 1989). These women are often painfully aware of how the difference between their child and other children is viewed by the community, and how their parenting role differs from that of other women (Bristol, 1984; Holroyd, 1974). This distress may intensify over time because their child's developmental deviations are increasingly obvious as the child grows up, and because community services often fail to meet the needs of older persons with autism (Bristol & Schopler, 1983; DeMyer &

Goldberg, 1983). Mothers of adolescents with autism report greater perceived stress than do mothers of normally developing young people of the same age (Fong & Harris, 1991).

Gill (1990) found that mothers of preschool children with autism experienced significantly greater stress than mothers of children with mental retardation or those whose children were developing normally. The mothers of children with autism characterized themselves as moderately depressed, women with mentally retarded children appeared to be mildly depressed, whereas the mothers of normally developing children fell in the nondepressive range. This pattern also emerged for measures of anxiety, somatic complaints, and emotional exhaustion in Gill's (1990) study. Interestingly, all three groups of mothers in her project reported high degrees of personal accomplishment in parenting. Although this score was highest for the mothers of normally developing children, the two groups of mothers of children with handicaps also reported considerable satisfaction in this domain.

Fathers are not exempt from the demands inherent in raising a child with autism, although, at least in traditionally structured families, they may escape some of the day-to-day distress because they are in the workplace for significant amounts of time. Work may provide men with a freedom not available to the woman who remains at home and offers fathers an alternative source of self-esteem beyond their role as parents. Nonetheless, fathers, too, share their wives' sense of frustration, loss, guilt and anger, although they may be less articulate in voicing these emotions than are their spouses (DeMyer, 1979; Wolf et al., 1989). Fathers often express concern about their wives' distress (DeMyer, 1979) and may feel especially burdened by the family's special financial requirements and the long-term needs of their developmentally disabled youngster (Lamb, 1983).

Given the stressful demands on mothers and fathers, it is not surprising to find reports that couples may experience marital distress linked to their child's special needs. Evaluation of this literature, however, reveals the considerable variability among respondents when describing their marriages. Several studies of parents of children with autism and other developmental disabilities have indicated that although raising a child with a serious developmental handicap has a negative effect on some marriages, it may strengthen others (e.g., DeMyer, 1979; Gath, 1978; Lonsdale, 1978). Morgan (1988) indicates that it is premature to draw conclusions about the impact of the child's autism on the marriage.

## Siblings

There is a small literature examining the effects of being a sibling of a child with autism. Mates (1990) identified little difference between his sample of siblings of children with autism and normative data. Similarly, McHale, Sloan, and

Simeonsson (1986) found few differences between siblings of children with autism and mental retardation and siblings of normally developing youngsters on self-report measures. However, they caution that close examination of their data reveals considerable variability in the data for the youngsters whose brother or sister had a handicapping condition. Some of these children described very positive, and others very negative, relationships with their siblings. These authors emphasize that having a brother or sister with a handicap need not invariably lead to a troubled sibling relationship but argue that it poses a significant developmental challenge for some youngsters. These issues can include the frustration of dealing with an unresponsive brother or sister, demands to be an auxiliary parent, the sacrifice of parental attention, discomfort caused by peer responses to the brother or sister's behavior, and similar difficult experiences. These problems may be intensified if the child with autism exhibits severe behavior problems that further diminish parent resources, place demands on the siblings to cope with aggressive or destructive behavior, or make it difficult for the sibling to bring friends home to be confronted by sometimes frightening behaviors of the child with autism.

Although there is good reason to believe that families who include a child with autism do experience greater stress than other families, it is nonetheless, also very important to remember that this impact is quite variable, and that some families may report considerable dysfunction, whereas others say that their functioning is not adversely affected, or in some cases that their family, marital, or personal functioning has been enhanced by the challenge of meeting the child's special needs. A compelling demand for professionals serving families who have a child with autism is to understand what differentiates the adaptive from maladaptively functioning family and how we might enable the less well-functioning family to improve its response to this family crisis.

## THE ABCX MODEL OF FAMILY FUNCTIONING

One potentially useful model of how families in general respond to stress was initially proposed by Hill (1949) and has been used by several researchers to better understand the complicated factors that influence family functioning (e.g., Bristol, 1987; McCubbin & Patterson, 1983; Wikler, 1981). This is the "ABCX" family crisis model in which A (a stressor) interacts with B (resources the family has available to meet the crisis) and with C (the family's definition of the stressful event) to produce X (the crisis). Variables B and C encompass a number of dimensions of family functioning that research has suggested may be important to understanding how families of children with autism cope with their child's special needs. For purposes of the present chapter, a relatively simple description of the ABCX theory will be sufficient; however, interested readers should note that the basic theory has undergone considerable elaboration (e.g., McCubbin & Patterson,

1983). In particular, provision has been made for the fact that families typically face not a single source of stress, but multiple events across time (e.g., Bristol, 1987).

In the ABCX model, A, the stressor, refers to any of the several events that impinge upon the family of the child with autism including the time of initial diagnosis, the severity of the child's symptoms, the child's starting school, the child's entry into adolescence, the child's turning 21 years of age, and so forth. Behavior problems such as self-injury, aggression, or destructiveness can be especially serious stressors. Variable B can include characteristics of the individual family members including psychological functioning, health, and finances; it can also include ways in which family members relate to one another including the marital interaction, sibling relationships, and the cohesiveness of the family as a whole. This variable can also refer to resources outside of the nuclear family such as formal and informal community support. It may sometimes be difficult to disentangle the cause and effect of some psychological characteristics such as depression or anxiety that might precede the discovery of the child's disability and be viewed as B variables or might emerge following this event and reflect the family's difficulty in coping (X variables).

Variable C, the family's perception of the event refers to the meaning the family members attach to the stressor. What is it that they say to themselves about their child's special needs? About the limitations they are experiencing as a family? Or, about what the child's special needs imply for that child and for the family in the years ahead?

The interplay of variables ABC determines whether the family will experience A (the stressor) as a crisis (X), and how effectively they cope with this event. Among the individual and family resources that researchers have examined as potentially important for coping with the needs of the child with autism are family cohesion, social support, coping strategies, and psychological hardiness. Measures of family and individual perception of the event have included assessment of the extent to which parents view the child's disability as catastrophic for the family and their degree of self-blame for the child's disability. These B and C factors have typically been examined as they relate to such outcomes (X variables) as depression, anxiety, marital adjustment, and parenting quality.

## Stresses for Families of Children with Autism

There are a number of potential crisis points across the life cycle of the family of a child with autism (Harris, Gill, & Alessandri, 1990). The notion of a family life cycle refers to the series of developmental challenges that occur in a family as children are born, start school, begin the differentiation process of adolescence, leave home, and so forth. These are normative events that create stress for most families, but that may be charged with exceptional demands when one member of the family has a disability such as autism. In addition to these normative events, the behavior problems of the child with autism may occur at any point in the cycle, serving as stressors in themselves, and intensifying the stress of normative events with which they cooccur.

An example of a normative life-cycle event made exceptional by the special needs of the child with autism would be the young person's twenty-first birthday. Parents describe their developmentally disabled child's twenty-first birthday as second only to the time of the child's diagnosis in degree of stress (Wikler, Wasow, & Hatfield, 1981). If the young adult is also engaged in disruptive, aggressive behaviors this transitional age may be made all the more difficult. As Wikler and her colleagues (1981) have noted, at times of transition, parents confront once again the sharp contrast between their child and others, and between their dreams for their child and the child's reality.

Each major event in the family's life cycle poses the potential for creating a crisis in family functioning. Whether, and to what extent, such a crisis arises, hinges upon Hill's (1949) other two variables, B (resources) and C (perceptions).

## Family and Individual Resources

Bristol (1987) used a variation of the ABCX model to assess the functioning of 45 families of children with autism or communication disorders seeking services from North Carolina's TEACCH program. Her results showed a significant positive relationship between both adequacy of social support, the use of active coping behaviors, and family adaptation. In addition, families who adapted less well were characterized by the presence of other family stresses, the mother's tendency to blame herself for the child's disability, and her definition of the child's disability as a family catastrophe. In a later study, Bristol and her colleagues (1988) reported that emotional support from one's spouse was significantly related to the quality of parenting a child with autism. Her work also suggests a relationship between family cohesion and adaptation (Bristol, 1984), although this may be a double-edged sword, with excessive cohesion merging into enmeshment that diminishes family functioning (Bristol, 1987).

One example of an individual psychological characteristic, classified as a B variable in Hill's (1949) format, is the quality of "hardiness" (e.g., Ganellen & Blaney, 1984; Kobasa, 1979). Hardy people are said to be resilient in the face of stress because of their sense of control, commitment, and challenge. These personal qualities in turn appear to influence the individual's perception of the stressor (Variable C).

Gill and Harris (1991) examined the extent to which hardiness might influence a woman's ability to cope with the stress of raising a child with autism.

We studied 60 mothers of children with autism, assessing their hardiness, depression, and somatic complaints. Consistent with our hypothesis, we found women who earned higher scores for hardiness were less likely to report somatic complaints and that those women who scored higher on the commitment subscale of the hardiness measure were least likely to voice symptoms of depression.

In the next study in this series, Gill (1990) included mothers of preschool-age children with autism, mental retardation, and normally developing children, thus enabling her to compare the impact of child rearing on these three groups. She found that both hardiness and social support were effective buffers of stress for these women and that there was a strong relationship between hardiness and social support, such that women with hardier attitudes also viewed themselves as having a more supportive social network.

## Perception of the Event

As the work of Bristol (1987) and Gill (1990) suggests, there appears to be a significant relationship between the family's perceptions of the child with autism and how the family adapts. The relationship between one's expectations and one's evaluations of the behavior of the young person with autism were examined by Fong (1991). She compared highly stressed mothers of adolescents with autism to mothers reporting low levels of subjective stress. The mothers were asked to watch brief videotaped vignettes of adolescents with autism doing routine tasks such as cutting vegetables and counting coins and to rate the tapes along several dimensions. The highly stressed women were more likely to view the scenes as physically or emotionally threatening than were the other women. Fong (1989) cites the example of a highly stressed woman fearing the adolescent chopping vegetables would cut himself and never be self-sufficient in this domain, whereas the less stressed woman might comment on the risk of being cut, but then add that mastery of the task would be an achievement for the young person. The same events can be construed very differently, depending upon the personal filter one brings to a situation.

In general it appears that the formal and informal social network available to a family, the cohesiveness of the family, the emotional support available in the marriage, and the cognitive/affective filter through which the family members view the child with autism are among the variables that can influence how families adapt to the child's special needs. Families that adapt less well are marked by depression, somatic complaints, marital discord, and a diminished sense of efficacy in the parenting role. These qualities may serve to diminish their effectiveness as behavior managers and thus lead to an increase in behavior problems, creating an ever-downward spiral of child misbehavior and parental despair.

## WORKING WITH FAMILIES OF NORMATIVE NEEDS

An awareness of some of the variables that influence functioning of families of children with autism makes it possible to consider educative, supportive, and therapeutic interventions that might enhance family functioning.

### Parent Training

One active coping strategy of documented efficacy for parents of children with autism is parent training to teach families the kinds of management procedures that will enable them to bring their child's disruptive behaviors under control and increase the parents' abilities to help their child master new, adaptive skills. Research on the effects of systematic parent training has shown consistently that parents can learn these skills and become more effective teachers for their children (e.g., Harris, Alessandri, & Gill, 1991; Kolko, 1984). Parents also report that training gives them more time for family recreation and leisure and less need to engage in "custodial" activities (Koegel, Schreibman, Johnson, O'Neill, & Dunlap, 1984). They also typically express satisfaction with the benefits of the training program (e.g., Harris, 1983; Kolko, 1984). Although not sufficient in itself, parent training appears to be one essential experience that should be available to every family of a child with autism. Families who are disorganized, or disengaged from one another, may have more difficulty benefiting from this training than those who are more cohesive. As a result, the disorganized family may need considerable help learning to manage their child's behavior.

### Support Groups

Another useful source of supportive/educative input for families of children with autism can be a support group that enables members to share their feelings, normalize their emotional responses, and enlarge their social networks to include other families who can lend a hand during difficult times. These groups, which are not intended to be therapy groups, but rather mutually supportive and educative groups, allow parents to explore the full gamut of emotional experiences related to their child's special needs. With an experienced facilitator, the group also offers opportunities for parents to explore and alter some of their cognitive attributions concerning their child and his or her role in the family.

Support groups that I have co-led have ranged over such diverse topics as the guilt parents feel about "neglecting" their other children, frustration and anger in dealing with members of the community or extended family who do not appear to understand their child's special needs, the difficulties of finding quality professional services for their child, resentment at having to subordinate one's needs to those of the child, and sorrow about their child's long-term needs for special care, even after the parents have died. Parents share with one another coping strategies they have found helpful, suggest alternative frameworks for understanding events, and sometimes provide tangible and intangible support for a member in the midst of a crisis. Although many of the activities of these groups should be under the control of the group members, it is probably best to have a trained person present to ensure the psychological safety of every member and respond in those instances when group members may feel overwhelmed by the needs of an individual.

The benefits of support groups need not be limited to parents. Sibling groups can also be helpful in exploring the issues confronted by children, including their jealous feeling about the attention their brother or sister with autism receives, concern about whether they might "inherit" the disease, anger at peers for their rejection of the brother or sister, protective feelings toward their parents, and so forth. As is the case for adults, these discussions aim at normalizing the emotional responses of the sibling, teaching effective coping responses, and providing factual information where that is lacking. "Parent training" is usually not appropriate for siblings, but giving them skills to enable them to play with their brother or sister may be of considerable benefit to the entire family (Harris, Alessandri, & Gill, 1991).

For some families enrolling their child in a good school program, providing parent training coupled with ongoing home consultation, and an optional support group are sufficient to enable them to cope effectively with their child's special needs. That does not mean they do not suffer episodes of sadness, anger, or grief, but rather that these events tend to be transient, responsive to support from friends and loved ones, and do not turn into chronic, gnawing discomfort or become manifested in maladaptive behaviors. None of us is exempt from pain, but those of us fortunate enough to cope well rebound from these episodes and resume a more stable, comfortable level of functioning.

## FAMILIES WITH SPECIAL NEEDS

Although families of children with autism do not suffer a higher degree of psychopathology than other families (e.g., Koegel, Schreibman, O'Neill, & Burke, 1983), nonetheless, on a purely statistical basis one would expect that some families will bring with them to the situation a preexisting psychological dysfunction. This dysfunction, compounded by the special needs of their child, especially if the child is difficult to manage, may create grave problems for some families. Such families may require several modes of intervention including treatment aimed specifically at their problems with addictive behavior, depression, anxiety, chaotic family functioning, and so forth, as well as treatment aimed at helping them deal with their child's special needs.

In addition to families who have a history of psychopathology, there are families who may have coped with their child's needs quite effectively until some additional stress such as the death of a spouse, loss of a job, marital discord, or the development of very-difficult-to-manage behavior on the part of the child placed them at increased risk for dysfunction. Such families may benefit from professional intervention beyond the parent training and support groups that should be routinely offered to all families. These additional interventions, although never losing sight of the special needs of the child with autism, must extend beyond the child to consider the functioning of the individual family members and the family as a whole.

## Marital Discord

One example of family disruption that can have a generalized impact on the functioning of the family of child with autism, and their ability to respond to their child's difficult to manage behavior, is marital discord. As noted above, feeling emotionally supported by one's spouse is a vital ingredient of adapting to the special needs of the child with autism (Bristol et al., 1988). Milgram and Atzil (1988) note that a mother's life satisfaction is enhanced when the father assumes his fair share of care for the child with autism. A woman with primary child-care responsibilities who does not feel supported by her spouse, and who is confronted by a self-injurious child, may find herself lonely, overwhelmed, and unable to cope with the child's exceptional needs.

In their work on depression in marriage, Beach, Sandeen, and O'Leary (1990) highlight the loss of social support suffered by the maritally discordant couple. Beach and his colleagues (1990) suggest a link between the loss of such experiences as marital cohesion, acceptance, and tangible assistance, and the depression of some couples in dysfunctional marriages. In fact, much of the focus of their empirically based therapy for maritally discordant, depressed couples is on the development of these vital aspects of social support.

The link between marital discord and depression might be especially problematic in the case of the couple who have a child with autism because the child's special needs, particularly if the child poses serious management problems, can serve as an additional stress that further heightens both the discord between the couple and each one's sense of despair. For example, discord may be intensified when their arguments focus on decisions about what is in the best interests of the child, and depression may be fueled by each parent's sense of failure in meeting the child's needs. As a consequence, the clinician who is treating a couple who have a child with autism and who complain of depression and marital distress may want to consider an approach such as that advocated by Beach and his colleagues (1990) with its emphasis on restoring the supportive aspects of the marital relationship. In the case of a family with a difficult-to-manage child, attention must also be paid to bringing these behaviors under control. Neither treating the relationship alone nor treating the child's behavior alone is likely to be as effective as addressing both issues.

## Family Cohesion

Just as cohesion, opportunities for emotional expression and acceptance, and the perception of tangible support from one's spouse are important for a couple, so are these qualities important for the family as a whole. Although it is essential to avoid enlisting siblings as auxiliary parents in the care of the child with autism, and important also that each member of the family retain a sense of himself or herself as a separate being, nonetheless, family cohesiveness contributes substantially to the well-being of the family. The challenge is to strike a balance between closeness and distance, between being a part of the family and being a separate person. There is, of course, a substantial range of healthy functioning along this dimension, and factors such as ethnicity and social class contribute to one's view of how close is "close enough" in family life. The clinician needs to assess the family, bearing in mind their cultural context, to determine the extent to which they may be enmeshed or disengaged as a unit, and how the members of the family experience these relationships. If there appears to be a dysfunctional balance within the family, one joins with the family in working toward a more adaptive level of individuation and integration (Minuchin, 1974). The assessment of cohesion may be based upon family interviews supplemented by an instrument such as the Family Environment Scale (Moos & Moos, 1981).

I have found some families with a chaotic, but warm environment especially difficult to treat, because the firm control that is in the best interests of the child with autism runs counter to their fundamental sense of how they wish to rear their children. Their warmth serves to counter the potential disadvantages of their disorganization for the normally developing child, but is insufficient for the autistic child.

## Maladaptive Perceptions

Altering the cognitive/affective filter through which members of the family view the needs of the child with autism is yet another avenue for bringing about change in individuals, or the family as a whole. As noted above, mothers who feel they are to blame for their child's disability, or who feel the child's needs constitute a catastrophe for the family, tend to reach a less-effective adaptation than those who hold a less-critical view (Bristol, 1987). These negative views can even color one's perception of relatively neutral events (Fong, 1991).

It is important to differentiate among several different kinds of maladaptive perceptions that might impact on family functioning. One is the belief that the family has no capacity to control the events in their lives and that they are helpless in the face of their child's needs. Such views may respond to efforts to teach parents to adopt a more "hardy" outlook as well as providing the family with skills that will enable them to gain better control over their child's behavior. Parent training is one way to improve a parent's sense of control over events in his or her life, although for some families such training might have to be woven into a highly supportive context and done in gradual increments in order to be effective. It may also be essential to teach parents how to utilize community resources and advocate on behalf of themselves and their child.

Another set of maladaptive perceptions are those that focus on such negative attributions as self-blame, a diminished sense of self-esteem, or a view of the child's disability as reflecting the meaninglessness of life. For persons with complaints of this nature the clinician may want to deal with the negative attributions using the same kinds of therapeutic procedures as one would use in response to negative statements from other domains (e.g., Beach et al., 1990; Peterson, 1982) but being alert to the realities of the impact of the child's autism. For some families the clinician's role might, in part, include helping them explore a more comforting outlook on life. For some such an outlook might be religious in nature, whereas for others it would involve another meaningful view of their purpose in life.

Finally, on a cautionary note, it is important to understand that some highly dysfunctional persons or families will resist efforts to engage them in a therapeutic process. Because therapy of all kinds is a collaborative venture, there may be situations where the concerned clinician will find himself or herself stymied. Under these conditions an educational focus on the child and an ongoing message of availability to the family may be all that can be accomplished. Fortunately, these families are relatively rare, and most parents, once convinced that something can be helpful to their child, will do what they can on the child's behalf.

## CONCLUSIONS AND SUMMARY

Parents of children with autism do not exhibit greater degrees of psychopathology than the population as a whole. Nonetheless, the child's special needs are a source of potent stress in their lives, and these family members do, on average, report more feelings of depression, somatic complaints, and marital discomfort than do their peers. Families whose children exhibit severe behavior problems may be especially vulnerable to the consequences of stress. There are some buffers that can help a family adapt to the special needs of the child with autism. Such buffers include a good social support network, family cohesion, and effective coping skills.

For some families, provision of adequate educational and professional services, including a good education for the child, training in management skills for the parents, and the availability of a supportive group for the parents and siblings can enable the family to function quite effectively. For other families who suffer some preexisting form of psychopathology, whose children pose exceptional problems, or who encounter additional stress from other sources, there may be a need for more specialized psychological treatments. Such treatments can include diminishing marital discord, helping the family establish an appropriate level of cohesiveness, and working with individuals to alter maladaptive negative attributions that are contributing to a diminished sense of control and efficacy as well as treating the child's difficult to manage behavior. Although the clinician would bring to these distressed families many of the same techniques that are useful for other individuals and families, the intervention process must also remain highly sensitive to the realities of the needs of the child with autism.

## REFERENCES

Beach, S. R. H., Sandeen, E. E., & O'Leary, K. D. (1990). *Depression in marriage.* New York: Guilford.

Bristol, M. M. (1984). Family resources and successful adaptation to autistic children. In E. Schopler & G. B. Mesibov (Eds.), *The effects of autism on the family* (pp. 289–310). New York: Plenum.

Bristol, M. M. (1987). Mothers of children with autism or communication disorders: Successful adaptation and the double ABCX model. *Journal of Autism and Developmental Disorders, 17,* 469–486.

Bristol, M. M., Gallagher, J. J., & Schopler, E. (1988). Mothers and fathers of young developmentally disabled and nondisabled boys: Adaptation and spousal support. *Developmental Psychology, 24,* 441–451.

Bristol, M. M., & Schopler, E. (1983). Stress and coping in families of autistic adolescents. In E. Schopler & G. B. Mesibov (Eds.), *Autism in adolescents and adults* (pp. 251–278). New York: Plenum.

DeMyer, M. K. (1979). *Parents and children in autism.* New York: Wiley.

DeMyer, M. K., & Goldberg, P. (1983). Family needs of the autistic adolescent. In E. Schopler & G. B. Mesibov (Eds.), *Autism in adolescents and adults* (pp. 225–250). New York: Plenum.

Fong, P. L. (1989). *Perceived stress in mothers of autistic adolescents.* Unpublished doctoral dissertation, Rutgers, The State University of New Jersey.

Fong, P. L. (1991). Cognitive appraisal in high and low stress mothers of adolescents with autism. *Journal of Consulting and Clinical Psychology, 59,* 471–474.

Fong, P. L., & Harris, S. L. (1991). *Perceived stress in mothers of autistic adolescents and mothers of nonhandicapped adolescents.* Manuscript submitted for publication.

Ganellen, R. J., & Blaney, P. H. (1984). Hardiness and social support as moderators of life stress. *Journal of Personality and Social Psychology, 47,* 156–163.

Gath, A. (1978). *Down's syndrome and the family—The early years.* London: Academic.

Gill, M. J. (1990). *The assessment of social support and individual characteristics as buffers against stress in mothers of handicapped and non-handicapped children.* Unpublished doctoral dissertation, Rutgers, The State University of New Jersey.

Gill, M. J., & Harris, S. L. (1991). Hardiness and social support as predictors of psychological discomfort in mothers of children with autism. *Journal of Autism and Developmental Disorders, 21,* 407–416.

Harris, S. L. (1983). *Families of the developmentally disabled: A guide to behavioral intervention.* Elmsford, NY: Pergamon.

Harris, S. L., Alessandri, M., & Gill, M. J. (1991). Training parents of developmentally disabled children. In J. L. Matson & J. A. Mulick (Eds.), *Handbook of mental retardation* (2nd ed., pp. 373–381). Elmsford, NY: Pergamon.

Harris, S. L., Gill, M. J., & Alessandri, M. (1990). The family with an autistic child. In M. Seligman (Ed.), *The family with a handicapped child* (2nd ed., pp. 269–294). Boston: Allyn & Bacon.

Hill, R. (1949). *Families under stress.* New York: Harper & Row.

Holroyd, J. (1974). The questionnaire on resources and stress: An instrument to measure family response to a handicapped family member. *Journal of Community Psychology, 2,* 92–94.

Kobasa, S. C. (1979). Stressful life events, personality, and health: An inquiry into hardiness. *Journal of Personality and Social Psychology, 37,* 1–11.

Koegel, R. L., Schreibman, L., Johnson, J., O'Neill, R. E., & Dunlap, G. (1984). Collateral effects of parent training on families with autistic children. In R. F. Dangel & R. A. Polster (Eds.), *Parent training: Foundations of research and practice* (pp. 358–378). New York: Guilford.

Koegel, R. L., Schreibman, L., O'Neill, R. E., & Burke, J. C. (1983). The personality and family-interaction characteristics of parents of autistic children. *Journal of Consulting and Clinical Psychology, 51,* 683–692.

Kolko, D. J. (1984). Parents as behavior therapists for their autistic child. In E. Schopler and G. B. Mesibov (Eds.), *The effects of autism on the family* (pp. 145–162). New York: Plenum.

Lamb, M. E. (1983). Fathers of exceptional children. In M. Seligman (Ed.), *The family with a handicapped child: Understanding and treatment* (pp. 125–146). New York: Grune & Stratton.

Lonsdale, G. (1978). Family life with a handicapped child: The parents speak. *Child Care, Health, and Development, 4,* 99–120.

Mates, T. E. (1990). Siblings of autistic children: Their adjustment and performance at home and in school. *Journal of Autism and Developmental Disorders, 20,* 545–553.

McCubbin, H. I., & Patterson, J. M. (1983). Family transitions: Adaptation to stress. In H. I. McCubbin & C. R. Figley (Eds.), *Stress and the family. Vol. I. Coping with normative transitions* (pp. 5–25). New York: Brunner-Mazel.

McHale, S. M., Sloan, J., & Simeonsson, R. J. (1986). Sibling relationships of children with autistic, mentally retarded, and nonhandicapped brothers and sisters. *Journal of Autism and Developmental Disorders, 16,* 399–413.

Milgram, N. A., & Atzil, M. (1988). Parenting stress in raising autistic children. *Journal of Autism and Developmental Disorders, 18,* 415–424.

Minuchin, S. (1974). *Families and Family Therapy.* Cambridge: Harvard University Press.

Moos, R., & Moos, B. (1981). *Family Environment Scale manual.* Palo Alto, CA: Consulting Psychologists Press.

Morgan, S. A. (1988). The autistic child and family functioning: A developmental-family systems perspective. *Journal of Autism and Developmental Disorders, 18,* 263–280.

Peterson, C. (1982). Learned helplessness and attributional interventions in depression. In C. Antaki & C. Brewin (Eds.), *Attributions and psychological change* (pp. 97–115). New York: Academic.

Schopler, E., & Mesibov, G. B. (1987). Introduction to neurobiological issues in autism. In E. Schopler & G. B. Mesibov (Eds.), *Neurobiological issues in autism* (pp. 3–11). New York: Plenum.

Wikler, L. (1981). Chronic stress of families of mentally retarded children. *Family Retardation, 30,* 281–288.

Wikler, L., Wasow, M., & Hatfield, E. (1981). Chronic sorrow revisited: Parent vs. professional depiction of the adjustment of parents of mentally retarded children. *American Journal of Orthopsychiatry, 51,* 63–70.

Wikler, L. M. (1986). Periodic stresses of families of older mentally retarded children: An exploratory study. *American Journal of Mental Deficiency, 90,* 703–706.

Wolf, L. C., Noh, S., Fisman, S. N., & Speechley, M. (1989). Brief report: Psychological effects of parenting stress on parents of autistic children. *Journal of Autism and Developmental Disorders, 19,* 157–166.

# 9

# The Impact of Stress and Anxiety on Individuals with Autism and Developmental Disabilities

JUNE GRODEN, JOSEPH CAUTELA, STACEY PRINCE, and JENNIFER BERRYMAN

Stress and anxiety have historically played a role in many theories of personality and behavior. Both psychoanalytic theorists and behaviorists have postulated that anxiety is the central component of neurotic disorders. Operant investigators, however, have been reluctant to use the concept of anxiety either as an explanatory concept or in a descriptive manner.

Although the construct of anxiety may be considered a psychological short-cut to describe a number of behaviors, it has proven useful in developing therapeutic strategies for producing significant behavior change. A number of behavioral therapeutic procedures, such as relaxation (Benson, 1975, 1984; Bernstein & Borkovec, 1973; Cautela & Groden, 1978; Groden, Cautela, & Groden, 1989; Jacobson, 1973), systematic desensitization (Wolpe, 1990), covert reinforcement (Cautela, 1970; Cautela & Kearney, 1986; Cautela & Kearney, 1993) and paradoxical intention (Ascher, 1980), have been developed to reduce behaviors subsumed under the concept of anxiety. These procedures have proven effective in reducing physiological arousal, decreasing verbal statements indicating fear or anxiety, and reducing avoidance of anxiety-provoking stimuli. A great deal of

JUNE GRODEN • The Groden Center, Inc., 86 Mount Hope Avenue, Providence, Rhode Island 02906. JOSEPH CAUTELA • Behavior Therapy Institute, 10 Phillips Road, Sudbury, Massachusetts 01776. STACEY PRINCE • Center for Clinical Research, University of Washington, Seattle, Washington 98195. JENNIFER BERRYMAN • State University of New York, Binghamton, New York 13902.

*Behavioral Issues in Autism*, edited by Eric Schopler and Gary B. Mesibov. New York, Plenum Press, 1994.

current literature has also focused on the related construct of stress: Descriptions of associated health risks and stress reduction techniques abound. (Benson & Proctor, 1987; Dohrenwend & Dohrenwend, 1974; McQuade & Aikman, 1974; Surwit, Williams, & Shapiro, 1982).

Although numerous books and articles have addressed stress and anxiety in the general population, very little has been written to address the implications of stress and anxiety for individuals with special needs. It is the contention of this chapter that the constructs of stress and anxiety have pragmatic value in understanding the behavior of persons with autism and developmental disabilities. We assert that many of the behaviors that are typically labeled as *autistic* or *stereotypic* are functionally related to the experience of stress and anxiety by individuals who lack a repertoire of appropriate coping mechanisms. We also contend that (1) like the general population, individuals with developmental disabilities are vulnerable to stressors; (2) the characteristics of autism and developmental disabilities may make this population even *more* vulnerable to the effects of stress and anxiety than the general population; and (3) research in the areas of stress and anxiety will greatly aid in the development of successful treatment strategies for this population.

## DEFINITION OF STRESS AND ANXIETY

Although stress and anxiety are terms often used interchangeably and will be considered together in this discussion, there is an important distinction to be made between them. The most widely accepted definition of stress is that put forth by Hans Selye (1974), who asserts that stress is the physiological reaction of the body to life situations that can be both happy events or unhappy events. The stress caused by happy or pleasant events is termed *eustress,* whereas stress brought about by unhappy events is termed *distress.* In either case, the physiological reactions that occur in the body can include muscle contraction, adrenal gland secretion, increased heart rate and blood pressure, increased perspiration, and inhibition of the digestive system. Stress occurs whenever a demand is placed on an organism to which the organism must respond by making an adjustment. In other words, the presence of stress indicates a disturbance of homeostasis in the individual, which may or may not be concurrent with the experience of anxiety.

The presence of anxiety, however, always indicates that the individual is experiencing stress. Although not stated explicitly by Wolpe (1958), his concept of anxiety includes three components: a subjective state inferred from verbal reports of the experienced level of anxiety; the extent of avoidance of anxiety-provoking stimuli or situations; and sympathetic nervous system arousal. Wolpe's original construct has remained the accepted definition of anxiety, with the additional component of nonverbal behaviors such as crying, whining, and visible muscle tension. Although the above four components are not always highly correlated in experimental investigations, most clinicians observe a high correlation of these components in their clients.

## STRESS AND STRESSORS IN THE GENERAL POPULATION

Although life events that serve as antecedents to stress, termed *stressors,* may differ on an individual basis, some of the more common stressors experienced by the general population include marriage, divorce, positive or negative changes in job status, birth of a child, fears, and pain.

Most individuals in the general population have developed a repertoire of coping strategies, or *buffers,* that enable them to handle stress effectively. These buffers differ on an individual basis, but can include talking to a professional or a friend; exercise; engaging in a favorite activity such as cooking or reading; and assertive responses.

## STRESS AND STRESSORS IN THE POPULATION WITH AUTISM AND DEVELOPMENTAL DISABILITIES

There are many indicators that suggest that persons with autism and other developmental disabilities experience a great deal of stress. The following section will contain excerpts from personal accounts from individuals with autism describing their stress; a description of the characteristics of autism that appear to exacerbate stress; physiological factors that contribute to stress; and external factors imposed on these individuals that intensify stress.

### Personal Statements from Individuals with Autism

Excerpts from the autobiographical accounts of two individuals with autism give anecdotal illustrations of the intense anxiety and stress these individuals experienced. In an autobiography, Tony W., a 22-year-old male with autism, stated that he "can't deal with stress, ... was very Nervous about everything, [and] Feared People and Social Activity Greatly" [sic] (Volkmar & Cohen, 1985, p. 50). Similarly, Temple Grandin, in her insightful autobiography, describes intense feelings of anxiety resembling panic attacks:

> Various stimuli, insignificant to most people, created a full blown stress reaction in me. When the telephone rang or when I checked the mail, I'd have a "stage fright" nerve attack. What if I didn't get any mail—or what if I did—and it was

something bad? The ring of the telephone set off the same reaction—panic. (Grandin & Scariano, 1986, p. 72)

These examples illustrate that persons with autism experience stress and that it is a significant problem in their lives. We are suggesting that the characteristics of persons with autism may also contribute to this stress and that the maladaptive and challenging behaviors that are exhibited may result from stressful experiences. This belief is based almost exclusively on clinical experience because there is a dearth of research literature in the field of autism that addresses this issue.

## Characteristics of Autism and Their Relationship to Stress

Numerous characteristics common to individuals with autism or developmental disabilities may create or intensify feelings of stress or anxiety. These characteristics include those that constitute stressors themselves and those that prevent the effective use of buffers.

One of the more prominent characteristics of autism is *communication deficits.* Between 28% (Wolff & Chess, 1965) and 61% (Fish, Shapiro & Campbell, 1966) of individuals with autism are essentially mute. Verbal individuals with autism also have communication difficulties. Their verbalizations may show abnormal or bizarre patterns, and they often fail to use language for effective social communication (Rutter, 1985).

Communication deficits are likely to expose these individuals to a great amount of stress if they are unable to effectively express their needs. Caregivers may be unable to discern when they are hungry, frightened, or suffering from pain. Lack of effective communication also precludes the use of coping mechanisms frequently used by the general population such as talking to and getting support from a friend.

Most individuals with autism show severe *deficits in social skills* (American Psychiatric Association, 1987; Kanner, 1943; Rutter, 1978), making it difficult for them to have positive interactions with others. Hobson (1986) also found that these individuals have difficulty interpreting emotions and suggests that this may contribute to their inability to understand others' emotions.

A large majority of all persons with autism also have *mental retardation* (American Psychiatric Association, 1987). Zetlin and Turner (1985) discovered that 84% of their sample with mental retardation experienced emotional problems during adolescence. Levine and Langness (1983) studied situational anxiety during athletic performance for individuals with and without mental retardation. They found that individuals with retardation experienced significantly more pregame anxiety than nonretarded individuals. The two groups also responded differently to anxiety. Nonretarded individuals responded to anxiety by increasing their activity levels, whereas retarded individuals reduced their activity level and played the game with less intensity. These results suggest that mental retardation increases the likelihood of experiencing stress and anxiety while decreasing the ability to cope effectively. Mental retardation and language deficits also contribute to an inability to understand verbal explanations. Thus, an individual with autism may be unable to understand his or her parent or his or her teacher's explanation of why an unpleasant event (e.g., a visit to the dentist) must occur.

*Low cognitive abilities* increase the frequency of failure, which has been shown to produce signs of anxiety in both the general population and persons with autism (Clark & Rutter, 1979; Finch, Montgomery, Kendall, & Morris, 1975). Difficulties with stimulus discrimination can also increase the frequency of failure. When given complex stimuli, many individuals with autism exhibit stimulus *overselectivity;* that is, they respond to only one component in a complex stimulus (Lovaas, Schreibman, Koegel, & Reim, 1971). Stimulus overselectivity can make it difficult for learning to occur, increasing the probability and frequency of failure.

Many individuals with autism appear to have *heightened sensitivity* and *irritability* due to perceptual aberrations (Ornitz & Ritvo, 1985). Auditory problems are most common, but visual, tactile, gustatory, olfactory, proprioceptive, and vestibular irregularities are also observed in this population. Young, Kavanaugh, Anderson, Shaywitz, and Cohen (1982) suggested that a deficit in the regulation of noradrenalin could be evidenced by "overreaction to minor stimuli; impaired discrimination and evaluation of stimuli; rushes of anxiety; disorganization of behavior; and avoidance of stimuli; particularly novelty, by withdrawing into oneself." Because of this heightened sensitivity, low-level stimuli generally ignored by most people may cause nervous system arousal in individuals with autism.

Another characteristic of autism is the *need to maintain sameness.* Minor changes in routine or environment that would not be anxiety-producing for a typical child can produce anxiety and intense behavior responses in individuals with autism. A child with autism may become distressed simply by having his or her seat at the dinner table changed (American Psychiatric Association, 1987). Ornitz and Ritvo (1985) described stimuli that elicit *fear* in persons with autism, such as sirens, vacuum cleaners, and barking dogs. They also noted severe intolerance to certain fabrics or foods. Bemporad (1976) interviewed a 31-year-old male who had been diagnosed by Kanner and found that he experienced a number of intense fears, including fear of children, dogs, and sudden noises.

*Ritualistic behavior* is another characteristic of autism. Just as individuals with obsessive-compulsive behaviors may become anxious when their ritual behaviors are interfered with, individuals with autism may experience great anxiety if their ritualistic behavior is interrupted or prevented (Rutter, 1985).

The incidence rate of *seizures* is higher in persons with autism. Deykin and MacMahon (1979) reported that the age-specific incidence rates of seizures were

3 to 28 times higher for children with autism than for children in the general population. Although occurrence of a seizure is a stressful event in itself, it may also be an indicator of stress or anxiety levels. Further research will be needed to investigate the relationship between anxiety and seizures for this population.

There are also external factors imposed on individuals with autism that add to stress. For example, the *special education or treatment* facility often has a high noise level due to the number of children who are disruptive or whose speech levels are unusually loud, which can be stressful to a person with autism.

The undesirable side effects of *punishment* are well documented in the literature, yet the use of aversives and punishment for persons with autism and other developmental disabilities has been widely accepted. These procedures include water squirts (Gross, Berler, & Drabman, 1982); gustatory aversives like tabasco sauce (Altmeyer, Williams, & Sams, 1985); time-out (Clark, Rowbury, Baer, & Baer, 1973; Calhoun & Matherne, 1975); electroshock (Ball, Sibbach, Jones, Steele, & Frazier, 1975; Birnbrauer, 1968; Foxx, McMorrow, Bittle, & Bechtel, 1986); and overcorrection (Foxx & Bechtel, 1982). Punishment procedures can produce signs of anxiety ranging from avoidance behavior to aggression (Azrin, Hutchinson, & Hake, 1963; Guess, Helmstetter, Turnbull, & Knowlton, 1987; Kazdin, 1975; Oliver, West & Sloane, 1974; Sulzer-Azaroff & Mayer, 1991).

## MALADAPTIVE BEHAVIORS AND THEIR RELATIONSHIP TO STRESS

Maladaptive behaviors (tantrum, aggression, self-injury, avoidance) exhibited by individuals with autism and developmental disabilities are frequently precipitated by stressful or anxiety-producing events and may in some cases serve to reduce the nervous system arousal typical of a stress reaction. In other words, these behaviors are used by the population with autism and developmental disabilities as alternatives to more effective buffers. We suggest that these behaviors, at least on some occasions, function as maladaptive coping strategies.

Because they are not always anxiety or stress related, it is important that clinicians conduct a functional analysis of a behavior in order to determine why an individual is exhibiting the problem behavior. Donnellan (Donnellan, Mirenda, Mesaros, & Fassbender, 1984) suggests that we analyze the communicative functions of aberrant behavior. Durand and Crimmins (1988) developed the Motivational Assessment Scale to help clinicians identify the function of a behavior. Their scale determines if the function of a behavior is to escape, or gain tangible reinforcement, social/attention, or stimulation. Iwata, Dorsey, Slifer, Bauman, and Richman (1982) have used functional analyses to identify the controlling variables of self-injurious behavior. Touchette, MacDonald, and Langer (1985) have used scatter plots to functionally analyze the maladaptive behavior exhibited by their clients. Future research utilizing functional analysis of behavior may indicate more clearly the relationship between the experience of stress and anxiety and the occurrence of maladaptive behavior.

*Self-injurious behavior (SIB)* occurs in only about 5% of psychiatric populations (Romanczyk, Colletti, & Plotkin, 1980). Schroeder, Schroeder, Smith, and Dalldorf (1978) found, however, that approximately 10% of the clients at a large state facility for persons with retardation exhibited this behavior. Most of those clients fulfilled the Rutter (1966) criteria for autism. The incidence rate of SIB was found to be even higher at a school for persons with autism. At the Groden Center, a treatment center for persons with autism, Groden, Berryman, and LeVasseur (1987) found that 49% of the clients exhibited some form of self-injury when they entered the program.

Several other investigators have linked the frequency of self-injurious behavior to the occurrence of painful or stress-producing conditions. While tracking the self-injurious behavior of a 10-year-old nonverbal child with autism, Groden (1984) found that the level of self-injury became extremely high immediately before the onset of painful middle ear infection (otitis media). DeLissovoy (1964) also found that there was a higher incidence of ear infection in a group of children who engaged in head-banging behavior than in a matched control group and concluded that head banging could be a form of escape from pain.

In another study (Carr, Newsom, & Binkoff, 1976), self-injurious behavior occurred at a high frequency in demand situations (a classroom, for example), and at a lower rate in low-demand conversational and free-play situations. These studies clearly suggest the possibility that self-injurious behavior is reinforced by the avoidance or termination of a stressful or aversive stimulus following an act of self-injury. It can be hypothesized, then, that self-injury is a distractor from pain, or that the pain of self-injury is less stressful because it is self-imposed, rather than externally controlled.

*Self-stimulatory behavior* also appears to be anxiety-related. Baumeister and Forehand (1973) demonstrated that stress, specifically frustration, can elicit self-stimulatory behavior in persons with mental retardation. Although individuals in the general population, as well as persons with special needs, exhibit self-stimulatory behaviors, Romanczyk, Colletti, and Plotkin (1980) found that self-stimulation in disturbed children is more intense, occurs more frequently, and presents different forms. They also found that self-stimulation may account for as much as 90% of the overt behavior displayed by severely retarded children.

Tantrums and aggression are frequently exhibited by persons with autism (Rutter, 1977). Upon entry at the Groden Center, 69% of the clients display tantrum behavior, and 74% display aggression (Groden, Berryman, & LeVasseur, 1987), generally during or immediately following stressful situations.

Future research is needed to substantiate the relationship between stress and anxiety and the occurrence of these behaviors. However, there is clearly a tendency for individuals with autism and developmental disabilities to respond to stressful or anxiety-producing situations with inappropriate behaviors rather than with effective coping mechanisms. Figure 1 depicts a flow chart that illustrates the chain of events that can result from adaptive versus maladaptive coping strategies.

In the adaptive model, the individual experiencing stress implements one of the buffer strategies in his or her repertoire, leading to decreased stress and/or increased effective coping behavior. The individual is likely to be positively reinforced by the results of his or her behavior, leading to a further reduction in stress. In contrast, the individual who exhibits the maladaptive model is disadvantaged in two ways: He or she cannot access the range of buffers available to the general populations, and he or she may possess the attributes of autism that cause him or her to be more prone to experiencing stress and anxiety. As a result of his or her inability to problem solve and/or reduce his or her level of stress, he or she engages in maladaptive coping behaviors that may include crying, yelling, self-stimulatory behavior, or more severe behaviors such as aggression and tantrums. These behaviors may also be functionally related to the stressor. For example, a child who is hungry, in pain, or just bored with the task at hand and who lacks the verbal skills to express such feelings may attempt to communicate

|  ADAPTIVE MODEL                  |  MALADATIVE MODEL                 |
| -------------------------------- | --------------------------------- |
| *(Exhibited by persons with good coping strategies)* | *(Exhibited by persons with poor coping strategies, especially by individuals with developmental disabilities)* |
| Stressors                        | Stressors                         |
| (promotion, death, separation,   | (taking criticism, changes,       |
| birth of a sibling, pain)        | inability to understand instruction, |
| ↓                                | external control)                 |
| Buffers                          | ↓                                 |
| (social networks, hardiness,     | Inability to Use Buffers          |
| internal locus of control        | (lack of friends, communication deficits, |
| ↓                                | lack of self-control)             |
| Adaptive Behaviors               | ↓                                 |
| (assertiveness, socializing,     | Maladaptive Behaviors             |
| exercise)                        | (aggression tantrum, self-injury, |
| ↓                                | stereotypic behaviors)            |
| Reinforcement                    | ↓                                 |
| ↓                                | Punishment                        |
| *Stress Reduction*               | ↓                                 |
|                                  | Increased Stress                  |

Fig. 1. Adaptive and maladaptive coping models.

through his or her aggressive, self-injurious, or tantrum behavior. Such behaviors, in turn, will frequently be punished, leading to an increase in stress, completing a loop of accumulating stress and anxiety.

## FOSTERING ADAPTIVE COPING STRATEGIES

Because stress and anxiety present many problems for individuals with autism and may often lead to other maladaptive behaviors, it is necessary for clinicians to identify procedures to reduce the amount of stress that persons with autism are exposed to, and to teach effective methods of coping with stress. The following is a synopsis of some of the strategies that can be employed to meet these goals.

### Social Skills Training

*Social skills training* is important for children and adults with autism. If one has acquired appropriate social skills, interaction with others is more positive and less anxiety-producing. A number of investigations have reported success with an ongoing social skills program for adolescents and adults with autism. Mesibov (1984) utilized individual sessions and group discussions, which include listening and talking, role playing, and appreciation of humor. McGee, Krantz, and McClannahan (1984) taught social skills in a more naturalistic setting, using two game situations for the assessment and training of positive and negative statements. Groden and Cautela (1987) demonstrated the efficacy of covert conditioning procedures in improving social skills in adolescents with autism. Carr and Durand (1985) have argued that teaching an individual appropriate, effective ways of communicating his or her needs may lead to the reduction or elimination of behaviors such as tantrums and aggression. For example, an individual who tears up her work when it is too difficult could be taught to ask her teacher for help. A specialized area of social skills training, assertiveness training, can help individuals with limited verbal skills learn to make appropriate verbal statements instead of using an inappropriate behavior to express their needs. A client who throws his work, for example, may learn to ask for a new task or a break.

### Increase of Positive Programs

In order to reduce maladaptive behaviors, LaVigna and Donnellan (1986) suggest that clinicians emphasize the use of positive programming procedures such as differential reinforcement of alternative behaviors, stimulus change, covert conditioning, and respondent conditioning procedures. As discussed above, although punishment produces signs of tension and anxiety, those procedures have been used extensively with this population.

Cautela (1984) also suggests increasing the general level of reinforcement by noncontingently increasing reinforcement. To help clinicians identify reinforcers for their clients, Cautela has developed a number of reinforcement survey schedules (Cautela, 1981).

## Self-Control

It is also important to teach individuals with special needs to *control their own behavior* and decrease dependence on external contingencies. Sulzer-Azaroff and Mayer (1991) contend that self-control procedures are very effective, and in addition they embody ethical and humanistic values.

## Relaxation

*Relaxation* procedures can improve self-management skills (Bruno-Golden, 1987) and have been used extensively to reduce anxiety-related problems in the general population, such as headaches (Benson, Klemchuk, & Graham, 1974); sleep disorders (Haynes, Woodward, Moran, & Alexander, 1974); test anxiety (Deffenbacher & Snyder, 1976; Russell & Sipich, 1973); speech anxiety (Gatchel, Hatch, Watson, Smith, & Gaas, 1977); and hypertension (Shoemaker & Tasto, 1975).

Relaxation has also been used effectively with persons with special needs. Clients with mental retardation have been treated for rat phobias (Peck, 1976), fear of adults (Matson, 1981a), fear of participating in community activities (Matson, 1981b), fear of riding in cars (Mansdorf, 1976), and acrophobia (Guralnick, 1973).

Cautela and Groden (1978) developed a relaxation program for persons with special needs. The program's goal is for clients to gain self-control by learning to make a relaxation response in place of the typical maladaptive behaviors he or she exhibits during stressful situations. The program has been used at the Groden Center for the past 10 years. Recent data indicate that 44% of the clients are able to relax when given a verbal cue by their teacher or therapist, and another 31% are able to use the procedure independently (Groden & Prince, 1988).

## Imagery and Cognitive-Based Procedures

*Imagery and cognitive-based procedures* also have been used extensively to reduce anxiety in the general population (Mavissakalian & Barlow, 1981), but clinicians have traditionally been reluctant to use them with individuals with low cognitive abilities.

Covert conditioning procedures (Cautela, 1970; Cautela, 1976; Cautela & Kearney, 1986) which rely heavily on imagery and other cognitive skills, have been adapted to the clients' low cognitive levels and used successfully at the Groden Center to treat a variety of problems, from poor social skills to tantrums and aggression in children and adults with mental retardation, autism, and severe behavior disorders (Groden, Berryman, & LeVasseur, 1987; Groden & Cautela, 1984; Groden, Cautela, & Groden, 1991). These investigators have found that imagery procedures can target specific or general situations that are stressful for a particular client and provide the individual with the opportunity to "practice" appropriate coping skills and behavior in that situation several times a day. Cognitive picture rehearsal, an adaptation in which clients look at photographs or simple drawings while the therapist/teacher describes the scene, was developed to help clients imagine the scenes more clearly. (Groden, Cautela, LeVasseur, Groden, & Bausman, 1993).

## Environmental Changes

Finally, there is agreement among clinicians and special educators that a child with autism or developmental disabilities learns best in a *structured environment* (Doherty & Swisher, 1978). Predictable, consistent routines may help reduce the stress and anxiety often experienced by individuals with autism who have a characteristic need to maintain sameness in their environments. The use of a concrete display of events in time, such as that provided by a picture schedule or sequence board is one strategy that can help the child with autism deal with changes in routine and may decrease the behavior problems arising from the child's confusion and resistance to change (Quinn & Beisler, 1986).

The preceding is only a partial list of the many procedures and strategies that can help individuals with autism and developmental disabilities cope effectively with stress and anxiety.

## CASE EXAMPLES

Three hypothetical case examples will be used as illustrations of the principles that have been advocated in this chapter.

> *Case 1.* Brad is 5 years old, unable to speak, but can use some picture communication cards. He has tantrum behavior whenever another child cries or is engaged in fighting or disruptive behavior. These are regarded as stress-

ful times for Brad. He is taught the relaxation response and practices it a few times a day. He is also taught to take a deep breath and relax whenever he hears another child crying or being disruptive. His teacher is taught to cue him to use relaxation at these times. He also has a picture imagery program in which he learns to continue his task or activity and ignore the behavior of other children. This is accomplished through a picture rehearsal program in the form of a storybook that he reviews a few times a day. The picture cards are used as cues when the situations occur in vivo.

*Case 2.* Mark, a person with autism, uses public transportation to get to his job each day. He reports that he gets especially anxious when he has to find a seat and that he worries frequently about losing his bus pass. He has a history of extreme violent responses when he gets anxious. Mark is taught the relaxation response and practices it while waiting for the bus. He is taught to find his seat by actually riding the bus and by role-playing practice with a staff member. He is also taught to carry enough money in case he loses his bus pass and to make a telephone call home in case he gets confused (alternative responses to violence). He practices these programs by role playing, by actually performing these behaviors in natural environments, and through listening and watching video- and audiotapes. He has learned to identify his own physiological reactions of stress (increased heart beat, increased stuttering, stereotypic rocking movements) and to use the relaxation response and assertiveness (e.g., asking for help) at these times.

*Case 3.* Jeremy is in a supported employment program. He has good verbal skills and holds a job in which he does office work such as filing, microfilming, and data entry. The job coach reported that he often loses his temper, talks in a loud voice, and exhibits stereotypic behaviors. When the job coach was instructed to do a behavioral analysis (Groden, 1989; O'Neill, Horner, Albin, Storey, & Sprague, 1990), he became aware that these behaviors occurred following the supervisor's corrective feedback, when he was asked to switch jobs, or if there was a change in the planned activity (e.g., lunch delay). Rather than removing him from the workplace or setting up consequence contingencies, we suggested that Jeremy's behavior was brought on by stress. Programs were instituted to reduce the stress induced by switching jobs, taking correction, and making schedule changes. Relaxation procedures were taught to Jeremy, and he was instructed to practice relaxation before beginning work (to reduce his general level of anxiety) and then to use the relaxation response when stressful events occurred. First the job coach would cue him when he recognized the antecedent situations (e.g., the supervisor correcting his work), and then Jeremy himself was taught to become aware of the antecedents and use relaxation as self control. In addition, Jeremy practiced scenes in imagery during therapeutic sessions outside of the workplace. In these sessions, he pictured the situations that were stressful, and he used the relaxation response. He might also learn to change his cognitions and say to himself, "Everyone makes errors; that's okay, I will do better next time." He also received social skills training with an emphasis on assertive responses. If, for example, he was asked to switch jobs, he might learn to say,

"Can I have an extra few minutes and then I will be ready to change?"

In each of these examples, the stress responses are being replaced with alternative, more adaptive responses. Problem behaviors are treated before they occur. A secondary effect occurs as a result of the job coach learning about the procedures. She learns to make more acute observations and intervene before the inappropriate situations occur, thus resulting in prevention of inappropriate behaviors.

## ADVANTAGES OF DESIGNING INTERVENTIONS TO REDUCE STRESS AND ANXIETY

There are many benefits to conceptualizing the many maladaptive behaviors of children and adults with special needs as being functionally related to the experience of stress. The advantages, which reach far beyond the pragmatic goal of reducing particular target behaviors, include, but are not limited to, the following:

- Individuals can learn to use adaptive coping mechanisms such as relaxation, imagery, and other self-control procedures when faced with stressful situations.
- As self-control is increased, dependence on external contingencies (e.g., contract or token systems, punishment) is reduced.
- As individuals learn to cope effectively with stress and reduce problem behaviors, independence, self-esteem, and personal dignity are enhanced.
- Effective transition to and maintenance in integrated community settings is facilitated as individuals learn to cope effectively with novel and stressful situations.

## IMPLICATIONS FOR FURTHER RESEARCH

The model presented in this chapter suggests several avenues for further inquiry:

- How can we develop and refine the means of measuring levels of stress and anxiety in the population with special needs? How useful are verbal reports and measures of physiological arousal and nonverbal behavior?
- What are the stressors involved in mainstreaming and integrating individuals with special needs? How do these stressors impact on the individuals we are serving?
- How can the stress-reduction techniques that have been successful with the nonhandicapped population be modified and adapted for the special needs population?

- To what extent can individuals with autism and developmental disabilities be taught to use self-control procedures to reduce stress and anxiety; that is, to what extent can the dependence on external contingencies be reduced?
- What is the effect of aversive procedures on stress and anxiety-related behaviors? Do punishment procedures produce or exacerbate behaviors related to stress and anxiety; that is, do they worsen the very conditions they are meant to alleviate?

## SUMMARY

In summary, we contend that individuals with autism and developmental disabilities do experience stress and anxiety at least as much as individuals in the general population. Further, one function of maladaptive behaviors, such as tantrums, aggression, and self-injury, is the reduction of stress and anxiety. The role of teachers and clinicians must include the design of interventions to teach adaptive coping strategies and reduce the effect of stress and anxiety. A focus on the reduction of stress and anxiety provides a rich framework for the analysis of problem behavior and research into effective interventions for a population that presents unique problems.

## REFERENCES

Altmeyer, B. K., Williams, D. E., & Sams, V. (1985). Treatment of severe self-injurious and aggressive biting. *Journal of Behavior Therapy and Experimental Psychiatry, 16*(2), 169–172.

American Psychiatric Association. (1987). *Diagnostic and statistical manual of mental disorders* (3rd ed., pp. 87–90). Washington, DC: Author.

Ascher, L. M. (1980). Paradoxical intention. In A. Goldstein & E. B. Foa (Eds.), *Handbook of behavioral interventions* (pp. 266–321). New York: Wiley.

Azrin, N. H., Hutchinson, R. R., & Hake, D. F. (1963). Pain-induced fighting in the squirrel monkey. *Journal of experimental analysis of behavior, 6,* 620.

Ball, T. S., Sibbach, L., Jones, R., Steele, B., & Frazier, L. (1975). An accelerometer-activated device to control assaultive and self-destructive behaviors in retardates. *Journal of Behavior Therapy and Experimental Psychiatry, 6,* 223–228.

Baumeister, A., & Forehand, R. (1973). Stereotyped acts. In N. R. Ellis (Ed.), *International review of research in mental retardation* (Vol. 6, pp. 55–96). New York: Academic.

Bemporad, J. R. (1976). Adult recollections of a formerly autistic child. *Journal of Autism and Developmental Disorders, 9,* 179–197.

Benson, H. (1975). *The relaxation response.* New York: Morrow.

Benson, H. (1984). *Beyond the relaxation response.* New York: Times Books.

Benson, H., Klemchuk, H. P., & Graham, J. R. (1974). The usefulness of the relaxation response in the therapy of headache. *Headache, 14,* 49–52.

Benson, H., & Proctor, W. (1987). *Your maximum mind.* New York: Random House.

Bernstein, D. S., & Borkovec, T. D. (1973). *Progressive relaxation training.* Champaign, IL: Research Press.

Birnbrauer, J. S. (1968). Generalization of punishment effects—A case study. *Journal of Applied Behavior Analysis, 1,* 201–211.

Bruno-Golden, B. (1987). Theoretical considerations and applications of relaxation training for children. *Journal of the Royal Society of Health, 107,* 51–54.

Calhoun, K. S., & Matherne, P. (1975). The effects of varying schedules of time-out on aggressive behavior of a retarded girl. *Journal of Behavior Therapy and Experimental Psychiatry, 6,* 139–143.

Carr, E. G., & Durand, V. M. (1985). Reducing behavior problems through functional communication training. *Journal of Applied Behavior Analysis, 18,* 111–126.

Carr, E. G., Newsom, C. D., & Binkoff, J. A. (1976). Stimulus control of self-destructive behavior in a psychotic child. *Journal of Abnormal Child Psychology, 4,* 139–153.

Cautela, J. R. (1970). Covert reinforcement. *Behavior Therapy, 1,* 33–50.

Cautela, J. R. (1976). The present status of covert modeling. *Journal of Behavior Therapy and Experimental Psychiatry, 7,* 323–326.

Cautela, J. R. (1981). *Behavior analysis forms for clinical intervention* (Vol. 2). Champaign, IL: Research Press.

Cautela, J. R. (1984). General level of reinforcement. *Journal of Behavior Therapy and Experimental Psychiatry, 15,* 109–114.

Cautela, J. R., & Groden, J. (1978). *Relaxation: A comprehensive manual for adults, children, and children with special needs.* Champaign, IL: Research Press.

Cautela, J. R., & Kearney, A. J. (1986). *The covert conditioning handbook.* New York: Springer-Verlag.

Cautela, J. R., & Kearney, A. J., (Eds.). (1993) *The Covert Conditioning Casebook.* Pacific Grove, CA: Brooks/Cole.

Clark, H. B., Rowbury, T., Baer, A. M., & Baer, D. M. (1973). Time out as punishing stimulus in continuous and intermittent schedules. *Journal of Applied Behavior Analysis, 6,* 443–455.

Clark, P., & Rutter, M. (1979). Task difficulty and task performance in autistic children. *Journal of Child Psychology and Psychiatry, 20,* 271–285.

Deffenbacher, J. L., & Snyder, A. L. (1976). Relaxation as self-control in the treatment of test and other anxieties. *Psychological Reports, 39*(2), 379–385.

DeLissovoy, V. (1964). Head banging in early childhood: Review of empirical studies. *Pediatrics Digest, 6,* 49–55.

Deykin, E. Y., & MacMahon, B. (1979). The incidence of seizures among children with autistic symptoms. *American Journal of Psychiatry, 136,* 1310–1312.

Doherty, L., & Swisher, L. (1978). Children with autistic behaviors. In F. D. Minifie & L. L. Lloyd (Eds.), *Communicative and cognitive abilities: Early behavioral assessment* (pp. 549–563). Baltimore: University Park.

Dohrenwend, B., & Dohrenwend, B. (1974). *Stressful life events: Their nature and effects.* New York: Wiley.

Donnellan, A. M., Mirenda, P. L., Mesaros, R. A., & Fassbender, L. L. (1984). Analyzing the communicative functions of aberrant behavior. *The Journal of the Association for Persons with Severe Handicaps, 9*(3), 201–212.

Durand, V. M., & Crimmins, D. B. (1988). Identifying the variables maintaining self-injurious behavior. *Journal of Autism and Developmental Disorders, 18*(1), 99–117.

Finch, A. J., Jr., Montgomery, L. E., Kendall, P. C., & Morris, T. (1975). Effects of types of failure on anxiety. *Journal of Abnormal Psychology, 84*(5), 583–585.

Fish, B., Shapiro, T., & Campbell, M. (1966). Long-term prognosis and the response of schizophrenic children to drug therapy: A controlled study of trifluroperazine. *American Journal of Psychiatry, 123,* 32–39.

Foxx, R. M. & Bechtel, D. R. (1982). Overcorrection. In M. Hersen & R. M. Eisler (Eds.), *Progress in Behavior Modification* (Vol. 13, pp. 227–288). New York: Academic.

Foxx, R. M., McMorrow, M. J., Bittle, R. G., & Bechtel, D. R. (1986). The successful treatment of a dually-diagnosed deaf man's aggression with a program that included contingent electric shock. *Behavior Therapy, 17,* 170–186.

Gatchel, R. J., Hatch, J. P., Watson, P. J., Smith, D., & Gaas, E. (1977). Comparative effectiveness of voluntary heart-rate control and muscular relaxation as active coping skills for reducing speech anxiety. *Journal of Consulting* & Clinical Psychology, 45(6), 1093–1100.

Grandin, T., & Scariano, M. M. (1986). *Emergence: Labeled autistic.* Novato, CA: Arena.

Groden, G. (1989). A guide for conducting a comprehensive behavioral analysis of a target behavior. *Journal of Behavior Therapy and Experimental Psychiatry, 20*(2), 163–169.

Groden, J. (1984). *Self-injurious behavior.* Paper presented at the New England Society for Behavior Analysis and Therapy, Boston, MA.

Groden, J., Berryman, J., & LeVasseur, P. (1987). *Relaxation as a treatment for stress and anxiety for children with special needs.* Paper presented at the Third Annual Conference on Behavior Disorders, Warwick, RI.

Groden, J., & Cautela, J. R. (1984). Use of imagery procedures with students labeled "trainable retarded." *Psychological Reports, 54,* 595–605.

Groden, J., & Cautela, J. R. (1987). *Procedures to increase social interaction among adolescents with autism: A multiple baseline analysis.* Unpublished manuscript, The Groden Center, Inc., Providence, RI.

Groden, J., Cautela, J. R., & Groden, G. (1989). *Breaking the Barriers: Relaxation procedures for people with special needs* (Video). Champaign, IL: Research Press.

Groden, J., Cautela, J. R., & Groden, G. (1991). *Breaking the Barriers II: Imagery Procedures for People with Special Needs* (Video). Champaign, IL: Research Press.

Groden, J., Cautela, J. R., LeVasseur, P., Groden, G., & Bausman, M. (1993). *Video Guide to Breaking the Barriers II.* Champaign, IL: Research Press.

Groden, J., & Prince, S. (1988). *The acquisition of relaxation skills by children and youth with developmental disabilities.* Paper presented at the Association for the Advancement of Behavior Therapy, New York, NY.

Gross, A. M., Berler, E. S., & Drabman, R. S. (1982). Reduction of aggressive behavior in a retarded boy using a water squirt. *Journal of Behavior Therapy and Experimental Psychiatry, 13,* 95–98.

Guess, D., Helmstetter, E., Turnbull, R. E., & Knowlton, S. (1987). *Use of aversive procedures with individuals who are disabled: A historical review and critical analysis.* Seattle, WA: Association for Persons with Severe Handicaps.

Guralnick, M. J. (1973). Behavior therapy with an acrophobic mentally retarded young adult. *Journal of Behavioral Therapy and Experimental Psychiatry, 4,* 263–265.

Haynes, S., Woodward, S., Moran, R., & Alexander, D. (1974). Relaxation treatment of insomnia. *Behavior Therapy, 5,* 555–558.

Hobson, R. P. (1986). The autistic child's appraisal of expressions and emotion. *Journal of Child Psychology and Psychiatry, 27*(3), 321–342.

Iwata, B. A., Dorsey, M. F., Slifer, K. J., Bauman, K. E., & Richman, G. S. (1982). Toward a functional analysis of self-injury. *Analysis and Intervention in Developmental Disabilities, 2,* 3–20.

Jacobson, E. (1973). *Teaching and learning, new methods for old arts.* Chicago: National Foundation for Progressive Relaxation.

Kanner, L. (1943). Autistic disturbance of affective contact. *Nervous Child, 2,* 217–250.

Kazdin, A. E. (1975). *Behavior modification in applied settings* (pp. 146–151). Homewood, IL: Dorsey.

LaVigna, G. W., & Donnellan, A. M. (1986). *Alternatives to punishment: Solving behavior problems with non-aversive strategies.* New York: Irvington.

Levine, H. G., & Langness, L. L. (1983). Context, ability, and performance: Comparison of competitive athletics among mildly retarded and nonretarded adults. *American Journal of Mental Deficiency, 87,* 528–538.

Lovaas, O. L., Schreibman, L., Koegel, R. L., & Reim, R. (1971). Selective responding by autistic children to multiple sensory input. *Journal of Abnormal Psychology, 77,* 211–222.

Mansdorf, I. J. (1976). Eliminating fear in a mentally retarded adult by behavioral hierarchies and operant techniques. *Journal of Behavioral Therapy and Experimental Psychiatry, 7,* 189–190.

Matson, J. L. (1981a). Assessment and treatment of clinical fears in mentally retarded children. *Journal of Applied Behavioral Analysis, 14,* 287–294.

Matson, J. L. (1981b). A controlled outcome study of phobias in mentally retarded adults. *Behavior Research and Therapy, 19,* 101–107.

Mavissakalian, M., & Barlow, D. H. (1981). *Phobia: Psychological and pharmacological treatment.* New York: Guilford.

McGee, G. G., Krantz, P. J., & McClannahan, L. E. (1984). Conversational skills for autistic adolescents: Teaching assertiveness in naturalistic game settings. *Journal of Autism and Developmental Disorders, 14*(3), 319–330.

McQuade, W., & Aikman, A. (1974). *Stress: What it is, what it can do to your health, how to fight back.* New York: Dutton.

Mesibov, G. B. (1984). Social skills training with verbal autistic adolescents and adults: A program model. *Journal of Autism and Developmental Disorders, 14*(4), 395–404.

Oliver, S. D., West, R. C., & Sloane, H. N., Jr. (1974). Some effects on human behavior on aversive events. *Behavior Therapy, 5,* 481–493.

O'Neill, R. E., Horner, R. H., Albin, R. W., Storey, K., & Sprague, J. R. (1990). *Functional analysis of problem behavior: A practical assessment guide.* Sycamore, IL: Sycamore Publishing.

Ornitz, E. M., & Ritvo, E. R. (1985). Perceptual inconstancy in early infantile autism. In A. M. Donnellan (Ed.), *Classic readings in autism* (pp. 142–178). New York: Teachers College Press.

Peck, C. I. (1976). Desensitization for the treatment of fear in the high level adult retardate. *Behavior in Research and Therapy, 15,* 137–148.

Quinn, K., & Beisler, J. (1986). *A curriculum for educating autistic students: A working draft.* Unpublished manuscript, Iowa Department of Public Instruction.

Romanczyk, R. G., Colletti, G., & Plotkin, R. (1980). Punishment of self-injurious behavior: Issues of behavior analysis, generalization, and the right to treatment. *Child Behavior Therapy, 2*(1), 37–54.

Russell, R. K., & Sipich, J. F. (1973). Cue-controlled relaxation in the treatment of test anxiety. *Journal of Behavior Therapy and Experimental Psychiatry, 4,* 47–49.

Rutter, M. (1966). Behavioral and cognitive characteristics of a series of psychotic children. In. J. K. Wing (Ed.), *Early childhood autism: Clinical, educational and social aspects* (pp. 51–81). London: Pergamon.

Rutter, M. (1977). Infantile autism and other child psychoses. In M. Rutter & L. Hersov (Ed.), *Child psychiatry: Modern approaches* (pp. 717–747). Oxford: Blackwell.

Rutter, M. (1978). Diagnosis and definition. In M. Rutter & E. Schopler (Eds.), *Autism: A reappraisal of concepts and treatment* (pp. 1–25). New York: Plenum.

Rutter, M. (1985). The treatment of autistic children. *Journal of Psychology and Psychiatry, 26*(2), 193–214.

Schroeder, S. R., Schroeder, C. S., Smith, B., & Dalldorf, J. (1978). Prevalence of self-injurious behaviors in a large state facility for the retarded: A three year follow-up study. *Journal of Autism and Childhood Schizophrenia, 8,* 261–269.

Selye, H. (1974). *Stress without distress*. Philadelphia: Lippincott.

Shoemaker, J., & Tasto, D. (1975). Effects of muscle relaxation on blood pressure of essential hypertensives. *Behavior Research and Therapy, 13,* 29–43.

Sulzer-Azaroff, B., & Mayer, G. R. (1991). *Behavior analysis for lasting change*. Fort Worth, TX: Holt, Rinehart & Winston.

Surwit, R., Williams, R., Jr., & Shapiro, Do. (1982). *Behavioral approaches to cardiovascular disease*. New York: Academic.

Touchette, P. E., MacDonald, R. F., & Langer, S. N. (1985). A scatter plot for identifying stimulus control of problem behavior. *Journal of Applied Behavior Analysis, 18,* 343–351.

Volkmar, F. R., & Cohen, D. J. (1985). The experience of infantile autism: A first person account by Tony W. *Journal of Autism and Developmental Disabilities, 15,* 47–54.

Wolff, S., & Chess, S. (1965). An analysis of the language of fourteen schizophrenic children. *Journal of Psychology and Psychiatry, 6,* 29–41.

Wolpe, J. (1958). *Psychotherapy by reciprocal inhibition*. Stanford: Stanford University Press.

Wolpe, J. (1990). *Practice of behavior therapy* (4th ed.). New York: Pergamon.

Young. J. G., Kavanaugh, M. E., Anderson, G. M., Shaywitz, B. A., & Cohen, D. J. (1982). Clinical neurochemistry of autism and associated disorders. *Journal of Autism and Developmental Disorders, 12,* 147–165.

Zetlin, A. G., & Turner, J. L. (1985). Transition from adolescence to adulthood: Perspectives of mentally retarded individuals and their families. *American Journal of Mental Deficiency, 89,* 570–579.

# 10

# Structured Teaching

## GARY B. MESIBOV, ERIC SCHOPLER, and KATHLEEN A. HEARSEY

## INTRODUCTION

Follow-up studies have consistently demonstrated that structured special educa-tional programs result in the most positive outcomes for youngsters with autism (Lockyer & Rutter, 1969; Rutter, Greenfeld, & Lockyer, 1967; Schopler, Mesibov, DeVellis, & Short, 1981). Although there are undoubtedly many reasons for this, one of the main explanations is that these special education programs are the only ones to provide the kind and amount of clarity and predictability that these children need to enhance their development (Bartak, 1978; Bartak & Rutter, 1973; Schopler, Brehm, Kinsbourne, & Reichler, 1971). Providing structure for children with autism helps them to organize themselves and respond more appropriately to their environments. Advantageous to most of us, structure is essential to the functioning of autistic children because of their deficits in organization and their inability to understand or successfully control their behavior without assistance, direction, and support.

The use of structured teaching as an intervention strategy has been central to the TEACCH Program since its inception in the middle 1960s. This chapter describes how structure is used and implemented in TEACCH-affiliated programs for children with autism and related communication handicaps. Physical organiza-tion, schedules, individual work systems, visual structure, and routines are specific

GARY B. MESIBOV, ERIC SCHOPLER, and KATHLEEN A. HEARSEY • Division TEACCH, School of Medicine, The University of North Carolina at Chapel Hill, Chapel Hill, North Carolina 27599-7180.

*Behavioral Issues in Autism*, edited by Eric Schopler and Gary B. Mesibov. New York, Plenum Press, 1994.

aspects of structure that have proven useful in classrooms for students with autism of all ages and levels of functioning. Structured teaching is the main approach at Division TEACCH for developing skills and minimizing behavioral difficulties.

## PHYSICAL ORGANIZATION

### Physical Layout

The physical layout of the classroom is important for students with autism. The use of consistent, visually clear areas and boundaries for specific activities enables students to better understand their environments and relationships between events. Teachers should consider the goals of their classrooms carefully and then designate a specific area for each major activity. The basic curriculum areas plus the needs of individual children with autism will be the major determinants of the classroom's physical structure.

Children with autism have difficulty differentiating between dissimilar events and seeing how distinct activities relate to one another. A clearly organized classroom highlights the specific activities and reinforces the important concepts. For example, if a visually clear location in the classroom is always used for individual work, a child will know what is expected when sent to that spot and can better understand the relationship between work and play if successful completion of an individual work activity is typically followed by play in a visually distinctive play area.

The physical layout of the classroom also can help students with autism by focusing their attention on the most relevant aspects of their tasks. Students with autism are often distracted by sights or sounds, making it difficult for them to identify or attend to relevant cues. Blocking out as many extraneous sights and sounds as possible can help them focus on the most relevant dimensions of their activities. Dividers minimize visual and auditory distractions. Bookshelves, window shades, the distribution of work areas around the classroom, and minimal use of decorations on the walls near individual work areas are other ways to minimize distractions.

### Selecting Work Areas

The natural setting must be considered when determining areas in a classroom. For example, work areas should not be placed near distracting mirrors or windows. If unavoidable, blinds or cardboard taped to the windows can eliminate the distractions. It is beneficial to have work areas near shelves or storage cabinets so that work materials are easily accessible. Built-in cabinets make ideal work area boundaries for this reason. Blank walls are also good locations for work areas. Facing students' tables or desks toward blank walls eliminates many distractions and helps students with autism to focus their attention on the relevant dimensions of their work activities. Places in the classroom where students spend independent time, such as play or leisure time, are best located away from exits so that students will not run away.

There are many considerations in arranging the work areas in a classroom. Although no physical space is perfect and most undesirable features can be modified, there are a few situations that might necessitate changing classrooms. A classroom with multiple exits (especially one to the outside) is undesirable for a student who is a runner. A classroom for intermediate students should not be located on a kindergarten hall. This situation decreases appropriate peer socialization opportunities and underscores the handicaps of the bigger, and obviously older, students. A classroom that is too small or one without adequate storage space is cluttered and uncomfortable, making it feel as if everyone is working on top of one another. This situation also makes it difficult for students to identify visual boundaries. Another high priority is the bathroom location. Toilet training lower-functioning students will be futile if there is a long distance between their classroom and the toilet. Even if students have independent bathroom skills, valuable classroom time should not be wasted walking to and from the bathroom if more convenient arrangements are possible.

Appropriate classroom work areas vary depending on the ages of the children in a class. For younger students, the pertinent learning areas are generally play, individual and independent work, snack, and self-help skills. There also might be a group area and a place for teaching prevocational skills. For older students, other areas, similar to those for younger children but emphasizing the unique needs of this group, should be established. These might include a leisure area, a workshop area, a domestic skills area, a self-help and grooming area, and a place for each student's independence training. Both younger and older students usually benefit from a transition area, a location in the classroom where all of the schedules are placed. Students go to the transition area to learn what the next activity will be. Transition areas are a concrete way of introducing consistency into the many changes that occur during the schoolday. All classrooms should also have places, such as cubbyholes, lockers, or special boxes, for students to put their personal belongings. The teacher's desk and work areas should be another separate place in the classroom.

## Boundaries and Needs of Students

Once the classroom and specific activity areas are selected, there are many ways to make visually clear boundaries: rugs, bookshelves, partitions, tape on the floor, and the arrangement of the furniture. For example, the carpeted section of the classroom often makes a pleasant leisure area. The workshop area may be outlined by shelves filled with materials and long work tables. A small throwrug can be placed in front of the sink to show students where to stand while washing their hands or the dishes.

In planning the physical structure of the classroom, it is also important to consider the unique needs of each individual student. For example, one work table might be opposite a blank wall with pieces of tape on the floor indicating where the chair is to be placed while the student is working. Another work area might be partitioned on two sides with dividers. A workshop area could be organized to meet the needs of several different students in a classroom; two sides of the workshop area could have shelves with materials for students who can obtain their own work independently, and the middle of the area could have a table and chair for those students who have mastered basic work skills and are now learning to work despite distractions. The amount of structure needed by each student is determined individually. As students learn to function more independently, the amount of physical structure used for them is tapered.

## SCHEDULES

Schedules are another essential part of classroom structure. By explaining to each student which activities will occur during the day and in what sequence, schedules—like the physical structure of the classroom—help students with autism to understand differences between discrete events and their relationships to one another. Schedules also help students anticipate and predict activities. Developing visually clear schedules for students that each understands at his or her own level of ability allows a teacher to communicate which discrete events will occur during the schoolday, when they can be expected to occur, and how they are related to one another (e.g., first work and then play).

Visually clear schedules assist students with autism for several reasons: (1) Many of these students have problems with sequential memory and the organization of time. (2) Receptive language difficulties make it hard for them to understand what they should be doing when given only oral directions. (3) Attentional problems are not as handicapping when information is presented visually because schedules provide a continuous opportunity for students to see what their activities will be.

Schedules help students to predict both daily and weekly events. This additional predictability diminishes their anxiety from not knowing what to expect and frustration from not knowing when a preferred activity will be available again. Problems with transitions that frequently plague students with autism also improve when meaningful schedules are used to enable students to anticipate upcoming activities. Schedules also can motivate some students to complete difficult or dreaded tasks because they can see on their schedules that more enjoyable activities will follow.

There are two types of schedules used simultaneously in TEACCH classrooms: the general classroom schedule and the individual student schedules. The overall classroom schedule outlines the day for the entire class. It does not indicate specific work activities for individual students but does show general work times, break times, and so forth. Table 1 is an example of a typical schedule for an intermediate age classroom.

This schedule shows when students are working and when they are engaged in other projects. Work times involve many different pursuits such as independent prevocational work, individual training on self-help skills, domestic chores, or jobs around the school. These specific activities are listed on the individual student schedules. The general classroom schedule is relatively consistent from week to week except when field trips, special events, or community training programs require adjustments.

The general classroom schedule is usually posted for everyone to see and use. It is often reviewed when students arrive in the morning or during a morning group session. The format may be written, as in Table 1, but some students might not comprehend a written schedule. For these students the same schedule might be illustrated with pictures or drawings representing each activity. For example, a picture of a desk or table might depict a work session. Such picture schedules can be arranged from top to bottom or from left to right on a large posterboard.

Individual schedules help students understand what to do during the activities listed on the general schedule. Individual schedules range from those created and administered by the teacher to those made up and followed by the students themselves. Irrespective of who generates them, however, the most important

Table 1. Typical Schedule for
Intermediate Age Classroom

| | |
|---|---|
| 8:30 | Student arrival, putting belongings away, greetings |
| 8:45 | Work session 1 |
| 9:30 | Work session 2 |
| 10:15 | Break |
| 10:30 | Leisure learning and school friends |
| 11:00 | Work session 3 |
| 11:45 | Prepare for lunch |
| 12:00 | Lunch |
| 12:30 | Outside or gym |
| 1:00 | Clean cafeteria tables and floors |
| 1:45 | Work session 4 |
| 2:30 | Dismissal |

aspect of these individual schedules is that they are meaningful to the students using them.

There are many ways to develop schedules so that each student, irrespective of cognitive ability, can understand what is represented. For some students who do not read, pictures can be used. For those students who cannot understand pictures, colors, numbers, or objects can be used to represent activities on their daily schedules. Some schedules require two or three activities to be completed within a time period, whereas others require only one completed activity before a break or reinforcement. Each individual schedule also needs balance, alternating desirable with less enjoyable student activities and physically demanding with less active pursuits.

As students begin to comprehend and use schedules, they learn how to follow directions and develop independence skills, both of which are necessary for successful functioning in adult community placements. Schedules also help them to predict and, in some small way, control their environments. Appropriate, individualized schedules are an important aspect of classroom structure that can have a substantial positive effect on the students in a program.

## INDIVIDUAL WORK SYSTEMS

Whereas a schedule tells each student the sequence of events during the day, a work system informs students of what they should do while in their independent work areas. The work system is central if students are to learn how to work independently of supervision. Work systems help students to know what is expected of them on their work activities, to organize themselves systematically, and to understand how to complete their tasks.

Individual work systems communicate four pieces of information to students: (1) what work they are supposed to do, (2) how much work there is, (3) how they will know when they have finished, and (4) what happens after the work is completed. Effective work systems are presented visually on a level that each child can understand. For example, a verbal, higher-functioning child might have a written work system with each task clearly labeled making it easy to locate. In the basket along with each task would be written instructions explaining the activity and its requirements. The verbal student would know what work to do by what was written on the work system corresponding to the label on one of the baskets in the work area. How much work would be determined by the number of items written on the child's work system for that particular time period. The child would know that the task was completed when all of the written directions had been carried out. There also should be a written explanation of what would happen after the task was completed.

Work systems can be developed for students at all levels of functioning.

Pictures, symbols, and numbers can communicate the same information to lower functioning students that words communicate to higher functioning ones. The visual structure of the tasks also can be helpful; visually clear tasks with a finite number of materials and distinct end points clarify what is expected and provide information on how they should be completed.

A work system for a lower functioning student might use pictures, symbols, colors, numbers, or objects. A child at this level might have a work system consisting of three circles of different colors going from top to bottom. Each circle would correspond to a circle on a box containing a visually clear task. The child would know what task to do by matching the color on the work system to a box with the same colored circle. The child would know how much work had to be done by the number of colored circles from top to bottom. If there were three circles, that would mean that there are three tasks to complete during the work session. The child would know that the work was completed when all three of the circles had been removed from the work system. Each circle would be removed as the child completed the work in the box with the corresponding colored circle. The consequence for the child after successfully completing the task might be represented by a picture at the bottom of the work system. It could be a picture of a computer indicating a computer game or of the art area indicating that the child was free to draw a picture.

Work systems make the concept of *finished* concrete and meaningful. This is an important advantage for students with autism. Not understanding the concept of *finished* makes working in a classroom laborious and tedious. Knowing how much work one has to complete and having a sense of how and when it will be accomplished can mean the difference between a child's working steadily or not at all.

## VISUAL STRUCTURE

Because students with autism have so much difficulty with communication, they do their best work when tasks are presented to them visually. Visual structure is therefore an important aspect of their tasks that can be achieved in a variety of ways such as visual clarity, visual organization, and visual instructions.

## Visual Clarity

Tasks with visually distinctive materials and patterns help students with autism identify the most important features of their materials. A sorting task can have visually clear shapes or colors that are especially interesting and attractive to the student working on it. If a table is to be cleaned, scattering extra dirt or crumbs makes it easier to understand the purpose of the chore by magnifying the difference between clean and dirty.

Visually clear tasks and materials help students with autism to learn effectively and function independently. What is visual is concrete and therefore easier for these youngsters to learn and understand. Visually clear materials are also more appropriate for the attention spans of students with autism because they allow latitude for when the students attend. If an assignment is presented verbally, a student with autism has to be listening to the relevant information at the precise moment when it is presented. With visual materials, students can look at them when they are ready because the materials remain available for as long as they are in their work areas.

Visual cues can also be a helpful way to label parts of the classroom that are important for students with autism to identify. Color coding the students' individual materials is a nice way of highlighting where their work areas are, what towels they should use, and where they should sit during a snack. Using name cards is another good way of identifying where activities occur for those students who can read. Strategic parts of the classroom can also be labeled with words if these are meaningful to the students in the class.

## Visual Organization

Visually organizing materials also facilitates learning in students with autism. A common problem among these students is an inability to modulate incoming stimuli. Students with autism are overwhelmed easily by sensory input, lacking the ability to control, simplify, or otherwise organize what is perceived through their senses. Visually organizing materials for them can help these students to process information more efficiently. For example, on a sorting task most students with autism perform more effectively when the materials are organized for them in small plastic cups, rather than spread out on a table in a big pile. Organizing materials into containers makes them easier for these students to manage and work with.

Another example of visual organization is helping students to modulate visual space on a domestic task like cleaning windows. If the windows are large, students with autism are often immobilized, unable to decide where or how to begin. Dividing the window into four visually distinct square sections makes the space smaller and more manageable. This subtle but important way of providing visual assistance often makes it possible for students with autism to complete tasks that were previously too complex.

## Visual Instructions

Visual instructions are helpful additions to work tasks. The most common example is a jig, which is a visual representation of how a task is to be carried out or where vital materials are to be placed. Jigs are helpful to students with autism because they provide instructions in the way that is easiest for them to understand. Jigs clarify task requirements, sequences, relevant concepts, and other important instructions. They are an essential tool for teaching students with autism to function in community-based settings without direct adult supervision.

An important advantage of jigs is that they are a mechanism for teaching students with autism to look for instructions, rather than following their general tendency to complete a task the way they think it should be. Following instructions is an essential skill for a student with autism because it allows the flexibility to respond to the inevitable changes that occur in community-based vocational settings. Capitalizing on their visual strengths by offering students with autism an unambiguous way of understanding our directions, jigs and other visual directions are powerful instructional devices that can be transferred to community-based settings and used by people with autism throughout their lives.

## ROUTINES

A final form of structure that is important for students with autism is routines. Routines are systematic and consistent ways of carrying out specific tasks. Struggling to understand what situations require and not organizing themselves easily or effectively, students with autism benefit from systematic routines. It is important that these routines be consistent enough to compensate for the students' problem-solving deficiencies but flexible enough to be useful in a variety of situations.

The first routine taught to these youngsters is a basic one of "first work and then play." This teaches them that their actions affect their environments and have consequences in their lives. "First-work-and-then-play" routines are useful in classrooms, in the workplace, and in most residential environments. Familiarity with this routine can be beneficial for students with autism.

"Left-to-right" and "top-to-bottom" are other routines that have long-lasting and far-reaching consequences. Students with autism are frequently immobilized when confronting new tasks with unfamiliar demands. Learning to approach all assignments in a left-to-right, top-to-bottom sequence gives them a systematic approach applicable to a multitude of tasks such as collating, washing dishes, mopping floors, sorting, reading, or writing.

Most children with autism develop stereotypical ways of approaching certain tasks. These can be amazingly steadfast though not necessarily productive. A child's need to touch each window five times before entering a school bus is a typical example of this. Because students with autism develop and follow routines in many of their activities, it is useful to redirect this tendency toward productive activities. By proactively developing productive and flexible routines for students with autism in important situations, their routines can be changed from distracting liabilities to valuable assets. Checking their schedules and following the directions from their work system are two routines that are especially important for effective community-based functioning.

## TEACHING METHODS

Other applicants of structure are the instructional techniques used by teachers. Providing directions for tasks, offering prompts, and delivering reinforcers are ways that teachers organize and structure the classroom experiences of their students.

### Directions

Directions explaining to students how to complete their tasks can be offered either verbally or nonverbally. In either case, the directions should be made easy to understand by individualizing them to each student's level of functioning. For verbal directions, this means using minimal language. By telegraphing their language, teachers help their students identify the most relevant parts of their instructions. For example, stating, "I want you to finish putting all these nuts and bolts together, and then, when you finish, you can go over to the play area and choose a toy to play with," boosts the chances a student will be confused. One could say as easily, "First finish nuts and bolts, then play." This telegraphic statement is more likely to be understood by a student with autism.

Directions can also be given nonverbally with contextual and visual cues. Ways of systematically presenting and positioning materials, using jigs, and providing meaningful written instructions have already been described and discussed. Providing only the materials that students will need for specific tasks will highlight the relevant materials for the students and also help their independent functioning. For example, having a glass cleaner, sink cleanser, toilet-bowl cleaner, and sponges sitting in a bathroom that is to be cleaned highlights what tasks should be done by the materials being used.

## Prompts

Teacher prompts can be helpful when teaching students new tasks. Students with autism learn more effectively when they accurately complete a task because successful task completion shows them precisely what to do and how to do it. Different types of prompts can be useful for students with autism. Physical prompts are used to guide student actions toward the completion of a task. For example, the teacher might assist a child in pulling up her pants after using the bathroom. A verbal prompt might remind a child with language to put a napkin on his or her lunch tray. Visual prompts, another way of assisting students with autism, take several different forms: the jigs and written directions mentioned earlier; color cards that students match to work boxes when retrieving their own work; or the words *PEANUT BUTTER* written in extra large letters to bring a student's attention to a jar.

Accompanying verbal directions with gestures as prompts often increases students' understanding. A teacher might point to the nuts and bolts from a work task and then to the play area while giving the directions "first work and then play." Before prompting a student with autism, it is important to have the student's attention. This does not mean that eye contact has to be established. Some students signal their attention by body orientation, a verbal response, or by stopping other activities. Teachers should be aware of how their students signal their attention and be sure they have captured it before delivering their prompts.

Prompts also can be gestural. For example, instead of telling the student to get a napkin, the teacher points to the napkin holder or to the empty space on the student's lunch tray. Modeling or demonstrating how something is done is another type of prompt. Prompts can be situational, too, such as the teacher saying, "Hi," to a visitor, which is a prompt to greet someone.

Teachers should be systematic in their use of prompts. If prompts are not offered clearly and consistently before a student responds incorrectly, they will be ineffective. For example, if a student is having difficulty adding the correct amount of detergent while washing dishes, the teacher must deliver the prompt before an error is made.

Teachers also must be conscious that they might be prompting their students unintentionally. In these situations, teacher and student positioning in the learning areas of the classroom can be crucial. Correct responses are frequently relayed to students by the slightest movement of the head or eyes of the teacher. Some students, generally referred to as prompt-dependent, will repeatedly glance at their teacher after each step of a task for validation and reassurance. While working with these students, teachers should position themselves beside or behind the students instead of in front of them. Thoughtful positioning minimizes the number of unintended prompts and cues.

## Reinforcers

Reinforcers are another way of structuring tasks for students with autism. Most of us are motivated to work because of a combination of praise from others, intrinsic satisfaction, and remuneration. Students with autism are generally not highly motivated by any of these. Teachers must discover what is motivating for their students and then teach them to work for these incentives. For example, if a teacher learns that a student is fascinated by sandpaper, that student's work times can be arranged so that sandpaper can be used in the workshop area after work is completed. For this student, the sandpaper is a meaningful and more motivating reward than the motivators traditionally used with nonhandicapped students.

Reinforcers can include many different items or activities. Some students are motivated by food or toys that they especially like; others are motivated by preferred activities. Some students are able to earn money or tokens throughout the day and trade them for reinforcers later on. There are also students with autism who are satisfied simply by completing their work accurately. These students need fewer external reinforcements as long as they are given a meaningful way of understanding when their work is successfully completed. Whenever possible, the type of reinforcer should be a natural consequence of the activity. For example, if making requests is being reinforced, the natural reward is the requested item. Praise and social reinforcers always should accompany more tangible rewards for students with autism. Pairing social and tangible reinforcers will increase the desirability of personal contact for these students and make people greater sources of reinforcement in the future.

Reinforcements must be used systematically if they are to be effective teaching tools. The frequency as well as the type of reinforcement should be individualized; some students need continuous reinforcement, whereas others only need intermittent reinforcement. Reinforcements should immediately follow the behavior or skill being learned, at least initially, so that the relationship between the two is clear to the student. A teacher can determine if the type and frequency of reinforcement are effective by assessing student interest and progress in the behavior being reinforced.

## SUMMARY

Structured teaching is a strategy developed to teach students with autism in classroom settings. Based on the needs, skills, and deficits of autism, it is a system for organizing the classroom, developing appropriate activities, and helping students with autism understand what is expected of them and how to function effectively. Focusing on their considerable visual skills and reliance on routines, structured teaching has been used effectively in the TEACCH Program for the past

20 years (Schopler, Mesibov, & Baker, 1982) to develop skills and minimize behavioral problems.

It is important to highlight that structured teaching is more than just an educational strategy. Based on the assumption that people with autism have behavioral difficulties because environments and teaching techniques are not based on their individualized needs, structured teaching is designed to minimize behavioral difficulties by creating meaningful environments that people with autism can understand and succeed in. When applied effectively, structured teaching also is a successful behavior management strategy. Structured teaching improves behavior proactively, by creating appropriate and meaningful environments that don't trigger the anxiety and frustration that typically cause people with autism to misbehave. If people with autism are to achieve their potential for community living and effective functioning, specialized teaching strategies like structured teaching must be an integral part of their educational programs.

## REFERENCES

Bartak, L. (1978). Educational approaches. In M. Rutter & E. Schopler (Eds.), *Autism: A reappraisal of concepts and treatment* (pp. 423–438). New York: Plenum.

Bartak, L., & Rutter, M. (1973). Special educational treatment of autistic children: A comparative study. I. Design of study and characteristics of units. *Journal of Child Psychology and Psychiatry, 14,* 161–179.

Lockyer, L., & Rutter, M. (1969). A five to fifteen year follow-up study of infantile psychosis. III. Psychological aspects. *British Journal of Psychiatry, 115,* 865–882.

Rutter, M., Greenfeld, D., & Lockyer, L. (1967). A five to fifteen year follow-up study of infantile psychosis. II. Social and behavioral outcome. *British Journal of Psychiatry, 113,* 1183–1199.

Schopler, E., Brehm, S., Kinsbourne, M., & Reichler, R. J. (1971). The effect of treatment structure on development in autistic children. *Archives of General Psychiatry, 24,* 415–421.

Schopler, E., Mesibov, G. B., & Baker, A. (1982). Evaluation of treatment for autistic children and their parents. *Journal of the American Academy of Child Psychiatry, 21,* 262–267.

Schopler, E., Mesibov, G. B., DeVellis, R. F., & Short, A. (1981). Treatment outcome for autistic children and their families. In P. Mittler (Ed.), *Frontiers of knowledge in mental retardation: Social, educational, and behavioral aspects* (pp. 293–301). Baltimore: University Park.

# IV

## Special Issues

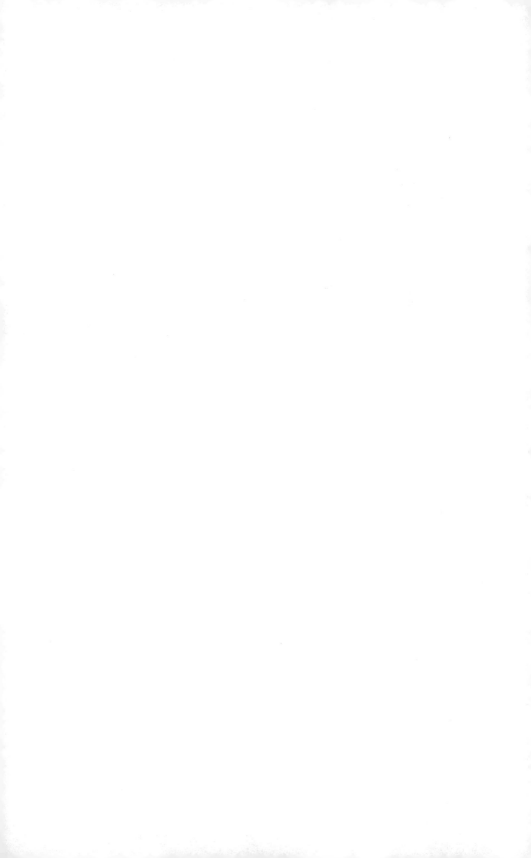

# 11

# Issues in the Use of Aversives

## Factors Associated with Behavior Modification for Autistic and Other Developmentally Disabled People

JOHNNY L. MATSON and JAY A. SEVIN

## INTRODUCTION

Nationally, professionals in the field of autism have been rocked by the controversy surrounding the use of punishment procedures also called aversives (Singh & Repp, 1993). The techniques in question have generally been discussed in the context of behavior modification strategies or learning-based technology, and psychologists and educators have been the primary groups involved. Behavior modification has had widespread application in the treatment of persons with autism (Van Houten, 1990). However, since the late 1980s the rhetoric surrounding these procedures has intensified. National agencies and policymakers have become involved in the debate over which procedures should and should not be considered acceptable to treat severe behavior problems of handicapped people (AAMD, 1987; Blake, 1988; Keyes, Creekmore, Karst, Crow, & Dayan, 1988; Matson, 1988). Given the broad implications of such a debate, the impact on the field has been considerable. A brief review of some of the major issues, including confusion over definition, conflict between advocates and professionals, concepts

JOHNNY L. MATSON and JAY A. SEVIN • Department of Psychology, Louisiana State University, Baton Rouge, Louisiana 70803.

*Behavioral Issues in Autism*, edited by Eric Schopler and Gary B. Mesibov. New York, Plenum Press, 1994.

as ideologies, data versus testimonials, age appropriateness as ideology, freedom of treatment choice, and professional control versus treatment by bureaucratic rule will be the primary focus of this chapter. Some likely outcomes and future directions of the aversives controversy will also be discussed.

## CONFUSION OVER DEFINITION

One means of illuminating the aversives issue is by way of a discussion of definitional problems. Confusion over the definition of an *aversive* procedure and different uses of the terminology have largely contributed to the debate. Many advocacy groups have defined an aversive as anything likely to produce psychological or physical pain. Unfortunately, this notion is insufficient in that it fails to take into account individual client differences. That is, this definition may fail to define what is aversive for a *particular* client. It is often difficult to determine what is painful to a client with autism because many persons with the most extreme problem behaviors are not verbal and cannot easily report pleasure or pain.

Furthermore, their overt demonstrations of emotion may differ substantially from the norm and may not be reliable indicators of distress. Thus, determinations of what is painful are typically made from the perspective of what is aversive *to the advocate* rather than the client. For example, proponents of this definition never define a hug or kiss from a child's parent as aversive. However, for a tactile defensive autistic child a hug may result in a great deal of distress. In contrast, self-injurious behaviors that most persons would consider extremely painful often do not appear to evoke pain in persons with developmental disabilities. Thus, one cannot state that "aversives" for developmentally disabled persons operate according to the same mechanisms we view in others, that is, pain.

A second definition commonly employed by advocacy groups lists as aversive any stimulus that most clients would avoid or escape from if given the opportunity (Johnston, 1988). This definition suffers from the same inadequacies as the previous definition. According to this criterion, mild electric shock devices such as the controversial Self-Injurious Behavior Inhibiting System (SIBIS) (Linscheid, Iwata, Ricketts, Williams, & Griffin, 1990) would certainly be classified as an aversive. In fact, in a recent survey of psychology students, SIBIS was rated as the most aversive of 20 behavior-reduction techniques (Allison & Silverstein, 1990). However, as noted by Allison (1990), early research has indicated that some clients actively seek out the SIBIS device (Linscheid et al., 1990). Again this definition fails to take into account individual differences and is not conducive to the construction of individualized treatment planning. It also fails to take into account that for many clients, aversiveness may not be correlated with intrusiveness.

An additional consideration involves the alternatives to using punishers. For some individuals, many of the alternatives to punishment may be the most psychologically and physically painful. Differential Reinforcement of Other Behavior (DRO) and Differential Reinforcement of Incompatible Behavior (DRI) are often characterized as the hallmarks for positive interventions. However, the effectiveness of a reinforcer depends on first producing or taking advantage of a naturally occurring deprivation state (Mulick, 1990). For example, in animal labs the common practice for many years has been to reduce rats' weights to 80% of free-feeding body weight before using edible reinforcers. Also, with autistic persons, edible stimuli are less likely to work as reinforcers if the client is not at all hungry; satiation is an important concern. Preferred sensory materials are less likely to be effective reinforcers if a child has unlimited access to other sensory stimuli in the environment. Reinforcement must be contingent. Thus, the typical practice is to remove items that are highly desired by the autistic person and to then only allow the person access to those items based on performance of certain skills (e.g., Charlop, Schreibman, & Thibodeau, 1985; McGee, Krantz, & McClannahan, 1983; Van Houten, 1990). It is difficult to see how this is such a positive method from the standpoint of decreasing discomfort, which is paramount to the definitions employed by advocacy groups.

A more appropriate definition of aversives is offered in the behavior modification literature. Learning theorists define stimuli in terms of the *effects* they have on behavior. An aversive is thus any stimulus that reliably increases the frequency of a response that precedes its removal or reliably decreases the frequency of a response that precedes its presentation (Coe & Matson, 1993). (Note that an aversive is not equivalent to punishment because an aversive could be used in either a negative reinforcement or punishment treatment paradigm.) Using this definition, aversives (and reinforcers) are empirically defined for each individual client, with the objective of establishing effective treatment strategies. Thus, the therapeutic value of a stimulus or a procedure is determined from the perspective of the client rather than that of the advocate. A procedure such as contingent restraint may function and be employed as an aversive with some clients (e.g., Azrin, Besalel,& Wisotek, 1982; Slifer, Iwata, & Dorsey, 1984) and as a reinforcer with others (Favell, McGimsey, & Jones, 1978). Unlike the previous two definitions, this one is treatment-oriented. It is optimal for determining strategies that will change behavior in predictable ways with individual clients.

Thus, confusion over terminology has been a prime issue in the debate. The different definitions discussed above would result in very different lists of procedures or stimuli classified as aversives. Whether something "appears" to be harmful or whether it is actually aversive and thus therapeutic may indeed be totally independent issues. The reader is referred to Mulick (1990) for additional discussion of definitional controversies and the issues involved in stimulus classification.

## CONFLICT BETWEEN ADVOCATES AND PROFESSIONALS

Advocacy had its roots in parental guardianship and the concerns of guardians for the rights and well-being of their children. Early efforts resulted in the development of the Association for Retarded Citizens, a national advocacy organization that began in the 1940s and expanded to over 100,000 members. Lobbyists were hired, and a national impact on programs and services resulted. This development was positive. However, as they reached adulthood, many handicapped persons no longer had parents or persons willing to accept the advocate role. Therefore, a second set of advocates emerged, professional advocates, many of whom were lawyers. Polemics brought about by adversarial relationships between developmental disabilities professionals and professional advocates were then transferred to the court system. Advocacy groups felt they served an important role, safeguarding the rights of developmentally disabled persons. Mental health professionals felt themselves most qualified to address the needs of clients in their charge.

This debate emerged largely because professionals were the primary contact people for handicapped persons. It was solidified by those advocates who saw normalization as a treatment and thus felt that a dramatic minimizing of the professional role was necessary. The unwillingness of many professionals to follow lawyer leadership was often viewed by advocates as self-serving (Guess, Turnbull, & Helmstetter, 1990). Many advocates rejected the need for behaviorally based programs and many other professional services. Professionals, who had found these programs to be beneficial and often critical to habilitation, opposed reductions in services. Controversy intensified with advocates' use of socially loaded, negative terms (e.g., referring to homogeneous grouping in classrooms and workshops, a common practice to facilitate learning, as "segregation").

Several issues began to emerge demonstrating the growing hostility between advocates and professionals. Controversies over the acceptability of various treatment procedures and over who should have the authority to determine acceptability were among these issues. Various national organizations became involved in the debate. Those groups who traditionally had served an advocacy role emphasized the need for legislative restrictions. This should be done to protect individuals from unnecessary professional involvement. Groups that took this position included the Association for Retarded Citizens (ARC), the Association for Persons with Severe Handicaps (TASH), and the American Association on Mental Retardation (AAMR).

Groups in opposition to such a restrictive approach, supporting professional input and decision making, were, of course, scientist/practitioners and their organizations. These groups felt that professionals who were experienced in treating handicapped individuals were most qualified to make treatment decisions. They felt the need to protect their clients from advocacy groups. The Association for

Advancement of Behavior Therapy (AABT), the American Psychological Association (APA), and the National Institute of Mental Health (NIMH) were groups that supported professional goals. This national debate has resulted in a polarization of the field. Several major differences in the two camps are evident and will be briefly reviewed.

## CONCEPTS AS IDEOLOGIES

Similar to the popular film *Star Wars,* a "galactic" battle of policymakers has emerged. The advocacy groups and scientist/professionals are the combatants. A brief review of the major points in the warring philosophies will be covered.

Major spokespersons for the advocates' side have been the initiators of the normalization movement. The concept of normalization has become very popular and is generally accepted by advocates and scientist/professionals alike. Problems arise around how best to achieve this goal. Advocates have largely endorsed a client-centered philosophy, reminiscent of the methods of Carl Rogers (1951). That is, a client should be treated with worth, kindness, and in a normal supportive fashion. This approach should bring about normal behavior. The scientist/practitioner view is that these goals while extremely important cannot be achieved in a normal fashion. With some persons abnormal means, such as behavior modification, are necessary to achieve normal behavior. In fact, deinstitutionalization and mainstreaming have seldom been effective in the absence of additional skills training (Emerson, 1985; Gresham, 1982). This clash of philosophies is not new and goes back at least to the Rogers–Skinner debate of the 1950s.

A frequent complaint of advocacy groups is that behaviorally-oriented professionals are inhumane. Culturally loaded terms have been employed by advocacy groups to portray behavioral researchers and clinicians as dangerous to the welfare of handicapped persons. Thus, homogeneous grouping to produce more efficient learning, which is backed by a wealth of scientific data (Matson, 1990), is referred to as *segregation.* Treatment strategies classified as punishment procedures in the operant literature have been called callous, dehumanizing (highly subjective terms), and unethical (without defining ethics).

Aversive procedures have also been mislabeled as "corporal punishment" (proposed by ACDD). These terms are employed to elicit an emotional, not a rational response. With such practices, the presumption of right and wrong is already established. It is done a priori, without systematic study. Issues are discussed in vague terms. Specific client issues are not addressed. Many advocates recommend that treatment procedures such as gentle teaching, use of scheduled activities, communication training, and positive procedures are not only preferable but more effective than other, more intrusive techniques (LaVigna & Donnellan,

1986). The research to support this position has generally been methodologically poor or has addressed treating relatively minor problems (e.g., in-seat behavior instead of self-injurious behavior).

The courts have been required to settle related disputes on a number of occasions. The principles outlined above have often come into question. The cases have routinely involved the most intrusive of behavioral methods and the most extreme problem behaviors. Two such cases were the Behavior Research Institute case in Massachusetts and the Phelan case in Michigan. Both cases received national attention, the former resulting in coverage on two of ABC's new programs, *20/20* and *Nightline*.

In the first case, extremely self-injurious and aggressive adult males were treated using reinforcers in conjunction with aversives, including contingent physical and mechanical restraint, overcorrection, and contingent water sprays to the face. In the latter case, SIBIS (Linscheid et al., 1990), a contingent electric shock device for self-injury, was at issue. In both cases the courts decided that these treatments were acceptable and could be used. The rationale for these decisions is largely based on a few premises.

First is the notion that a database from the scientific community is an important qualifier when establishing the legitimacy of a treatment. This assumption has been upheld by courts time and time again (e.g., the BRI and Phelan cases). Despite the lack of research supporting non-data-based or minimal data-based programs, advocacy groups have continued to assert that certain targeted data-based programs are not necessary (Guess, Helmstetter, Turnbull, & Knowlton, 1986; LaVigna & Donnellan, 1986). They have continued to attempt to pass laws against procedures they view as unacceptable. Their position is based largely upon views that research is not important (e.g., one "expert therapist" in the advocacy camp indicates that these are issues of the heart and not data). Further, an amazing amount of misinformation (Guess et al., 1986) is present to support the advocacy position and is addressed below.

Some key arguments have been made by advocates in opposition to aversives. One argument has been that aversive procedures are not necessary; that is, nonaversive procedures if correctly employed are just as effective as aversives with all clients (Donnellan, LaVigna, Negri-Shoultz, & Fassbender, 1988). As noted by Allison (1990), to entirely abolish the use of aversive techniques, one would have to demonstrate that in no case was an aversive procedure successful where nonaversive procedures failed. However, a number of well-controlled studies have documented the successful treatment of aberrant behaviors using reinforcers and aversives where reinforcement procedures alone had previously failed (Azrin, Belasel, & Wisotek, 1982; Jordan, Singh, & Repp, 1990; Matson & Keyes, 1990). The efficacy of aversive procedures in treating severely life-threatening behaviors has been documented over and over again in the literature (Linscheid et al., 1990; Matson, 1990; Matson & DiLorenzo, 1984; Matson & Taras, 1989);

and it appears that aversive procedures are necessary reductive techniques for some clients.

A second assumption is that such procedures do not meet community standards. Curiously, however, there are no data to support this position. Several surveys on corporal punishment have been conducted. Typically, the majority of parents include methods of corporal punishment among intervention strategies rated as acceptable for their own children (Heffer & Kelley, 1987; Kelley, Grace, & Elliot, 1990). Ironically, then, what little we do know seems to contradict the assumption that the general population is in opposition to such methods. Rather, it would appear that the advocate position falls outside the mainstream.

A third argument frequently made is that punishment procedures do not result in generalization or maintainence of treatment gains (Guess et al., 1986). This point has largely been untested. In a 20-year review of all published studies in referred journals examining self-injury and aggression in developmentally disabled persons, rarely was punishment alone a treatment (Matson & Taras, 1989). Punishment was almost always combined with reinforcement. Thus, the proper statement would be that the combined reinforcement and punishment methods did not result in generalization and maintenance. Even this statement, however, is inaccurate because effective generalization and maintenance of treatment gains using aversives in conjunction with reinforcers have been documented in several studies (Matson & Taras, 1989). Although more work is certainly needed, criticisms based on lack of generalization data are to some degree out of context. Given the serious nature of self-injury and aggression, the state of the art has been the development of methods to produce some suppression of problem behaviors at some point in time. Only now are we beginning to study generalization and maintenance as primary research questions and to determine the least restrictive yet effective treatment for a given problem.

Fourth, it is frequently stated that punishment procedures typically result in more negative side effects than what is observed with reinforcement techniques. In our review of the literature (Matson & Taras, 1989), the level of positive side effects was universally very high for all techniques. This was true even for contingent electric shock where 96% of the reported side effects were positive.

Although not tested to date, it would appear that an issue more relevant to side effects might be the effectiveness of the intervention. Thus, a technique with 95% effectiveness is likely to produce fewer adverse side effects than a treatment with 20% effectiveness. Further, the rapidity with which positive effects occur will most likely be associated with intensity and frequency of negative side effects. That is, a number of parameters are likely to produce side effects. Given the often complex relationships among behaviors, side effects are likely to covary across the parameters noted above and with others as well. This issue is complicated, and at present we have very few answers. However, as with the previously discussed points, the small amount of information we do have seems to run contrary to the advocate views on the topic.

Fifth, it has been argued that we should not use aversive procedures with the developmentally disabled because we would not use them with convicted criminals. (The implicit assumption in this statement is that convicted criminals are the lowest of us and deserve less.) Those who support a scientific perspective would not take such an approach. Intrusive behavioral measures as treatment (e.g., contingent water mist or movement suppression time-out) are not used with convicted criminals because these people are not engaging in head banging or hand biting or other severe forms for self-injury that have proved treatable with aversion procedures. The argument that a procedure that is inappropriate for one group is necessarily inappropriate for all groups rests on faulty logic. We do not, for example, do open heart surgery with persons who have healthy hearts. Different problems require different interventions.

A sixth argument has been that major organizations such as the American Association on Mental Retardation (AAMR) and the Autism Society of America (ASA) do not support the use of aversives. However, this supposition is misleading (Blake, 1988; Keyes, Creekmore, Karst, Crow, & Dayan, 1988). The AAMR and the ASA have not taken votes of their memberships on these issues. In fact, those surveys that have been conducted suggest the opposite. For example, in a poll of 55 psychologists of the AAMR in Louisiana, 57% supported the use of aversives (Keyes et al., 1988). Sixty-four percent of those questioned felt that procedures that resulted in visible pain should not be banned, and 78% of the respondents supported continued research into aversive therapies as methods of behavior management. Only 29% of the psychologists felt that aversive procedures should be labeled as inhumane.

The authors concluded that psychologists in the AAMR are in substantial disagreement with the position statement of the AAMR against aversives. Further, 81% of doctoral-level respondents concluded that there was not sufficient research to conclude that all complex behavior problems can be effectively managed using only nonaversive procedures. In general, greater levels of direct contact with severe problem clients and higher educational degrees were among the respondent characteristics associated with opposition to the banning of aversive procedures (Keyes, Creekmore, Karst, Crow, & Dayan, 1988).

A poll of the executive board of the Autism Society of America found that a majority did not support a ban on aversives, although the organization at one time had such a policy position. Board votes, decisions by executive directors, reports from special committees, and similar internal mechanics often dictate policy. There is nothing wrong with these methods, and they are common. However, accepting executive or committee decisions as representative of the entire membership in many instances will be inaccurate.

## DATA AND TESTIMONIALS

In the field of developmental disabilities, non-research-based methods have commonly been discussed in considering treatment effectiveness. It is argued here that a data-based approach is preferred and constitutes a "consumer report" for interventions with developmentally delayed persons. Good methodology and the ability to obtain reliable and valid conclusions are critical.

Unfortunately, in the history of the field, testimonials have largely maintained equal status, particularly for the advocates, as a means of establishing treatment effectiveness. Videotaped vignettes, comments by parents that a treatment was effective, and anecdotal remarks by caregivers are no substitute for controlled studies. This does not mean that such comments are insignificant. Anecdotal reports may draw attention to important issues, generate interest in the development of new intervention strategies, and encourage empirical study of treatment procedures by professional researchers. Nevertheless, the efficacy of a treatment procedure must be established through controlled studies. It is the ethical responsibility of the therapist to employ procedures that have been empirically validated as effective.

## AGE APPROPRIATENESS AS IDEOLOGY

The behavioral model emphasizes skill acquisition and the shaping of complex skills from existing behaviors. Target goals are accomplished through the use of chaining, fading, reinforcement, and other behavioral procedures applied according to learning principles. Discrete skills are identified, task-analyzed, and broken into smaller steps that are trained in a highly structured and systematic fashion. There are numerous studies that have been conducted demonstrating the value and effectiveness of this method (Matson, 1990). The primary objective is to enhance self-sufficiency.

"Age appropriateness" is a developmental model endorsed by many advocacy groups and used extensively throughout the United States. It hinges on the belief that clients' esteem may be enhanced, aberrant behaviors decreased, and performance facilitated by using work-and-leisure materials that are appropriate for persons of normal intelligence with the same chronological age. The ideology of age appropriateness is based on developmental progressions of persons without developmental disabilities. It emphasizes the importance of acceptance by same-age normal peers. To date there is no research to support the viability of age appropriateness as a treatment approach. The use of age-appropriate materials may prove to be an effective adjunctive intervention strategy. However, at present, there are no data to support its effectiveness, and thus reliance on these methods should be discouraged.

## FREEDOM OF TREATMENT CHOICE

The scientist/practitioner position on aversives is that they should always be used with positive procedures and only when positive procedures alone are impractical or likely to be ineffective (Matson & Dilorenzo, 1984; Van Houten, Axelrod, Bailey, Favell, Foxx, Iwata, & Lovaas, 1988). Further, they should only be used when target problems are severe (typically extreme aggression or self-injury), and thus the "costs" of the treatment are outweighed by the "benefits." It is argued that the broadest possible range of interventions should be available. Although positive procedures are always preferred, for some clients positive procedures alone are not effective (Jordan et al., 1990; Matson & Keyes, 1990). It is felt that it is unethical to purposefully withhold an effective treatment for life-threatening behavior. As discussed by Konarski (1990), moral and ethical considerations often constitute the greatest arguments for using aversive procedures with some clients.

Those opposed to aversives feel that such methods should not be available components of treatment. Advocacy groups typically take this position for one of two reasons. First, they feel such methods are too intrusive. They argue that there is too much potential for abuse of these methods (Guess et al., 1986). Thus, the risks outweigh the benefits. Second, the effectiveness of aversive procedures is called into question. It is argued that these methods are not normative, do not generalize or maintain, and that positive procedures are always adequate. As noted, the factual information available at this time largely does not support this latter position. The former argument is far more compelling and more difficult to refute.

## PROFESSIONAL CONTROL VERSUS TREATMENT BY BUREAUCRATIC RULE

The advocate position is one supportive of government involvement. Advocacy groups propose that aversive procedures require regulation. They argue that treatment regulation cannot be achieved through professionals, thus making governmental regulation the only recourse.

Scientist/practitioners support the notion that they, with the input of parents, should regulate their own professions. They argue that developmental disabilities professionals are uniquely qualified to determine least restrictive yet effective interventions. Where regulation is necessary, it should be conducted by professionals with applied skills and treatment experience. Governmental bodies have often regulated treatments without taking into account the empirical literature; they attempt to change the laws of behavior with a vote. It is argued that the principles of learning theory and the effectiveness of an intervention for a particular client are laws of nature, just as the existence of gravity is a law of nature and cannot be changed by a vote. Furthermore, governmental regulation takes the right of treatment selection out of the hands of parents and guardians, who are most likely to have the client's interests at heart.

## FUTURE DIRECTIONS

There are a substantial number of factors that separate the advocacy and professional camps. Some have argued that taken at its simplest, the advocacy/professional division might best be conceptualized as ideology versus science (Mulick, 1990). As discussed, definitional controversies, treatment philosophies, importance assigned to empirical research, and opposing views about treatment regulation are all issues central to the aversives debate. These differences are formidable. Because both camps believe they are fighting for the welfare of developmentally disabled persons, it is unlikely that current divisions will be shortlived. Thus, one likely trend is that the debate will continue for some time. However, a number of other outcomes are likely in the next few years that will change the landscape of treatment for developmentally disabled persons.

A second trend is toward more complex and refined intervention packages. The aversives issue has been a primary factor in the rapid advancement of treatment technology in this area. Research has been funded by national agencies on the topic, and the study of least-restrictive effective procedures has become a national priority. The development of a considerable variety of studies and procedures has resulted. Initial emphases were on training behaviors incompatible with a given inappropriate behavior (e.g., self-injury or aggression). These goals have been achieved for a large number of clients via shaping and differential reinforcement procedures. These continue to be some of the primary goals of treatment for persons with developmental disabilities.

Two other dimensions have been added as means of further decreasing aberrant behaviors. One dimension focuses on building a range of prosocial skills. The second area involves environmental restructuring and control of antecedent events that promote adaptive and prevent maladaptive behavior, making contingent strategies less important for some clients.

Among the skill-building areas, social skills has perhaps been the most extensively studied topic. Social skills training has been applied in educational settings (Brown & Shaw, 1986), institutions (Foxx, McMorrow, & Mennemier, 1984), and community and natural environments (Senatore, Matson, & Kazdin,

1982; Wildman, Wildman, & Kelly, 1986). The general notion that mentally retarded persons have handicaps in social adaptation has further reinforced the opinion that this treatment is necessary for a range of problems and in a variety of settings. It has become a very common treatment component (Marchetti & Campbell, 1990).

Another treatment component emphasized in recent years has been self-control methods. Clients are taught skills that will allow them to manage their own behavior. Initial attempts at self-control training can be found in the early self-management and independence training literature (Matson, Marchetti, & Adkins, 1980). More recently, self-control methods have been applied in the treatment of aggression. For example, Benson (1986) and Benson, Rice, and Miranti (1986) have successfully employed an anger management program with mentally retarded persons. This program is likely to prove beneficial for autistic persons also. The approach emphasizes not only teaching the client to modify outward behaviors but also ruminative thoughts that lead to outbursts. Similarly, Cole, Gardner, and Karan (1986) used a treatment package to control aggression that included self-monitoring, self-evaluation, and self-consequenting. Even more recently, self-management techniques have been applied in the treatment of stereotypies of autistic clients (Koegel & Koegel, 1990).

The restructuring of antecedent conditions is also an area receiving considerable attention. Often referred to as behavioral diagnostics, it emphasizes that no single psychological mechanism underlies recurring aggression problems (Gardner & Cole, 1988). Environmental and personal factors that are determinants of problem behaviors are targeted for change. A three-step process is used to determine the motivators of problem behaviors and to indicate how best to re-arrange or otherwise modify problem behaviors. These factors include (1) gathering information relative to those variables that potentially contribute to the likelihood of the aggression; (2) developing client-specific causes of problem behaviors; and (3) developing client-specific interventions.

Gardner and Cole (1990) propose a method to identify aggression via a multicomponent model. They divide the causes into three major factors: (1) events that instigate and/or increase the probability of occurrence; (2) events that strengthen and maintain behavior; and (3) events that decrease behavior. The model attempts to look at all possible factors likely to produce aggression (e.g., a workshop supervisor reprimands the client in the presence of peers, over-crowding, high noise level [antecedents], and being allowed to escape from the work setting [consequences]). Models of this sort have been instrumental in ensuring a more broad-based and effective means of dealing with problem behaviors.

A third trend is the better regulation of aversives. It is our view that the inclusion of aversive procedures as possible components in treatment programs for some clients should continue. However, there is a need for better delineating who is qualified to administer these interventions. State regulations, for example, might help determine qualified personnel. Input from professionals in the field will be necessary to accomplish this goal. Being a licensed psychologist or board-certified psychiatrist does not necessarily ensure that a person has the skills needed to administer behavioral interventions for extreme problem behaviors. These certifications are overly broad and often do not address clinical competencies. Some very positive steps such as the development of treatment teams and human rights committees have been useful in establishing a checks-and-balances system for intervention.

## CONCLUSIONS

The relative infancy of the field of applied behavior analysis is most certainly a major factor in the debate on aversives. As a technology for behavior change has emerged, so have questions about which interventions are likely to be acceptable. There are a number of parallels in the medical technology field pertaining to genetic engineering, artificially prolonging life after brain death, and other issues regarding the interface of technology and social mores. Most likely these issues will be resolved in time with additional debate. In the meantime, controversies over these highly volatile issues are likely. Efforts by advocacy groups to stop aversive procedures will continue. However, given the range of effective interventions that presently exist, it is highly unlikely that these efforts will result in a total ban on aversive interventions.

## REFERENCES

AAMD position statement on aversive therapy. (1987). *Mental Retardation, 25,* 118.

Allison, D. B. (1990). On the limits of further empirical evidence for deciding the debate over aversive techniques. *The Behavior Therapist, 13,* 147–148.

Allison, D. B., & Silverstein, J. M. (1990). *Quantifying treatment aversiveness: An empirical approach.* Paper to be presented at the meeting of the Association for Behavior Analysis, Nashville, TN.

Azrin, N. H., Belasel, V. A., & Wisotek, I. E. (1982). Treatment of self-injury by a reinforcement plus interruption procedure. *Analysis and Intervention in Developmental Disabilities, 2,* 105–113.

Benson, B. A. (1986). Anger management training. *Psychiatric Aspects of Mental Retardation Reviews, 5,* 51–55.

Benson, B. A., Rice, C. J., & Miranti, S. V. (1986). Effects of anger management training with mentally retarded adults in group treatment. *Journal of Consulting and Clinical Psychology, 54,* 728–729.

Blake, A. (1988). Aversives: Are they needed? Are they ethical? *Autism Research Review, 2,* 1–8.

Brown, G. S., & Shaw, M. (1986). Social skills training in education. In C. Hollin & P. Trower (Eds.), *Handbook of social skills training* (Vol. 1, pp. 59–78). New York: Pergamon.

Charlop, M. H., Schreibman, L., & Thibodeau, M. G. (1985). Increasing spontaneous verbal responding in autistic children using a time delay procedure. *Journal of Applied Behavior Analysis, 18,* 155–166.

Coe, D. A. & Matson, J. L. (1993). On the empirical basis for using aversive and nonaversive therapy. In N. N. Singh and A. C. Repp (Eds.), *Severe behavior problems in developmental disabilities: Issues in non-aversive therapy.*

Cole, C. L., Gardner, W. I., & Karan, O. C. (1986). Self-management training of mentally retarded adults presenting severe conduct difficulties. *Applied Research in Mental Retardation, 6,* 337–347.

Donnellan, A. M., La Vigna, G. W., Negri-Shoultz, N., & Fassbender, L. L. (1988). *Progress without punishment.* New York: Teachers College Press.

Emerson, E. B. (1985). Evaluating the impact of deinstitutionalization on the lives of mentally retarded people. *American Journal of Mental Deficiency, 90,* 277–288.

Favell, J., McGimsey, J., & Jones, M. (1978). The use of physical restraint in the treatment of self-injury and as positive reinforcement. *Journal of Applied Behavior Analysis, 11,* 225–241.

Foxx, R., McMorrow, M., & Mennemeir, M. (1984). Teaching social/vocational skills to retarded adults with a modified table game. An analysis of generalization. *Journal of Applied Behavior Analysis, 17,* 343–352.

Gardner, W. I., & Cole, C. L. (1988). Conduct disorders: Psychological therapies. In J. L. Matson (ed.), *Handbook of behavior modification with the mentally retarded* (2nd ed., pp. 225–248).

Gresham, F. M. (1982). Misguided mainstreaming: The case for social skills training with handicapped children. *Exceptional Children, 48,* 422–433.

Guess, D., Helmstetter, E., Turnbull, H. R., III, & Knowlton, S. (1986). *Use of aversive procedures with persons who are disabled: An historical review and critical analysis* (Monograph). Seattle: The Association for Persons with Severe Handicaps.

Guess, D., Turnbull, H. R., III, & Helmstetter, E. (1990). Science, paradigms, and values: A response to Mulick. *American Journal on Mental Retardation, 95,* 157–163.

Heffer, R. W., & Kelley, M. L. (1987). Mothers' acceptance of behavioral interventions for children: The influence of parent race and income. *Behavior Therapy, 2,* 153–163.

Jordan, J., Singh, N. N., & Repp, A. C. (1989). An evaluation of gentle teaching and visual screening in the reduction of stereotypy. *Journal of Applied Behavior Analysis, 22,* 9–22.

Kelley, M. L., Grace, N., & Elliot, S. N. (1990). Acceptability of positive and punitive discipline methods: Comparisons among abusive, potentially abusive, and nonabusive parents. *Child Abuse & Neglect, 14,* 219–226.

Keyes, J. R., Creekmore, W. N., Karst, R., Crow, R., & Dayan, M. (1988). AAMR position statement on aversive therapy: The controversy. *Mental Retardation, 26,* 314–318.

Koegel, R. L., & Koegel, L. K. (1990). Extended reductions in stereotypic behavior of students with autism through a self-management treatment package. *Journal of Applied Behavior Analysis, 23,* 119–127.

Konarski, E. A., Jr. (1990). Science as an ineffective White Knight. *American Journal on Mental Retardation, 95,* 169–171.

LaVigna, G. W. & Donnellan, A. M. (1986). *Alternatives to punishment: Solving behavior problems with non-aversive strategies.* New York: Irvington.

Linscheid, T. R., Iwata, B. A., Ricketts, R. W., Williams, D. E., & Griffin, J. C. (1990). Clinical evaluation of the Self-Injurious Behavior Inhibiting System (SIBIS). *Journal of Applied Behavior Analysis, 23,* 53–78.

Marchetti, A. G., & Campbell, V. A. (1990). Social skills. In J. L. Matson (Ed.), *Handbook of behavior modification with the mentally retarded* (2nd ed., pp. 333–350). New York: Plenum.

Matson, J. L. (1988). *IARET Newsletter, 1,* 1.

Matson, J. L. (Ed.). (1990). *Handbook of behavior modification with the mentally retarded.* (2nd ed.). New York: Plenum.

Matson, J. L., DiLorenzo, T. M. (1984). *Punishment and its alternatives.* New York: Springer-Verlag.

Matson, J. L., & Keyes, J. B. (1990). A comparison of DRO to movement suppression time-out and DRO with two self-injurious and aggressive mentally retarded adults. *Research in Developmental Disabilities, 11,* 111–120.

Matson, J. L., Marchetti, A., & Adkins, J. A. (1980). Comparison of operant and independence training procedures for mentally retarded adults. *American Journal of Mental Deficiency, 84,* 487–494.

Matson, J. L., & Taras, M. E. (1989). A 20 Year review of punishment and alternative methods to treat problem behaviors in developmentally disabled persons. *Research in Developmental Disabilities, 10,* 85–104.

McGee, G. G., Krantz, P. J., Mason, D., & McClannahan, L. E. (1983). A modified incidental-teaching procedure for autistic youth: Acquisition and generalization of receptive object labels. *Journal of Applied Behavior Analysis, 16,* 329–338.

Mulick, J. A. (1990). The ideology and science of punishment in mental retardation. *American Journal on Mental Retardation, 95,* 142–156.

Rogers, C. R. (1951). *Client-centered therapy: Its current practice, implications and theory.* Boston: Houghton-Mifflin.

Senatore, V., Matson, J. L., & Kazdin, A. E. (1982). A comparison of behavioral methods to train social skills to mentally retarded adults. *Behavior Therapy, 13,* 313–324.

Singh, N. N., & Repp, A. C. (1993). *Severe behavior problems in developmental disabilities: Issues in non-aversive therapy.*

Slifer, K. J., Iwata, B. A., & Dorsey, M. F. (1984). Reduction of eye gouging using a response interruption procedure. *Journal of Behavior Therapy and Experimental Psychiatry, 15,* 369–375.

Van Houten, R. (1990). Emotional problems II: Autism. In J. L. Matson (Ed.), *Handbook of behavior modification with the mentally retarded.* (2nd ed., pp. 421–437). New York: Plenum.

Van Houten, R., Axelrod, S., Bailey, J. S., Favell, J. E., Foxx, R. M., Iwata, A., & Lovaas, O. I. (1988). The right to effective behavioral treatment. *Journal of Applied Behavior Analysis, 21,* 381–384.

Wildman, B. G., Wildman, H. E., & Kelly, W. J. (1986). Group conversational-skill training and social validation with mentally retarded adults. *Applied Research in Mental Retardation, 7,* 443–458.

# 12

# Some Characteristics of Nonaversive Intervention for Severe Behavior Problems

## GLEN DUNLAP, FRANK R. ROBBINS, and LEE KERN

### INTRODUCTION

Among the most salient of developments in intervention for people with autism and other developmental disabilities has been the emergence of nonaversive orientations to the treatment of problem behavior. This salience has been reflected in numerous books and articles (e.g., Evans & Meyer, 1985; Horner, Dunlap, Koegel, Carr, Sailor, Anderson, Albin, & O'Neill, 1990; LaVigna & Donnellan, 1986; Meyer & Evans, 1989; Repp & Singh, 1990), resolutions by advocacy and professional organizations (see Singh, Lloyd, & Kendall, 1990), federally sponsored conferences (e.g., Horner & Dunlap, 1988), and research efforts designed to develop more precise and effective procedures.

Nonaversive approaches have achieved prominence for many reasons. Arguments in support of nonaversive interventions have been based on ethics, civil rights, and indications that positive procedures (as opposed to aversive procedures) are more likely to produce durable changes in a manner that is acceptable in typical community settings and that contributes to enriched lifestyles for people with disabilities (Guess, Helmstetter, Turnbull, & Knowlton, 1987). Although the controversy surrounding the use of aversive procedures continues (e.g., Iwata, 1988; Mulick, 1990; Repp & Singh, 1990), the debate has been constricted

GLEN DUNLAP • Florida Mental Health Institute, University of South Florida, Tampa, Florida 33612-2399.    FRANK R. ROBBINS • Early Childhood Learning Center, 150 Fearing Street, Amherst, Massachusetts 01002.    LEE KERN • Children's Seashore House, Biobehavioral Unit, 3405 Civic Center Boulevard, Philadelphia, Pennsylvania 19104.

*Behavioral Issues in Autism*, edited by Eric Schopler and Gary B. Mesibov. New York, Plenum Press, 1994.

recently to the most serious (e.g., life-threatening) behaviors, and in general, there is broad agreement that nonaversive approaches represent the favored orientation for addressing problem behaviors exhibited by people with autism and mental retardation (Horner & Dunlap, 1988; National Institutes of Health, 1990).

The purpose of this chapter is to offer a description of nonaversive interventions and their use with developmentally disabled populations. The intent is to present an overview and a sampling of the empirical basis for procedures that rely on positive behavioral support. We do not attempt to elaborate upon the arguments in favor of or against nonaversive (or aversive) procedures. These points have been made in numerous forums (see, in particular, Repp & Singh, 1990, for a diverse collection of essays on all aspects of the controversy). Rather, we seek to describe some of the foundations and trends that comprise nonaversive interventions.

In this first section of the chapter, we define the subject matter and offer a brief summary of the empirical literature. The following sections, which make up the majority of the chapter, are devoted to a discussion of three themes that characterize continuing developments in nonaversive intervention. These themes are (1) functional assessment and the use of hypotheses to design hypothesis-based interventions, (2) an emphasis on antecedent and curricular manipulations, and (3) considerations of personal control and choice-making opportunities.

## Definition and Overview

The term *nonaversive intervention* has created some confusion because it has different meanings when used by different people (Horner, Dunlap et al., 1990). In this chapter, we will use the term in its broad and most common connotation, as it is applied in familiar reference to the body of positive procedures for reducing problem behaviors. Nonaversive intervention refers to a very diverse collection of strategies that have in common the following characteristics: (1) They avoid the use of punishment procedures that produce pain, tissue damage, or social humiliation; (2) they explicitly seek to develop or increase the occurrence of desirable behaviors as an essential element in the reduction of problem behaviors; and (3) they are implemented with a pervasive concern for the rights and dignity of the individual, and with a consideration that the procedures should be acceptable to the general populace when they are applied in public environments (Horner, Dunlap et al., 1990).

Nonaversive interventions tend to be proactive in the sense that they are typically applied when the problem behavior is not occurring (Carr, Robinson, & Palumbo, 1990; Carr, Robinson, Taylor, & Carlson, 1990; Meyer & Evans, 1989). This differs from reactive strategies, including punishment operations, which are designed to suppress responding through contingent application of an aversive stimulus. In addition, nonaversive strategies often include specific instructional objectives that have the goal of teaching alternative responses as replacements for the problem behavior (e.g., Durand, 1990; Evans & Meyer, 1985). Nonaversive approaches may also include preventive measures. These typically involve removing or ameliorating those environmental events that serve to evoke or set the occasion for the problem behavior (e.g., Touchette, MacDonald, & Langer, 1985). Differential reinforcement techniques (LaVigna & Donnellan, 1986) also constitute important elements of the nonaversive armamentarium. Finally, a very substantial, but underrecognized, component of nonaversive intervention has to do with lifestyle enrichment. This pertains to a diversity of changes that may affect the way that a person lives, works, plays, and socializes. For example, lifestyle modifications may include a change of residence, a move to an integrated classroom, a different job, an expansion of opportunities for outdoor recreation, the development of new friendships, or any combination of related lifestyle factors. These kinds of changes are difficult to operationalize in a catalog of techniques (and they are difficult to evaluate experimentally), but they represent a significant feature of the nonaversive approach (e.g., Meyer & Evans, 1989; Berkman & Meyer, 1988).

The empirical basis for nonaversive strategies has developed substantially over the past years (Carr, Robinson, Taylor, & Carlson, 1990; Dunlap, Ferro, & dePerczel, in press; LaVigna & Donnellan, 1986), however it is important to recognize certain limitations of the existing literature. First, most nonaversive interventions involve multicomponent and highly individualized manipulations that are not well-suited for evaluation by standard experimental methodologies. Second, many nonaversive stategies are designed to influence problem behavior in an indirect manner (e.g., by increasing the frequency of a desirable alternative). In contrast to those manipulations that treat problem behavior with powerful and direct (e.g., suppressive) measures, such indirect effects may be less immediate and thus less amenable to the design requirements of within-subject methodologies. Although there are nonaversive techniques that provide for immediate reductions in the rate of problem behavior (e.g., Singer, Singer, & Horner, 1987; Winterling, Dunlap, & O'Neill, 1987), some of the strategies that produce the most durable effects may take longer to produce elimination of serious problem behaviors. Third, the emergence of a strong emphasis on nonaversive approaches has been present for less than a decade. In comparison with the literature on punishment, this is a brief time with which to establish a compelling empirical foundation.

Nevertheless, the empirical foundation that does exist offers a variety of strategies for reducing even the most serious of problem behaviors. Differential reinforcement procedures, including differential reinforcement of other behaviors (DRO) and differential reinforcement of incompatible behaviors (DRI), are well-documented operations that involve the scheduling of positive reinforcement at times when the problem behavior is not occurring. The literature describes a large number of specific differential reinforcement schedules (LaVigna & Donnellan, 1986), all of which have been documented to reduce problem behaviors in at least some circumstances. A related set of strategies relies on instructional techniques, as well as reinforcement, to teach responses that are intended to increase a person's effectiveness in daily activities. Such teaching strategies include training in instruction following (e.g., Russo, Cataldo, & Cushing, 1981), self-management (e.g., Gardner & Cole, 1984; Koegel & Koegel, 1990; Shapiro & Klein, 1980), communication (e.g., Carr & Durand, 1985; Horner & Budd, 1985), or even specific skills such as toy play (e.g., Santarcangelo, Dyer, & Luce, 1987). Several authors have argued that skill development is an essential aspect of nonaversive intervention (Evans & Meyer, 1985), that it already has a rich scientific foundation, and that it is likely to become even more prominent as researchers adopt additional methodologies for investigating proactive and preventive approaches to behavior management (e.g., Dunlap, Johnson, & Robbins, 1990).

Other general stategies that have acquired empirical support involve the manipulation of antecedent stimuli to increase the probability of desirable behaviors and decrease problem responses (e.g., Touchette et al., 1985). These approaches involve identifying the circumstances that evoke different patterns of behavior and then modifying those circumstances in order to promote adaptive, and prevent undesirable, responding. The kinds of stimuli that can be manipulated include those that are present in the immediate environment as well as more distal (and setting) events that may increase the probability of behavior problems. The literature on such stimulus-based interventions has been produced, almost entirely, within the most recent decade. Nevertheless, numerous studies have shown that such approaches can be very effective in eliminating serious problem behaviors (Carr, Robinson, Taylor, & Carlson, 1990). Several advances and directions in this area are discussed in a later section of this chapter. Finally, it is important to reiterate that much nonaversive intervention involves multiple components and that, thus far, the documentation of these multifaceted strategies is largely in the form of case studies (e.g., Berkman & Meyer, 1988).

Although the support for nonaversive approaches is growing steadily, there is not a sufficient database to assert that *all* problem behaviors in all contexts can be fully and durably eliminated through nonaversive environmental interventions. Of course, this is a statement that applies to any orientation to treatment, whether it be based on psychopharmacology, contingent aversives, or any other approach. In addition, it must be stressed that nonaversive intervention does not always represent a simple or consistently straightforward process. In cases that are characterized by very severe topographies and long and complicated learning histories, the nonaversive approach can require a level of creativity and tenacity that is at least as demanding as other perspectives (e.g., Turnbull & Turnbull, 1990). In these most challenging of cases, nonaversive intervention may require ongoing assessment and many levels and phases of intervention (e.g., Berkman & Meyer,

1988) that can be difficult for service systems to engineer. In order to achieve durable improvements in the problem behaviors and the lifestyles of these most intransigent cases, any approach (including the nonaversive orientation) will require structural modifications in the way that environments provide habilitative support as well as systems that are designed for individualized assessment and ongoing efforts of prevention and intervention (Dunlap et al., 1990; Horner, Dunlap et al., 1990). Still, the point remains that nonaversive interventions are supported by substantial (and increasing) efficacy data, and they also avoid many of the harmful or stigmatizing effects that may be produced by more intrusive methods.

As an orientation, nonaversive intervention is just now acquiring a consistent definition and clear directions for continued development (Horner, Dunlap et al., 1990). In the remainder of this chapter, we develop three themes that appear to characterize much of the current status (and future development) of nonaversive approaches.

## FUNCTIONAL ASSESSMENT AND HYPOTHESIS-DRIVEN INTERVENTION

Perhaps the most important perspective, integral to the discussion of non-aversive intervention, concerns the growing emphasis and improving technology for conducting functional assessments of problems such as aggression and self-injurious behavior. The term *functional assessment* denotes the identification of antecedent and consequent events that occasion and maintain the behavior (Lennox & Miltenberger, 1989). Once completed, a functional assessment should result in three important outcomes. The problem behavior should be operationally described and measured, both occurrence and nonoccurrence of the behavior should be predictable in relation to specific times and situations, and the purpose or function of the behavior should be clearly identified (O'Neill, Horner, Albin, Storey, & Sprague, 1990). The primary goal is to achieve a thorough understanding of the problem behavior in relation to the environment prior to commencing with intervention. With this understanding, interventions can be designed that are consistent with the causes of the behavior problem and, thus, be more effective (Carr, Robinson, & Palumbo, 1990).

The major purpose of a functional assessment is the elucidation of the function of the problem behavior, or the identification of functional relationships between events in the environment and the behavior. When behavior problems are associated with environmental variables, one (or more) of three general hypotheses (or functions) is generally postulated. These include positive reinforcement, negative reinforcement, and "automatic" or sensory reinforcement (e.g., Carr 1977). Studies have shown that problem behaviors are sometimes maintained by positive reinforcement in the form of social attention (Iwata, Dorsey, Slifer, Bauman & Richman, 1982), or tangibles such as food or access to certain activities.

For example, Horner and Budd (1985) reported on an individual whose problem behaviors were determined to represent attempts to access food during snack time. Other research has demonstrated that a number of students' behavior problems are maintained by negative reinforcement. Weeks and Gaylord-Ross (1981) presented data on three individuals whose self-injurious and aggressive behaviors were functionally related to increased task difficulty. Finally, some behavior emitted by persons with autism and related handicaps seem to be maintained by sensory or "automatic" reinforcement. Inferential data supportive of this hypothesis can be drawn from studies that report high levels of problem behavior for some students when they are left without social or activity stimulation (e.g., Iwata et al., 1982) and from other work that reports decreases in stereotypic behavior when the sensory consequences are removed (Rincover, 1978).

Although the process of conducting a functional assessment often takes many forms, the procedures can be grouped under the general headings of informant-based methods, direct observation methods, and experimental analysis (Lennox & Miltenberger, 1989). In general, methods such as interviews and observations in the natural environment are used to develop viable *hypotheses* regarding functional relationships between environmental events and challenging behaviors. Methods of experimental analysis, or a "true" functional analysis (Iwata, Vollmer, & Zarcone, 1990), can serve to empirically *test* or validate hypotheses such that the presence of functional relationships can be firmly established.

## Informant-Based Methods

Informant-based methods that include questionnaires, interviews, and rating scales can be used as a starting point for conducting a functional assessment. The purpose of this information-gathering process is to develop hypotheses regarding the factors that may elicit and maintain problem behaviors. In this context, a number of instuments have been developed that rely on the reporting of parents, teachers, or other persons knowledgeable about the individual with behavioral challenges. The Functional Analysis Interview Form (O'Neill et al., 1990) can be administered to an individual with knowledge regarding the behavior problem of interest or can be utilized as a questionnaire. This form contains a series of questions that elicit information concerning the physical and environmental events that are associated with problem behavior and adaptive responding. The Motivation Assessment Scale (MAS) (Durand & Crimmins, 1988) is a 16-item rating scale that specifically examines the role of social attention, escape, tangible rewards, and sensory stimulation as possible maintaining factors for behavior problems. The MAS provides potentially important information and only takes a few minutes to administer, score, and interpret. Data obtained during this process should lead to hypotheses about *potential* functional relationships, as hypotheses advanced must be tested more rigorously before they can be stated with certainty.

## Direct Observation Methods

Direct observation methods are often used to gain a better understanding of behavior problems and provide further refinement of hypotheses developed through informant-based methods. Many teachers and other professionals have employed some form of antecedent–behavior–consequence (A-B-C) assessment. An A-B-C assessment is accomplished through recording environmental events that occur temporally contiguous to the behavior problem in question (e.g., Cooper, Heron, & Heward, 1987). O'Neill et al. (1990) have developed a modified version of an A-B-C form that makes this process more systematic and allows for clearer summarization and detection of patterns. In the same vein, Touchette et al. (1985) developed a "scatter plot" technique that attempts to discover relationships between various times of day and frequencies of target behavior. Once such information is obtained, additional (experimental) analyses can be conducted to establish the presence of true functional relationships between specific events and the occurrence of problem behavior.

## Experimental Analysis

Experimental analysis (or "hypothesis testing") involves systematically manipulating aspects of the environment such that functional relationships suggested by nonexperimental data can be confirmed. These procedures were pioneered by Iwata et al. (1982) in research that described analog manipulations designed to delineate the reinforcers (e.g., positive, negative, or sensory reinforcement) that maintained self-injurious behavior. Other authors (e.g., Carr & Durand, 1985; Steege, Wacker, Berg, Cigrand, & Cooper, 1989) have used very similar techniques to distinguish the functions of other serious behavior problems. Although these procedures often result in the identification of true functional (or causal) relationships, they are othen time consuming and costly. This has led some researchers to attempt to streamline the process such that it may be accomplished in the context of an outpatient clinic setting requiring shorter periods of time (Wacker, Steege, Northup, Reimers, Berg, & Sasso, 1990), or by completing experimental manipulations in the natural context over a limited number of school days (Dunlap, Kern-Dunlap, Clarke, & Robbins, 1991).

The functional assessment process is designed to (1) delineate functional relationships between antecedent and consequent events and problem behaviors and (2) provide information about these relationships that can be used to design and implement strategies to ameliorate behavior problems. Failure to link assessment to intervention can result in ineffective interventions (Carr, Robinson, & Palumbo, 1990) that are characterized as being *reactive* in nature and tend to be based on the topography of the behavior problem rather than its presumed function. For example, if a student's intense aggression is elicited by difficult, language-based tasks (i.e., it is maintained by escape from the difficult task), a seclusion time-out program will not only be ineffective but will likely exacerbate the problem behavior. An effective alternative, suggested by a functional assessment, would be to simplify the task or to teach the student to request assistance. Similarly, for an individual whose hand biting is maintained by sensory consequences, teaching the person to request assistance will be unproductive as well as ineffectual. Instead, this individual might benefit from a more adaptive, and innocuous, means of generating sensory stimulation (e.g., by using her hands to manipulate age-appropriate toys).

It is important to emphasize that functional assessment procedures are by no means a "cookbook" for easily solving all behavior problems. Although in many cases this process will be fairly straightforward, some of the challenging behaviors exhibited by people with autism and related disabilities are quite complex and difficult to understand. In these cases, the process of functional assessment and hypothesis development can be arduous and lengthy. For example, Dunlap et al. (1991) reported that the initial phase of information gathering and hypothesis development involved extensive obervation, interviews, and team meetings over a 5-week period of time. However, once the hypotheses were developed, they were tested and confirmed over period of only 4 days. The hypotheses then led to program recommendations that resolved the long-standing, serious disruptive behaviors of an adolescent female.

Functional assessment and the development of hypothesis-based interventions represent an essential foundation of nonaversive behavior management. The process is fundamental for the prescription of interventions that respond to the idiosyncratic pragmatics of problems behaviors. The range of possible prescriptions is as extensive as the number of people who exhibit such behaviors, and the interventions may take many different forms. However, the interventions may be categorized. In the following sections, we discuss two broad categories of interventions that represent increasing emphasis in nonaversive behavioral support.

## ANTECEDENT AND CURRICULUM-BASED INTERVENTIONS

A second major trend in the area of nonaversive behavior management is increased attention to antecedent stimuli. Through the process of functional assessment, stimuli or setting events that influence or control problem behavior can often be identified. In addition to consequences, a wide variety of antecedent events has been associated with the occurrence of problem behavior. These may include temporally contiguous events such as noise level, instructional commands, crowding (McAfee, 1987), task materials, or schedule predictability. Sometimes, however, problem behaviors may be associated with more complex and temporally distant events (e.g., Wahler & Graves, 1983), such as missing breakfast, social exchanges at an earlier time, or pain associated with sinus problems. Antecedent or curriculum-based interventions focus on identifying stimuli associated with both desirable as well as undesirable behaviors. These stimuli can then be arranged so that the presentation of those controlling nonproblematic behaviors is increased while the presentation of those controlling problem behavior is reduced or ameliorated.

A number of recent studies have successfully identified and manipulated antecedent or setting factors to reduce or eliminate problem behavior. Many of these studies have been conducted with individuals with severe cognitive impairments, in addition to challenging behavior problems. Touchette et al. (1985) demonstrated the process of functional assessment and subsequent antecedent manipulation to reduce self-injurious behavior of an adult man with autism. By using a scatterplot, they were able to identify a specific time period during the day associated with high rates of self-injurious behavior. One element that was different during this time period was the staff member working one-to-one with the man. In order to test this hypothesis, reversals were conducted by manipulating staff schedules. It was found that the particular staff member was indeed associated with high rates of self-injury. Self-injury occured primarily in the presence of this staff member, regardless of the time of day. Because the absence of the staff member was associated with low levels of problem behavior, a simple intervention involving schedule manipulations was readily suggested.

Winterling et al. (1987) used "task variation" to reduce problem behavior in three individuals with autism. In this study, repeated presentations of a single instructional task resulted in high rates of disruptive and self-stimulatory behavior. When the target instructional task was interspersed with a variety of previously acquired tasks, disruptive behavior was substantially reduced. In addition, acquisition of the target task was improved when tasks were varied (Dunlap, 1984).

Using a related strategy, Singer et al. (1987) used "pretask requests" to reduce transition difficulties. Children's inappropriate behaviors during transitions from play to instructional periods were reduced by presenting brief instructions associated with high levels of compliance prior to the instruction to transition. Specifically, children were asked to perform a number of simple tasks, such as "Give me five" prior to the instruction to transition. After presenting these pretask requests, transition performance was greatly improved. Horner,

Day, Sprague, O'Brien, and Heathfield (1991) used similar procedures in instructional contexts to reduce aggression and self-injury among learners with severe disabilities.

## Curriculum-Based Interventions

As is suggested by several of the studies discussed above, the manipulation of antecedent events often involves curriculum-based interventions. In this sense, the goal of curricular interventions is to make changes related to specific tasks so that problem behavior is reduced. These changes include altering the instructional demands, the difficulty of task assignments, the instructional materials, or the response to be performed (e.g., Carr & Durand, 1985; Gaylor-Ross, 1982; Weeks & Gaylord-Ross, 1981). An advantage of curricular interventions is that alternative behaviors or responses can be strengthened. By focusing on increasing competencies and adaptive behavior skills, modifications can be made that will result in lifestyle enrichment for individuals with disabilities.

Curriculum-based interventions often represent broadened procedures addressing an individual's lifestyle in a comprehensive manner. Because severe behavior problems are usually complex and may not be maintained by a single variable, successful interventions often require multiple concurrent manipulations. For example, it is possible that an intervention for one individual could simultaneously require changes in the schedule of reinforcement, additional staff training, curriculum changes to target functional skills, new options for augmentative communication, and an increase in the number of social contacts. Although the effects may be difficult to replicate experimentally because of the highly individualized nature of this type of intervention, a growing number of case descriptions are contributing relevant information to the design and implementation of such comprehensive interventions (Berkman & Meyer, 1988; Dunlap et al., 1991; LaVigna, Willis, & Donnellan, 1989).

In a comprehensive intervention involving multiple components and requiring significant lifestyle modifications, Berkman and Meyer (1988) were able to virtually eliminate self-injury and substantially increase desirable behavior in a nonverbal man who was described as developmentally disabled and psychotic. The first component of the intervention was designed to alter the stimulus conditions that were associated with self-injury. This was accomplished primarily by avoiding institutional settings, in which the man had resided for more than 37 years, and by introducing new circumstances that did not have a history associated with problem behavior. The second component involved teaching alternative behaviors that were functional for community-based activities. These included self-management, communication, daily living, and employment skills. The third component was to provide an array of choice-making opportunities ranging from what to wear to the determination of the daily acitivity schedule. Although the process of implementation was extensive and lengthy, the combination of these multiple intervention components resulted in a durable reduction of problem behavior as well as significant lifestyle enhancement.

The major advantages of antecedent interventions is that they are proactive in nature and that they often produce rapid behavior change (Carr, Robinson, Taylor, & Carlson, 1990). In addition, antecedent and curriculum-based interventions can be designed such that alternative, prosocial behaviors replace problem behaviors. By identifying and developing appropriate and functional skills, successful adjustment is increased, and problem behavior is decreased.

## INCREASING PERSONAL CONTROL AND CHOICE

A third theme that is gaining increasing attention in the literature on nonaversive behavior management has to do with the extent to which people with disabilities are able to exert control over their environment. This theme may be summarized as follows: (1) People with autism and similar disabilities typically have few opportunities and few capabilities for controlling their surroundings in acceptable ways, (2) many problem behaviors can be viewed as efforts to control or manipulate circumstances in the environment, and (3) if a person's opportunities and capabilities for controlling the environment in acceptable ways are increased, there should be concomitant decreases in the occurrence of problem behaviors. This theme, of course, has great pertinence to the enhancement of personal lifestyles, but in this chapter the concern is principally with the ways in which personal control and the effective expression of preferences can influence the occurrence of problem behavior.

Many authors have noted in recent years that the lives of people with severe disabilities are characterized by very little choice over events that affect their daily lives (O'Brien, 1987; Shevin & Klein, 1984). It is typical that people with severe disabilities have virtually no say about such things as with whom they associate, where they live, where they work, or what they do for recreation. Choices tend to be very limited, even with regard to relatively minor concerns such as the sequence with which routines are completed, what to eat for breakfast, what to wear to school, how long to stay in bed, or what activity to engage in for exercise. People with severe disabilities tend to live lives that are passive in the sense that they are provided few options and rarely make decisions or even participate in the process of social decision making.

The observation that problem behaviors can be interpreted as attempts to control the environment is supported by substantial research, much of which concerns the delineation of specific functions, or purposes, that govern the behavior problem. For example, many instances of problem behavior have been related to the attention that the behavior evokes (Iwata et al., 1982; Lovaas & Simmons, 1969). In these instances, the problem behavior "controls" the actions of other people by securing their attention. Other occurrences of problem behavior have been identified as serving to terminate (or escape) an unpleasant activitity (Carr, Newsom, & Binkoff, 1976; Weeks & Gaylord-Ross, 1981). In such situations, the behavior problem "controls" or arranges the environment in such a way that the disliked activity is no longer present. Several other controlling functions have been described (e.g., Donnellan, Mirenda, Mesaros, & Fassbender, 1984); however the essential point is that this body of research has shown that when a problem behavior is successful in changing the environment in a particular and predictable manner, that behavior is reinforced and thus maintained. Conversely, if the problem behavior is ineffective in predictably controlling the environment, the behavior will extinguish. This, of course, is a perspective that has occupied the field of behavior management for many years. Current orientations, however, have altered the manner with which this perspective is applied. In particular, the motivation for controlling a person's environment has been endowed with greater legitimacy, and an emphasis has been placed on procedures for empowering people to exercise control in more acceptable and adaptive ways.

Two features characterize these procedures. The first is that the procedures develop and/or encourage communicative responses that may operate on (or control) the social environment, and the second is that the procedures provide assurance that the communicative responses do, in fact, work regularly to produce the desired control. The literature describes two sets of procedural operations, both of which share the above features: functional communication training and choice making.

## Functional Communication Training

Functional communication training (Carr & Durand, 1985; Durand, 1990) is a process through which the function of a particular problem behavior is identified and then a functionally equivalent, communicative alternative is established and reinforced. The process begins with a functional assessment that specifies the purpose of the problem behavior (Carr, Robinson, & Palumbo, 1990; Lennox & Mitlenberger, 1989). Although the purpose is always assumed to be some kind of controlling function, the specific function varies across people and contexts (Haring & Kennedy, 1990). When the function is identified, a communicative alternative is selected that has the potential for controlling the environment in a way that is functionally equivalent to the problem behavior (Carr, 1988).

For example, if a difficult task evokes hitting and kicking because aggression has been effective in removing task demands, then a functionally equivalent expression might be for the person to communicate, "I want a break," or "I need assistance because the task is too difficult." The form of the communication depends upon the abilities of the person. Some people might be taught to use speech, whereas others might be taught to use a manual sign, gesture, or idiographic picture card. The main point is that the expression must communicate the message (and exert the control) that was conveyed by the problem behavior. After the communicative topography is established, measures must be taken to insure that the message is indeed funcitonal; that is, the communication must work effectively to produce predictable changes in the behavior of other people. If the communicative alternative is effective and efficient, there is a probability that the use of the alternative will increase and that the problem behavior will be reduced (Horner, Sprague, O'Brien, & Heathfield, 1990). In this manner, the person's problem behavior is decreased because the person is given the means, the opportunity, and the power for increased control over her or his surroundings.

## Preference and Choice Making

A second set of operations that relate to control has to do with expressions of preference and choice making. Reasearch in this area has shown that people with severe and profound disabilities (including autism) can (1) learn to express preferences among stimuli when provided with concrete choice options (e.g., Dyer, 1987; Green, Reid, White, Halford, Brittain, & Gardner, 1988; Wacker, Wiggens, Fowler, & Berg, 1988); (2) perform more successfully when they make choices among preferred rewards (Dyer, Dunlap, & Winterling, 1990); and (3) display reduced levels of problem behaviors when they are provided opportunities to select choices from menus of rewards and/or task activities (Dunlap et al., 1991; Dyer et al., 1990; Parsons, Reid, Reynolds, & Bumgarner, 1990).

Systematic assessments of preference have been demonstrated to be important in identifying reinforcing stimuli for people whose disablilities prevent them from volunteering such information through speech or other commonly interpreted means (e.g., Green et al., 1988; Pace, Ivancic, Edwards, Iwata, & Page, 1985; Parsons & Reid, 1990). These assessments typically involve presenting various stimuli (e.g., foods, toys) and observing whether some preference is indicated through approach responses, smiles, or other displays of positive affect. Those stimuli that are associated with the most positive of these indications are then used as rewards. Systematic assessments of reinforcers have been found to be more effective than arbitrary reinforcer selections and, in fact, have been shown to be more accurate than the opinions of caregiving staff (Green et al., 1988). An important aspect of this type of assessment is that, in effect, the choice of rewards is made by the person whose behavior is to be rewarded. In an extension of this line of research with students described as autistic, Dyer (1987) demonstrated that reinforcers selected on the basis of the students' preference were associated with reduced levels of stereotypic responding.

Dyer and her associates (1990) conducted a study to examine the influence of choice-making opportunities on the seriously disruptive behavior of students with autism and mental retardation. In this study, three learners who exhibitied aggression, self-injury, and tantrums were exposed to instructional activities in two experimental conditions. In one of the conditions, the students were asked to work on tasks that were selected by the teachers. When the students were successful, they earned rewards that were also identified by the teacher. In the choice-making condition, the same tasks and rewards were available, but in this phase the students were allowed to select which tasks they would work on and which rewards they would earn.

The investigation produced a number of interesting results. First, the choice-making condition was consistently associated with reduced levels of problem behaviors. This outcome was especially clear with the more serious behavior problems, such as physical aggression. The data from the choice-making condition also showed that the students varied their selections; that is, they did not perseverate on a specific task or reward. Finally, it is important to note that the students' rates of correct responding were approximately equal across the two conditions. In other words, the students were as productive in the choice condition as they were in the no-choice condition.

Although the results of Dyer et al. (1990) are encouraging, there is still little empirical information regarding the effects of increased choice making on the behavior of people with autism and other severe disabilities. It is possible that too much latitude could lead to deleterious outcomes if options are not managed in a responsible manner. For example, it is probable that many people, if given the opportunity, would choose to avoid difficult school or work activities in favor of preferred recreation or "free" time. Clearly, there must be some restriction on the range of choices available (as there are for all people). A challenge for research has to do with expanding methods for providing choices and for increasing the control that people with disabilities have over their own environments. Part of this challenge will involve an optimal balance between the enhancement of choice making and insurance that people with disabilities receive productive educational/habilitative programming (Bannerman, Sheldon, Sherman, & Harchik, 1990).

Although there are many questions to be resolved, the connection between control (e.g., choice making) and the occurrence of problem behaviors is a phenomenon that has been demonstrated repeatedly and that has important implications for nonaversive intervention. As we have discussed, investigations have shown that procedures designed to empower people to exert greater control over their surroundings are associated with reduced levels of problem behavior. This message is essential because it indicates a strategy of behavior management that is not only effective and nonaversive but is also habilitative and respectful of a person's rights to live with a measure of dignity and autonomy.

## SUMMARY

Nonaversive intervention is a complex assortment of behavioral supports that is guided by an emphasis on dignity and a commitment to lifestyle enrichment for people with disabilities. In this chapter, we have attempted to summarize the current basis for nonaversive intervention. We have stressed the importance of functional assessment and the need to use empirical information as a guide for designing behavioral programs. The increasing role of antecedent manipulations and opportunities for choice making were discussed as developments and illustrations of the proactive alternatives to restrictive programming. We have also emphasized that the behavior problems of persons with autism can be quite complex and may require extensive preintervention analysis. Finally, it is important to emphasize that the breadth of nonaversive options will continue to expand with increasing research and innovative assistance for people with autism and related disabilities.

ACKNOWLEDGMENT

Preparation of this manuscript was supported by Cooperative Agreement No. G0087C0234 from the National Institute on Disability and Rehabilitation Research. However, the opinions are those of the authors, and no official endorsement should be inferred.

## REFERENCES

Bannerman, D. J. Sheldon, J. B., Sherman, J. A., & Harchik, A. E. (1990). Balancing the right to habilitation with the right to personal liberties: The rights of people with developmental disabilities to eat too many doughnuts and take a nap. *Journal of Applied Behavior Analysis, 23,* 79–89.

Berkman, K. A., & Meyer, L. H. (1988). Alternative strategies and multiple outcomes in the remediation of severe self-injury: Going "all out" nonaversively. *Journal of the Association for Persons with Severe Handicaps, 13,* 76–86.

Carr, E. G. (1977). The motivation of self-injurious behavior: A review of some hypotheses. *Psychological Bulletin, 84,* 800–81616.

Carr, E. G. (1988). Functional equivalence as a mechanism for response maintenance. In R. H. Horner, G. Dunlap, & R. L. Koegel (Eds.), *Generalization and maintenance: Lifestyle changes in applied settings* (pp. 221–241). Baltimore: Paul Brookes.

Carr, E. G., & Durand, V. M. (1985). Reducing behavior problems through functional communication training. *Journal of Applied Behavior Analysis, 18,* 111–1226.

Carr, E. G., Newsom, C. D., & Binkoff, J. (1976). Stimulus control of self-destructive behavior in a psychotic child. *Journal of Abnormal Child Psychology, 4,* 139–153.

Carr, E. G., Robinson, S., & Palumbo, L. W. (1990). The wrong issue: Aversive versus nonaversive treatment. The right issue: Functional versus nonfunctional treatment. In A. C. Repp & N. N. Singh (Eds.), *Perspectives on the use of nonaversive and aversive interventions for persons with developmental disabilities* (pp. 362–379). Sycamore, IL: Sycamore Press.

Carr, E. G., Robinson, S., Taylor, J. C., & Carlson, J. I. (1990). Positive approaches to the treatment of severe behavior problems in persons with developmental disabilities: A review and analysis of reinforcement and stimulus-based procedures. *Monograph of the Association for Persons with Severe Handicaps, Number 4.* Seattle, WA: TASH.

Cooper, J. O., Heron, T. E., & Heward, W. L. (1987). *Applied behavior analysis.* Columbus, OH: Merrill.

Donnellan, A. M., Mirenda, P. L., Mesaros, R. A., & Fassbender, L. L. (1984). Analyzing the communicative functions of aberrant behavior. *Journal of the Association for Persons with Severe Handicaps, 2,* 201–212.

Dunlap, G. (1984). The influence of task variation and maintenance tasks on the learning and affect of autistic children. *Journal of Experimental Child Psychology, 37,* 41–64.

Dunlap, G., Ferro, J., & dePerczel, M. (in press). Nonaversive behavioral intervention in the community. In E. Cipani & F. Spooner (Eds.), *Curricular and instructional approaches for persons with severe handicaps.* New York: Allyn & Bacon.

Dunlap, G., Johnson, L. F., & Robbins, F. R. (1990). Preventing serious behavior problems through skill development and early intervention. In A. C. Repp & N. N. Singh (Eds.), *Perspectives on the use of nonaversive and aversive interventions for persons with developmental disabilities* (pp. 273–286). Sycamore, IL: Sycamore Press.

Dunlap, G., Kern-Dunlap, L., Clarke, S., & Robbins, F. R. (1991). Functional assessment, curricular revision, and severe behavior problems. *Journal of Applied Behavior Analysis, 24,* 387–397.

Durand, V. M. (1990). *Functional communication training: An intervention program for severe behavior problems.* New York: Guilford.

Durand, V. M., & Crimmins, D. B. (1988). Identifying the variables maintaining self-injurious behavior. *Journal of Autism and Developmental Disorders, 18,* 99–117.

Dyer, K. (1987). The competition of autistic stereotyped behavior with usual and specially assessed reinforcers. *Research in Developmental Disabilities, 8,* 607–626.

Dyer, K., Dunlap, G., & Winterling, V. (1990). The effects of choice-making on the serious problem behaviors of students with developmental disabilities. *Journal of Applied Behavior Analysis, 23,* 515–524.

Evans, I. M. & Meyer, L. H. (1985). *An educative approach to behavior problems.* Baltimore: Paul H. Brookes.

Gardner, W. I., & Cole, C. L. (1984). Aggression and related conduct difficulties in the mentally retarded: A multicomponent behavior model. In S. E. Breuning, J. L. Matson, & R. P. Barrett (Eds.), *Advances in mental retardation and developmental disabilities* (Vol. 2, pp. 41–84). Greenwich, CT: JAI.

Gaylord-Ross, R. (1982). Curricular considerations in treating behavior problems of severely handicapped students. In K. D. Gadow & T. Bialer (Eds.), *Advances in learning and behavioral disorders* (Vol. 1, pp. 193–224). Greenwich, CT: JAI,.

Green, C. W., Reid, D. H., White, L. K., Halford, R. C., Brittain, D. P., & Gardner, S. M. (1988).

Identifying reinforcers for persons with profound handicaps: Staff opinion versus systematic assessment of preferences. *Journal of Applied Behavior Analysis, 21,* 31–43.

Guess, D., Helmstetter, E., Turnbull, H. R., & Knowlton, S. (1987). *Use of aversive procedures with persons who are disabled: An historical review and critical analysis.* Seattle: The Association for Persons with Severe Handicaps.

Haring, T. G., & Kennedy, C. H. (1990). Contextual control of problem behavior in students with severe disabilities. *Journal of Applied Behavior Analysis, 23,* 235–243.

Horner, R. H., & Budd, C. M. (1985). Teaching manual sign language to a nonverbal student: Generalization of sign use and collateral reduction of maladaptive behavior. *Education and Training of the Mentally Retarded, 20,* 39–47.

Horner, R. H., Day, M., Sprague, J., O'Brien, M., & Heathfield, L. T. (1991). Interspersed requests: A nonaversive procedure for decreasing aggression and self-injury during instruction. *Journal of Applied Behavior Analysis, 24,* 265–278.

Horner, R. H., & Dunlap, G. (Eds.). (1988). *Behavior Managment and Community Integration for Individuals with Developmental Disabilities and Severe Behavior Problems.* A monograph of the Research and Training Center on Community-Referenced Behavior Management, Eugene, OR: University of Oregon.

Horner R. H., Dunlap, G., Koegel, R. L., Carr, E. G., Sailor, W., Anderson, J., Albin, R. W., & O'Neill, R. E. (1990). Toward a technology of "nonaversive" behavioral support. *Journal of the Association for Persons with Severe Handicaps, 15,* 125–132.

Horner, R. H. Sprague, J. R., O'Brien, M., & Heathfield, L. T. (1990). The role of response efficiency in the reduction of problem behaviors through functional equivalence training: A case study. *Journal of the Association for Persons with Severe Handicaps, 15,* 91–97.

Iwata, B. A. (1988). The development and adoption of controversial default technologies. *The Behavior Analyst, 11,* 149–157.

Iwata, B. A., Dorsey, M. F., Slifer, K. J., Bauman, K. E., & Richman, G. S. (1982). Toward a functional analysis of self-injury. *Analysis and Intervention in Developmental Disabilities, 2,* 1–20.

Iwata, B. A., Vollmer, T. R., & Zarcone, J. H. (1990). The experimental (functional) analysis of behavior disorders: Methodology, applications, and limitations. In A. C. Repp & N. N. Singh (Eds.), *Perspectives on the use of nonaversive and aversive interventions for persons with developmental disabilities* (pp. 301–330). Sycamore, IL: Sycamore Press.

Koegel, R. L., & Koegel, L. K. (1990). Extended reductions in stereotypic behavior of students with autism through a self-management treatment package. *Journal of Applied Behavior Analysis, 23,* 119–127.

LaVigna, G. W., & Donnellan, A. M. (1986). *Alternatives to punishment: Solving behavior problems with nonaversive strategies.* New York: Irvington.

LaVigna, G. W., Willis, T. J., & Donnellan, A. M. (1989). The role of positive programming in behavioral treatment. In E. Cipani (Ed.), *The treatment of severe behavior disorders* (pp. 59–83). Washington, DC: American Association on Mental Retardation.

Lennox, D. B., & Miltenberger, R. G. (1989). Conducting a functional assessment of problem behavior in applied settings. *Journal of the Association for Persons with Severe Handicaps, 14,* 304–311.

Lovaas, O. I., & Simmons, J. Q. (1969). Manipulation of self-destruction in three retarded children. *Journal of Applied Behavior Analysis, 2,* 143–1557.

McAfee, J. K. (1987). Classroom density and the aggressive behavior of handicapped children. *Education and Treatment of Children, 10,* 134–145.

Meyer, L. H., & Evans, I. M. (1989). *Nonaversive intervention for behavior problems: A manual for home and community.* Baltimore: Paul H. Brookes.

Mulick, J. A. (1990). The ideology and science of punishment in mental retardation. *American Journal on Mental Retardation, 95,* 142–156.

National Institutes of Health. (1990). Treatment of destructive behaviors in persons with developmental disabilities (consensus development statement). *Journal of Autism and Developmental Disorders, 20,* 403–429.

O'Brien, J. (1987). A guide to lifestyle planning: Using the Activities Catalog to integrate services and natural support systems. In B. Wilcox & G. T. Bellamy (Eds.), *A comprehensive guide to the Activities Catalog* (pp. 175–189). Baltimore: Paul Brookes.

O'Neill, R. E., Horner, R. H., Albin, R. W., Storey, K., & Sprague, J. R. (1990). *Functional analysis: A practical assessment guide.* Sycamore, IL: Sycamore Press.

Pace, G., Ivancic, M., Edwards, G., Iwata, B., & Page, T. (1985). Assessment of stimulus preferences and reinforcer values with profoundly retarded individuals. *Journal of Applied Behavior Analysis, 18,* 249–255.

Parsons, M. B., & Reid, D. H. (1990). Assessing food preferences among persons with profound mental retardation: Providing opportunities to make choices. *Journal of Applied Behavior Analysis, 23,* 183–195.

Parsons, M. B., Reid, D. H., Reynolds, J., & Bumgarner, M. (1990). Effects of chosen versus assigned jobs on the work performance of persons with severe handicaps. *Journal of Applied Behavior Analysis, 23,* 253–258.

Repp, A. C., & Singh, N. N. (Eds.). (1990). *Perspectives on the use of nonaversive and aversive interventions for persons with developmental disabilities.* Sycamore, IL: Sycamore Press.

Rincover, A. (1978). Sensory extinction: A procedure for eliminating self-stimulatory behavior in psychotic children. *Journal of Abnormal Child Psychology, 6,* 299–310.

Russo, D. C., Cataldo, M. F., & Cushing, P. J. (1981). Compliance training and behavioral covariation in the treatment of multiple behavior problems. *Journal of Applied Behavior Analysis, 1,* 21–35.

Santarcangelo, S., Dyer, K., & Luce, S. C. (1987). Generalized reduction of disruptive behavior in unsupervised settings through specific toy training. *Journal of the Association for Persons with Severe Handicaps, 12,* 38–44.

Shapiro, E. S., & Klein, R. D. (1980). Self-management of classroom behavior with retarded/disturbed children. *Behavior Modification, 4,* 83–97.

Shevin, M., & Klein, N. K. (1984). The importance of choice-making skills for students with severe disabilities. *Journal of the Association for Persons with Severe Handicaps, 9,* 159–166.

Singer, G. H. S., Singer, J., & Horner, R. H. (1987). Using pretask requests to increase the probability of compliance for students with severe disabilities. *Journal of the Association for Persons with Severe Handicaps, 12*(4), 287–291.

Steege, M. W., Wacker, D. P., Berg, W. K., Cigrand, K. K., & Cooper, L. J. (1989). The use of behavioral assessment to prescribe and evaluate treatments for severely handicapped children. *Journal of Applied Behavior Analysis, 22,* 23–33.

Touchette, P. E., MacDonald, R. F., & Langer, S. N. (1985). A scatter plot for identifying stimulus control of problem behavior. *Journal of Applied Behavior Analysis, 18,* 343–351.

Turnbull, A. P., & Turnbull, H. R. (1990). A tale about lifestyle changes: Comments on "Toward a technology of 'nonaversive' behavioral support." *Journal of the Association for Persons with Severe Handcaps, 15,* 142–144.

Wacker, D., Steege, M., Northup, J. Reimers, T., Berg, W., & Sasso, G. (1990). Use of functional analysis and acceptability measures to assess and treat severe behavior problems: An outpatient clinic model. In A Repp & N. N. Singh (Eds.), *Perspectives on the use of nonaversive and e interventions for persons with developmental disabilities* (pp. 331–348). Sycamore, IL: Sycamore Press.

Wacker, D. P., Wiggins, B., Fowler, M., & Berg, W. K. (1988). Training students with profound or multiple handicaps to make requests via microswitches. *Journal of Applied Behavior Analysis, 21,* 331–343.

Wahler, R. G., & Graves, M. G. (1983). Setting events in social networks: Ally or enemy in child behavior therapy. *Behavior Therapy, 14,* 19–36.

Weeks, M., & Gaylord-Ross, R. (1981). Task difficulty and aberrant behavior in severely handicapped students. *Journal of Applied Behavior Analysis, 14,* 449–463.

Winterling, V., Dunlap, G., & O'Neill, R. (1987). The influence of task variation on the aberrant behavior of autistic students. *Education and Treatment of Children, 10,* 105–119.

# 13

# The Eden Decision Model

## A Decision Model with Practical Applications for the Development of Behavior Decelerative Strategies

PETER F. GERHARDT and DAVID L. HOLMES

## INTRODUCTION

Individuals with developmental disabilities have tremendous needs and often require intensive, lifelong intervention (Schopler & Mesibov, 1983) in such diverse areas as self-care and related life skills, functional communication skills, social skills, independent living skills (e.g., bill paying), and the use of adaptive work or mobility devices. Behavioral and educational methods of training have been found to be most effective in this effort (Schopler, Mesibov, & Baker, 1982). In addition, there is often the need to reduce certain dangerous or problematic behaviors.

In contrast to the need to develop life-relevant skills, this latter need has resulted in great controversy (e.g., Gardner, 1989; Gerhardt et al., 1992; Griffith, 1986; Guess, Helmstetter, Turnbull, & Knowlton, 1987; Holmes & Gerhardt, 1989; LaVigna & Donnellan, 1986; Van Houten, Axelrod, Baily, Favell, Foxx, Iwata, & Lovaas, 1988) between proponents of nonaversive interventions and proponents of "full-range behavior modification" (D. L. Holmes, personal communication, 1990). These latter professionals, including the present authors, concur with Schopler (1990) in his assertion that "optimum individualized treatment

PETER F. GERHARDT and DAVID L. HOLMES • The Eden Services, 1 Logan Drive, Princeton, New Jersey 08540.

*Behavioral Issues in Autism*, edited by Eric Schopler and Gary B. Mesibov. New York, Plenum Press, 1994.

for each child is best determined by parent and professional collaboration and consideration of the best available specific treatment options" (p. 10). The intent of this discussion, however, is not to present a comprehensive analysis of this controversy. Instead, the focus is on the one component óf the debate on which there exists agreement between proponents of the conflicting arguments; that is, the need to conduct a comprehensive functional analysis of the problematic behavior prior to the implementation of any intervention strategy, aversive or nonaversive.

Previous authors (e.g., Evans & Myer, 1985; Groden, 1989; O'Neill et al., 1990; Parrish, Iwata, Dorsey, Bunck, & Silfer, 1985; Touchette, MacDonald, & Langer, 1985) have proposed strategies for the development of a functional analysis in both the clinical and the applied setting. The Eden Decision Model (EDM), expands upon some of these earlier frameworks in data collection and assessment by utilizing staff perceptions as to the function of a particular behavior as the impetus behind the development of a data-based functional analysis along five interrelated but distinct components: (1) determination of need; (2) analysis of environmental conditions (3) analysis of curricular conditions; (4) differential reinforcement; and (5) analysis of behavior maintenance conditions—development of an aversive decelerative procedure.

## COMPONENT I—DETERMINATION OF NEED

Component I of the EDM, as depicted in Figure 1, calls for a data-based determination of need. This is necessary in order to validate subjective perceptions that an identified behavioral excess warrants attention as it is (1) harmful to the individual or to others; (2) highly interfering with the work or learning process; or (3) restricting the individual's access to the community in some significant way.

Determination of need is achieved by first defining the identified behavior in operational terms. Any behavior is an observable event and, as such, can be described in terms that are concrete, factual, and free from inferences (Powers & Handleman, 1984). The definition must also meet the criteria of objectivity and clarity as demonstrated by measurable reliability. Failure to define a behavior in accurate operational terms results in diminished reliability in the identification of the behavior, reducing the consistency with which the behavior may be addressed. Ultimately, this can only result in the failure of any intervention strategy.

Following the development of the operational definition, the determination of need process requires that a baseline, or preintervention, measure be recorded. The exact length and topography of the baseline (e.g., time sample, frequency count, durational analysis, interresponse time, etc.) is, in large part, a factor of the nature of the defined behavior (Foster, Bell-Dolan, & Burge, 1988). Reliability measures,

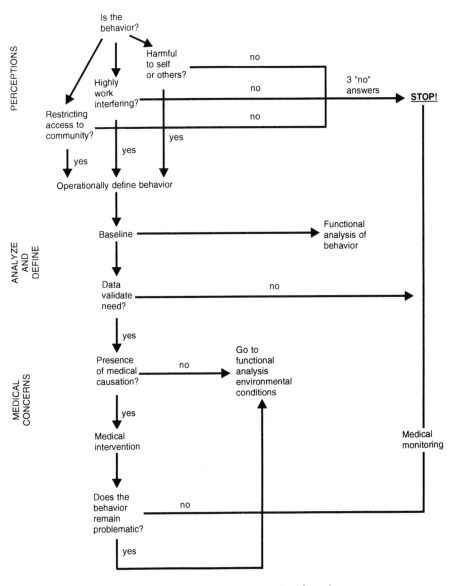

Fig. 1. Component I—Determination of Need

recorded throughout the baseline, ensure the accuracy of the data. A well-developed baseline procedure provides for a reliable quantitative representation of a stable rate of responding of a defined behavior over time.

## Baseline Recording and the Applied Functional Analysis

In applied settings, a truly clinical functional analysis (e.g., Iwata, Dorsey, Slifer, Bauman, & Richman, 1982) of the defined behavior may not always be practical or possible. In such instances, the EDM employs an applied functional analysis in conjunction with the baseline procedure. The direction and scope of the applied functional analysis or baseline procedure is one drawn from staff perceptions as to the function of the behavior and a review of the questions posed in the five components of the EDM.

For example, should perceptions suggest that the behavior was primarily maintained as an attempt to control a noisy, distracting environment, data collection during the applied functional analysis or baseline procedure might focus on such concerns as number of people in the environment, noise level in the environment, presence or absence of idiosyncratic distractors, and an assessment of the individuals' ability to appropriately control the level of activity in their environment. Different perceptions would result in a data-collection process focusing on entirely different areas of potential behavioral correlates suggested by the EDM.

For the EDM, the applied functional analysis or baseline procedure incorporates two complementary strategies. The first is the scatter plot recording system as described by Touchette, MacDonald and Langer (1985). Using this system, data may be quickly and reliably coded as a factor of any two variables of interest (e.g., noise level and number of people in environment). Although most behavioral excesses will require more than one coded assessment to even partially determine their function, the scatter plot system appears to remain relatively efficient for the purposes of the EDM. Secondly, an anecdotal log or A-B-C (antecedent–behavior–consequence) analysis (Bijou, Peterson, Harris, Allen, & Johnson, 1969) is suggested as a complementary procedure throughout the applied functional analysis or baseline period. Information recorded in this log may include descriptions of the various environmental conditions (i.e., place, activity, other staff or clients in area, etc.) that, although not being coded as part of the scatter plot system, may be associated with the defined behavior as well as information regarding which conditions appear to not be associated with the behavior. Other potentially relevant information such as hours of sleep, appetite, meal content, perceived affect, and clothes worn may also be recorded as part of this ongoing log. Both strategies should be extended as long as necessary to initially obtain stable and accurate information and, later, significant reductions in the defined behavior.

This period of analysis, it should be noted, is not necessarily a period free from interaction or even intervention. Positive reinforcement, corrective feedback, and prompting should continue so as not to interrupt the teaching or learning process. In addition, in the case of severe aggressive or self-injurious behaviors, interventions intended as "crisis management" including response interruption, blocking, or restraint may be necessary in order to ensure the safety of the individual during the analysis.

If the applied functional analysis or baseline data fail to validate the perceptions that the defined behavior warrants the development of an intervention strategy (i.e., the behavior does not occur frequently or with enough severity to be dangerous, interfere with work or learning, or significantly restrict community access), the EDM process is discontinued. If the converse is true and the data confirms the perceptions, the EDM assessment continues.

## Medical Concerns

As part of the initial analysis, the EDM calls for an evaluation of the possibility that the defined behavior may be the result of an untreated medical condition (Gunsett, Mulick, Fernald, & Martin, 1989). Inquiry of this nature is considered of specific importance in cases where the defined behavior (1) is new to the individual's behavioral repertoire; (2) is actually a significant increase in a previously identified behavior; or (3) appears to be somewhat independent of external reinforcing conditions or stimuli. Possible medical conditions to be evaluated include, gastric disturbances or ulcers, constipation, ear infections, or headaches, allergies, dental problems, and so on.

It bears noting that rarely will the data collected during analysis provide a clear indication of a potential medical causation. A good deal of data interpretation is often necessary. For example, gastric problems may be indicated by an increased behavioral frequency within 1½ hours before or after meals, with possibly, certain meals producing a greater response than others. A similar behavior pattern, however, may also be indicative of very distinct food preferences, may be in response to the increased activity in the environment during meal times, or may be related to other events or activities scheduled around meal times. In any case, all potential medical causes (such as listed in Table 1) need to be investigated and eliminated before any other intervention strategy can be developed or implemented.

If a medical causation is identified and an effective medical intervention is implemented, the EDM assessment stops while ensuring the availability of on-

Table 1. Component I—Intervention Strategies

| Data-based conclusion that defined behavior is not problematic |
|---|
| Medical interventions related to: |
| Presence of body aches (ear infections, headaches, etc.) |
| Allergies |
| Colds or flu |
| Gastric problems |
| Constipation |
| Physical insult (cuts, abrasions, blisters, etc.) |
| Dental problems |
| Difficulties associated with menstruation, etc. |

going medical monitoring. If no medical causation is discovered, or if an appropriate medical intervention has been implemented but the defined behavior remains problematic (i.e., is maintained through external reinforcement conditions), the EDM requires a stepwise analysis of the data collected during the applied functional analysis or baseline procedure. The first level of analysis, if appropriate, is Component II—Functional Analysis of Environmental Conditions.

## COMPONENT II—FUNCTIONAL ANALYSIS OF ENVIRONMENTAL CONDITIONS

Once the need for the development of an intervention strategy has been determined, the EDM provides for an analysis of any data collected relevant to the conditions present in the physical environment that may be associated with the display of the defined behavior. In order to design intervention strategies that are appropriate and effective, there needs to be an awareness of the various characteristics of the physical environment that may predict the presence or absence of such a behavior (Simpson & Regan, 1986). As shown in Figure 2, Component II of the EDM calls for an assessment of both the characteristics of the physical environment (primary and secondary environmental considerations) as well as the individual's ability to respond to these conditions (interaction considerations).

### Primary Environmental Considerations

In assessing the primary environmental conditions, the core question presented by the EDM is "Is the individual's environment physically uncomfortable?" Particular attention is to be given to such conditions as heat, light, and other environmental necessities such as correctly fitting clothing, the level of physical

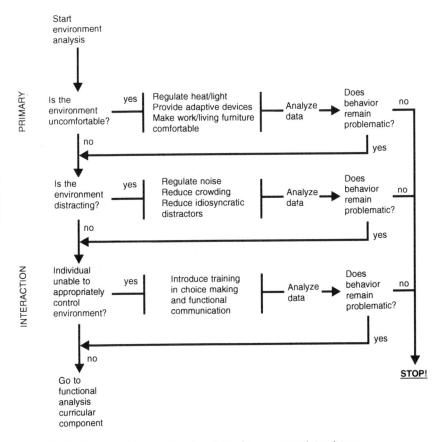

Fig. 2. Component II—Functional Analysis of Environmental Conditions

comfort present in the work or living area (i.e., wood or cloth furniture as opposed to metal furniture), and the availability of necessary adaptive devices.

Some of the relevant information available from the applied functional analysis or baseline data at this point could include whether or not the defined behavior occurs more frequently in a certain room or area (e.g., by a drafty window), in response to physically challenging situations (e.g., fine motor tasks), or when the individual is not in possession of a preferred item (i.e., dressed in a nonpreferred manner or served a nonpreferred meal). Possible intervention strategies at this point range from the simple (i.e., moving the individual away from the drafty window or not serving a particular meal) to the slightly more complex (i.e., developing functional adaptive devices and training clients in their use).

## Secondary Environmental Considerations

The EDM defines secondary environmental conditions as those that may distract or confuse the individual. These would include excessive noise, over-crowding, or a cluttered work space. In addition, potentially confusing or inconsistent staff interactions that may be associated with the display of the behavior are assessed as a secondary environmental condition.

As before, information obtained during the applied functional analysis or baseline procedure should provide an indication as to the potential relationship between these conditions and the behavior. Intervention strategies related to secondary environmental considerations would include the regulation, to the extent possible, of noise or overcrowding; the control of idiosyncratic distractors (e.g., music, presence or absence of preferred reinforcers); and staff training on the importance of appropriate and consistent staff–client interactions. A systematic evaluation of the basic environmental conditions associated with a particular behavior can result in a number of relatively simple strategies and environmental modifications through which the behavior may be reduced (Hart & Risley, 1976).

## Environmental Interaction Considerations

The environmental interaction considerations of Component II go beyond the actual physical conditions of the environment and assess the ability of each individual to effectively and appropriately respond to these conditions. In other words, "Can the individual communicate his/her responses to the environment in a functional and appropriate manner?" As communication skills appear to interact to some degree with the development and maintenance of all other skills, the expansion of an individual's limited communication repertoire is essential if long-term successful programming for an individual is to be provided (Donnellan, Mirenda, Mesaros, & Fassbender, 1984). This expansion may be accomplished through the development and implementation of teaching programs that introduce the use of functional communicative alternatives (e.g., Differential Reinforcement of Communicative Behaviors—DRC) to the defined behavior. As functional communicative alternatives are made available, the need for the continued display of the behavior may be reduced (Carr & Durand, 1985).

Examples of relevant information available from the applied functional analysis or baseline procedure would include indications of whether the behavior occurs more frequently in high-demand situations; whether it occurs more frequently during periods of low available reinforcement or attention; whether it occurs in response to frustrated needs or desires (e.g., someone else has an individual's personal property); or whether the behavior occurs more frequently in response to situations where the individual is unable to exercise control (e.g., scheduling changes, meal choices, etc.). Primary intervention strategies include the teaching of the appropriate communicative response (i.e., "help," "I want _____," "pay attention to me," or "go away"). The introduction of choice-making training, delayed reinforcement (tolerance) training, relaxation training, and the development of schedules that afford the individual opportunity for input into his/her daily routine may be additional effective intervention strategies at this point.

Following a completed analysis of the environmental conditions and the implementation of any related intervention strategies, such as those listed in Table 2, the defined behavior is examined relative to baseline rates. Should the data indicate that the behavior has been significantly reduced, the EDM assessment stops, and current intervention strategies proceed while monitored. If the behavior has not been significantly reduced, the EDM process may require additional analysis; that of potential curricular or demand correlates to the behavior. This is the intent of Component III—Functional Analysis of the Curricular Component.

It should be noted that although the format of the EDM, as presented in this text, is as an assessment tool where continuation from one component to the next based on an examination of the data associated with a particular strategy, a more functional and practical use of the EDM may lie in the development of multi-element intervention packages designed to address more than one aspect of an individual's environment at one time. An example of the EDM used in this manner is presented in the accompanying case study.

Table 2. Component II—Intervention Strategies

| |
|---|
| Provide necessary light or heat as indicated |
| Provide necessary adaptive devices and training in their use |
| Provide comfortable work/living furniture |
| Regulate noise |
| Reduce crowded conditions |
| Reduce idiosyncratic distractors |
| Provide preferred, idiosyncratic environmental conditions preferred clothes, music, arrangement of work materials, etc. |
| Provide task and reinforcer choices |
| Introduce Functional Communication Training |
|     Yes/no |
|     Stop |
|     Help |
|     Pay attention to me |
|     Requests for preferred items or activities, etc. |

## COMPONENT III—FUNCTIONAL ANALYSIS OF THE CURRICULAR COMPONENT

The completion of a functional analysis of the environmental conditions along with the implementation of any associated intervention strategies helps ensure an environment that is capable of maintaining appropriate, adaptive behavioral responding. If the defined behavior remains problematic, in Figure 3 the EDM calls for an analysis of the individual's curriculum as it may relate to the defined behavior. Although they may not be viewed as behavior management tools, educational planning, assessment, and implementation are crucial for developing functional skills and supplanting time otherwise invested in nonfunctional or problematic behaviors (Simpson, Regan, Sasso, & Noll, 1986).

The core question in the analysis of the curricular component is, "Does a task precipitate the behavior?" The answer, as before, is referenced to the data collected (based on staff perceptions) during the applied functional analysis or baseline

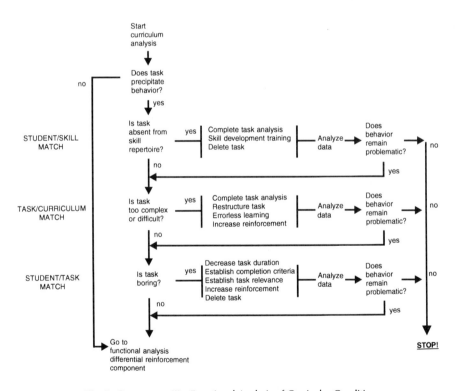

Fig. 3. Component III—Functional Analysis of Curricular Conditions

procedure. If a task(s) does precipitate the display of the behavior, the EDM proposes the development of an appropriate intervention strategy based on the examination of the following three programmatic "matches": (1) individual-to-skill match; (2) task-to-curriculum match; and (3) individual-to-task match.

## Individual-to-Skill Match

In assessing the individual-to-skill match, the primary concern is whether or not a particular skill is present in an individual's response repertoire. For the purposes of the EDM, skill is defined as being present if it can be reliably displayed with minimal prompting across environments. An easy, but often false, assumption is that an individual will have a particular skill in their repertoire because they possess similar skills or may even have displayed the skill itself on occasion. Relevant data obtained during the EDM assessment process could include the identification of specific tasks associated with the behavior, durational assessments, and formal skill assessments or inventories.

If a skill cannot be documented as present, an intervention strategy based on teaching the skill or its prerequisite components should be developed. In some cases, another alternative would be to delete the problematic task from the individual's programmatics. Two cautions must be noted with regard to task deletion. First, task deletion must be accomplished in an way that does not inadvertently negatively reinforce (through termination of an unpleasant task contingent on the behavior) the behavior. Second, prior to task deletion, a determination must be made that the deleted task is not one that is essential for the future independent functioning of the individual. For example, although a color-matching program might be a candidate for deletion, a toothbrushing program would not.

## Task-to-Curriculum Match

The second match is the task-to-curriculum match that asks, "Does a task, when assessed in the context of an individual's current curriculum, appear to be of significantly greater complexity or difficulty than the remainder of the curriculum tasks?" For example, is a sustained effort of up to ½ hour required for the problem task, whereas other tasks require a sustained effort of less than 10 minutes? Is the problem task a multistep packaging job requiring the chaining of four different skills (i.e., collecting items, collating related literature, packaging materials, and packing completed items in shippers), which were not previously chained? In both cases, the prerequisite skills may be within an individual's repertoire, but they are being required in a more complex manner than had come to be expected. Examples of relevant data available from the EDM process would include a durational analysis, an assessment of task sequencing, and anecdotal task descriptions.

Intervention strategies based on the restructuring of the task may be effective in this case. Restructuring may include a reworking of the individual task analysis, an introduction of errorless learning paradigms, or simply an increase in the delivery of functional, reliably identified reinforcement (e.g., Green, Reid, White, Halford, Brittain, & Gardner, 1988; Pace, Ivancic, Edwards, Iwata, & Page, 1985).

## Individual-to-Task Match

The final curricular analysis is an assessment of the individual-to-task match. The core question in this phase is, "Is the task boring or simply disliked?" Although boredom itself may be a difficult construct to assess, manipulation of variables that may be associated with boredom is relatively simple. These variables include (but are not limited to) decreasing task duration, developing a completion criteria for the task (providing the individual with input into when a task is completed), providing alternative tasks, establishing a functional relevance of the task to an individual's environment, increasing reinforcement associated with the task, or if necessary, discontinuing the task. Alternate techniques such as demand-fading (Iwata, 1987) and counterconditioning paradigms may also be considered in order to increase individual task acceptance and preference.

On completion of the functional analysis of the curricular component and the implementation of any related intervention strategies (Table 3), the defined behavior is again examined in relation to the baseline rate of responding. If the behavior has been significantly reduced, the EDM assessment stops, and all intervention strategies continue to be implemented and monitored. If the behavior has not been reduced, the decision-making process proceeds to Component IV—Differential Reinforcement.

## COMPONENT IV—DIFFERENTIAL REINFORCEMENT

With the possible exception of the communication-based interventions proposed in Component II, all strategies up to this point are "preemptive" in nature. That is to say, they represent attempts to decrease the defined behavior by manipulating the stimulus conditions associated with the behavior. If, however the data indicate that these strategies have not reduced the behavior, "postemptive," or reactive, strategies need to be considered. In Component IV (Figure 4), the EDM provides for the development and implementation of procedures

Table 3. Component III—Intervention Strategies

| |
|---|
| Complete appropriate, individualized task analysis |
| Skill development training |
| Restructure task |
| Implement errorless learning condition |
| Increase task-related reinforcement |
| Decrease task duration |
| Establish completion criteria |
| Establish task relevance to individual's environment |
| Delete task (if appropriate) |
| Undertake data-based reinforcement assessment |
| Demand fading |
| Counterconditioning |

involving the delivery of structured differential reinforcement (DRO, DRL, DRI, DRA, etc.).

Before continuing, two terms used in the EDM need to be clearly defined. *Reinforcement* is defined as any stimulus that, when presented contingent on the display of a behavior, increases the probability that the behavior will be displayed again. An aversive, on the other hand, is defined as any stimulus that, when presented contingent on the display of a behavior, decreases the probability that a behavior will be displayed again (Azrin & Holz, 1966). By definition, then, differential reinforcement procedures include both a reinforcement component (praise or other reinforcement for desired behavior) and an aversive component (absence or withdrawal of reinforcement for nondesired behavior) (Matson & DiLorenzo, 1984). In order to avoid definitional confusion therefore, Component IV provides for the assessment of differential reinforcement procedures independent from other procedures, including those that may be functional aversives or implemented as crisis-management techniques (e.g., response interruption, response cost, or nonexclusionary time-out).

## Assess

The EDM presents three considerations relevant to the implementation of a differential reinforcement-alone (DR-Alone) procedure. First, are there external reinforcing conditions present that are maintaining this behavior? DR-Alone may not, in some cases, be effective if the defined behavior is self-stimulatory in nature (e.g., Harris & Wolchick, 1979; Koegel & Koegel, 1989) and maintained through perceptual reinforcement (Lovaas, Newsome, & Hickman, 1987). Second, are

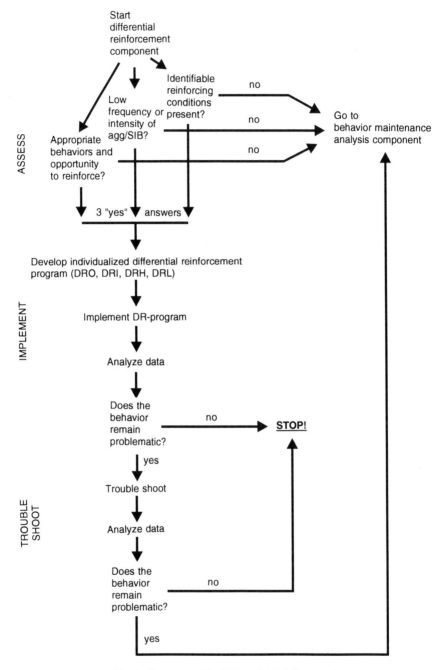

Fig. 4. Component IV—Differential Reinforcement

there other, more appropriate behaviors within an individual's response repertoire, and is there the opportunity to reinforce them? If alternative behaviors do not exist, or the frequency of the defined behavior is so high as to greatly limit opportunities for reinforcement, alternative strategies to DR-Alone may need to be considered. Third, if the defined behavior involves aggression or self-injury, is the behavior infrequent enough or of low enough intensity that DR-Alone would not compromise the individual's right, as well as the right of others, to work and live in a safe environment? If this right would be jeopardized, alternate strategies need to be considered (Van Houten et al., 1988). Alternate strategies would range from teaching a desired alternate response prior to implementing DR-Alone to combining differential reinforcement with certain potentially more intrusive strategies as discussed in Component V.

## Implement and Trouble Shoot

Assuming conditions appropriate to the use of DR-Alone exist, an individualized program may be developed and implemented as indicated in Table 4. Data are analyzed, and the effectiveness of the intervention is assessed. If DR-Alone has not produced a significant reduction in the defined behavior, the EDM calls for the "trouble-shooting" of the current intervention. Program parameters including duration of reinforcement interval and the value of the available reinforcement should be evaluated as a trouble-shooting measure. In addition, the reliability and consistency of the program staff in the implementation of the DR-Alone procedure needs to be assessed.

Following trouble-shooting, indicated changes are made, and the intervention is reimplemented. If there is a significant reduction in the behavior, the development process stops and the revised DR-Alone procedure remains in effect and continues to be monitored. If there has not been a significant decrease, trouble-shooting may again be implemented. If, however, there appears to be a need for an additional intervention strategy in combination with DR-Alone procedure, the

Table 4. Component IV—Intervention Strategies

Complete data-based reinforcement assessment
Develop DRO, DRI, DRA, DRL, or DRH with appropriate reinforcement interval
Trouble shoot
   Intervals of appropriate duration
   Reinforcement functional and appropriate
   Appropriate alternate behaviors being reinforced
   Staff compliance with program
Reimplement program

EDM proceeds to its final assessment component: Component V—Development of an Aversive Decelerative Procedure.

## COMPONENT V—DEVELOPMENT OF AN AVERSIVE DECELERATIVE PROCEDURE

Having progressed through Components I–IV of the EDM, the probability is high that the following statements are valid: (1) The individual is living and working in an environment that is safe, comfortable, and, to the extent possible, free from unnecessary distractions; (2) the individual either has been or is currently being taught strategies that provide for appropriate environmental input and control; (3) the individual is being instructed in a manner commensurate with his/her abilities while being presented with appropriate, ongoing curricular challenges; and (4) functional reinforcement is available to the individual on a regular basis. All four of these statements must be true if the introduction of any of the aversive strategies presented in Component V is to result in long-term behavior change and is to be effectively faded at later date.

In Component V (Figure 5), the use of aversive procedures is to be considered given the ineffectiveness of the previous, less intrusive strategies associated with Components I–IV. When selecting an aversive procedure, the following three conditions should be met: (1) The procedure is one that, through a thorough review of the relevant literature, is assumed that it will be effective; (2) the procedure that is chosen must not negatively effect other, more appropriate behaviors; and (3) the procedure that is chosen must be less intrusive and disruptive than the defined behavior itself (Holmes & Holmes, 1987).

### Maintained by Positive Reinforcement—Attention

For the EDM, the information available from the applied functional analysis that relates to the addition of an aversive strategy (Table 5) comes from the answer to the question, "What are the reinforcement conditions maintaining the behavior?" If the data indicate positive reinforcement (attention-seeking behavior— occurs during times of reduced staff or peer interaction) as the behavior maintenance condition, a strategy may be chosen from those options that manipulate the positive reinforcement associated with the display of the defined behavior. These options would include extinction or planned ignoring, time-out, nonexclusionary time-out, visual screening, and the various response cost or token earn procedures, all of which are implemented with related teaching programs and differential reinforcement procedures. Further, all appropriate environmental and curricular modifications would remain in effect.

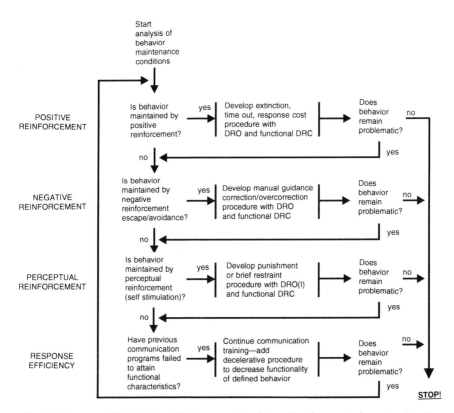

Fig. 5. Component V—Behavior Maintenance Conditions Development of an Aversive Procedure

## Maintained by Negative Reinforcement—Escape

In the case where the defined behavior is maintained as an escape response (negative reinforcement—occurs to terminate a task demand or nonpreferred stimulus), a strategy may be chosen that is designed to negate the efficacy of such an escape. These options may include response interruption, simple correction or putting through, positive practice overcorrection, negative practice overcorrection, or restitutional overcorrection. Again, all procedures are implemented with related teaching and differential reinforcement procedures while previously developed environmental and curricular modifications remain in effect.

Table 5.  Component V—Intervention Strategies[a]

| |
|---|
| Extinction or planned ignoring |
| Time-out |
| Nonexclusionary time-out |
| Response cost |
| Visual screening |
| Response interruption |
| Correction or manual guidance |
| Positive practice overcorrection |
| Restitutional overcorrection |
| Brief physical aversive |
| Physical or mechanical restraint |

[a]All strategies implemented with complementary teaching and
reinforcement strategies.

## Perceptual Reinforcement

If the behavior is one that is determined to be maintained primarily as a self-stimulatory response and maintained by the reinforcement provided by the behavior itself, a more "classic" aversive or punisher may be the appropriate option. Such options may include verbal reprimands, physical aversives (e.g., a light tap on the hands), visual screening, or brief restraint in the form of response-interruption procedures. Overcorrection procedures may also be considered as potentially appropriate intervention strategies for such behaviors.

## Inadequate Response Efficiency

Lastly, as an additional somewhat specialized case, the EDM addresses the situation in which a functionally equivalent response is present in the individual's repertoire, but the defined behavior remains a more efficient means of communicating this response. Under these circumstances, the EDM provides for the use of an aversive procedure that is designed to decrease the efficiency of the defined behavior thereby increasing the efficiency of the equivalent response. For example, the verbal request, "I need a break," would result in a break being granted, whereas a behavior such as the throwing of work materials would result in an appropriately chosen aversive procedure. In this case, the functional communication training may be regarded as the primary agent of behavior change, whereas the aversive procedure is available as a secondary or backup behavior-change strategy that is expected to be faded quickly.

In all cases, the effectiveness of the chosen procedure is assessed according to the data. Trouble-shooting is undertaken as necessary and, if the program is effective, the procedure proceeds while being continually monitored. On maintained low rates of the defined behavior, structured attempts are to be made at fading the use of the aversive procedure while continuing the use of differential reinforcement and any related teaching programs. The environmental and curricular conditions of Components II and III continue to be assessed regularly to ensure that conditions that are necessary to support appropriate behavioral responding are maintained. Should the defined behavior remain problematic following trouble-shooting, the defined behavior is again assessed in line with the entire EDM, and new strategies are developed and implemented.

## EDM CASE STUDY

### Individual Description

At the time of assessment, Oscar was a 29-year-old adult male with autism who functioned in the severe range of mental retardation. Oscar was verbal, but articulation difficulties often made comprehension difficult. He was, however, generally able to express most of his wants, needs, and interests. Oscar resided in a community group home for individuals with autism and was employed in a sheltered employment setting.

### Determination of Need

Oscar entered the Eden Work Education Resource Centers (WERCs) program with a history of severe and directed aggression. Initially, aggression was brought under control through the use of relaxation training for times during which Oscar appeared anxious (anxious or anticipatory behaviors); a token-earn system for time on task and use of appropriate communication, and a restraint procedure for any occurrences of aggression or attempts at aggression. An EDM assessment was indicated, however, as the frequency of aggression had increased over previous weeks to a level where safety concerns became a factor. Aggression and anxious/anticipatory behaviors were defined as:

Aggression—any directed biting, kicking, grabbing, hitting, or scratching of others, not to include any accidental or social contact.
Anxious behavior—the taking of rapid short breaths or the repetition of the same question or statement more than twice within 2 minutes.

As a result of staff input regarding the defined behaviors, the applied functional analysis or baseline procedure consisted of the following measures: frequency of aggressive episodes; duration of time until calm following an aggression; an anecdotal assessment of the "intensity" of each episode of aggression; frequency with which Oscar was offered the option to relax; day of the week; number of people in the environment; time of day; and activities or curricular demands. An A-B-C log was also maintained to supplement this information. During the assessment, a medical evaluation was completed that failed to identify any potential medical correlates to Oscar's increased aggression.

Data collected during the assessment validated staff reports of a need to modify Oscar's existing behavioral programming. Aggression, during assessment, occurred at a rate of approximately 3 episodes per week (Figure 6), whereas anxious behaviors were displayed approximately 21 times per week (Figure 7). Following 9 weeks of assessment, the data collected on the potential environmental correlates to aggression were analyzed in accordance with the EDM.

## Environmental Conditions

Two particular staff perceptions were validated by the applied functional analysis or baseline data. First, Oscar was far more likely to aggress whenever there were more than 20 people in his immediate environment (Figure 8). Thirty-five percent of all aggressions were associated with this level of crowding. As Oscar spent only 8 to 10% of his time at this level of crowding, this finding was considered especially significant. Second, aggressions appeared to be associated with those times when Oscar worked in the kitchen (Figure 9). As lunch, a high-aggression activity was also a high-crowding activity; the decision was made to address crowding as the primary correlate to aggression and kitchen activities as a secondary correlate. (It bears noting that this outcome was contrary to staff predictions. Prior to assessment, staff perceptions were that kitchen tasks were the primary correlate to aggression. Crowding, although viewed as possibly related, was not predicted as a primary correlate. This highlights the importance of a data-based assessment in determining the function of a behavior.)

As a result of this initial analysis, functional escape training was initiated to address Oscar's difficulty with crowds. Functional escape training consisted of prompting Oscar to request to leave the room when there were more than 10 people in his environment. The option to escape was also offered in place of relaxation if staff perceived the overall level of activity in the environment as potentially disturbing to Oscar.

Functional escape training was introduced in Week 10, resulting in a 66% reduction in the frequency of aggression with, oddly, no related reduction in anxious behavior (Figure 6 and Figure 7). Of particular interest is that Oscar only once accepted the opportunity to leave the situation. It seems possible that he perceived leaving the situation as a form of punishment and therefore, less desirable than remaining in the stressful, crowded situation.

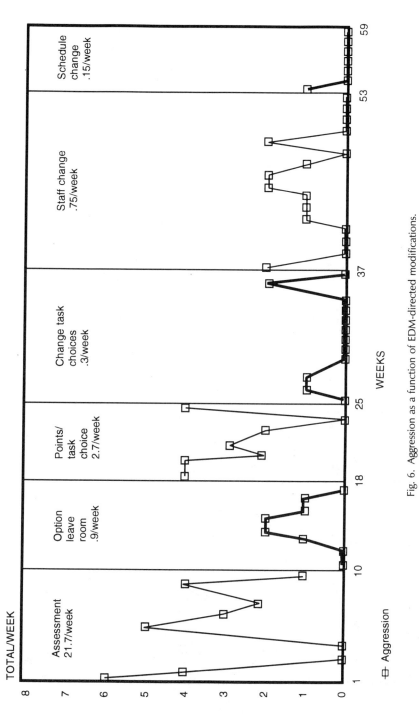

Fig. 6. Aggression as a function of EDM-directed modifications.

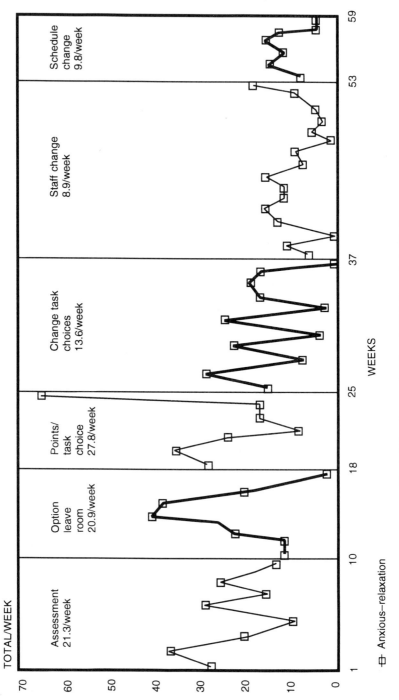

Fig. 7. Relaxation as a function of EDM-directed modifications.

## Curricular Considerations

At this point, the continuation of the applied functional analysis procedure throughout functional-escape training provided clearer support for kitchen-associated activities (i.e., lunch prep and lunch cleanup) as now being the primary correlates of aggression. A review of the ongoing data in accordance with the elements of Component III suggested two possible explanations for kitchen activities precipitating aggression. According to the A-B-C log, on a number of occasions across program, Oscar had declined to chose a reinforcer to work as part of his token system. Apparently his reinforcement menu was no longer functionally defined. Second, although all problematic kitchen activities were previously documented as within Oscar's repertoire, they simply appeared to be nonpreferred (boring?) activities.

Working on these data-based assumptions, two complementary strategies were introduced at this point in addition to continuing to offer Oscar the opportunity to escape crowded situations. Oscar's token program was modified in such a way so that he would earn points for each task completed. The longer, or more complex the task, the greater its point value. In conjunction, a reinforcer assessment was used to identify a broader array of functional secondary reinforcers for which Oscar could cash in points. Second, to address the potential boredom, task-choice options were introduced into all kitchen-related activities. This allowed Oscar to choose his kitchen activity from a variety of tasks, each of which was assigned a specific point value.

In Week 18, the point-earn system and task-choice procedure were implemented. Aggression returned to levels equal to those obtained during the initial assessment, with no change in the frequency of anxious behaviors (Figures 8 and 9). Initially, a return to the previous token system and a suspension of the task-choice procedure was considered in an attempt to reduce the frequency of aggression. However, the decision was made to continue with the changes while additional data were collected. The intent was to effectively modify either or both procedures in such a way as to reduce both aggression and anxious behaviors.

In Week 25, based on information obtained from the continued A-B-C log, the choice-making procedure was modified such that a greater array of shorter tasks was made available, and the nature of some of the task choices were modified (e.g., prepare chile or sandwiches). With the introduction of this change, the frequency of aggression was reduced such that there were only four episodes over the next 12 weeks. In addition, for the first time, a drop in the frequency of anxious behaviors was evidenced, indicating a general lowering of Oscar's overall level of anxiety (Figures 8 and 9).

Two additional changes, not related to the EDM or ongoing assessment, are noted on the graph and deserve attention. First, in Week 37 Oscar's teacher-job coach left, resulting in higher rates of aggression during the training and transition of new staff. Although higher than during the previous

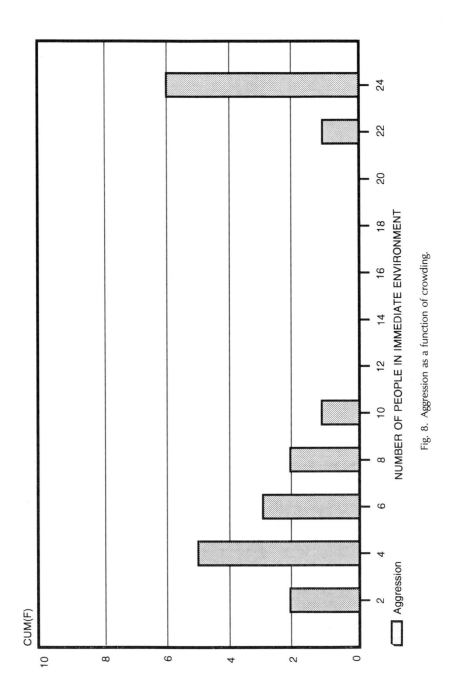

Fig. 8. Aggression as a function of crowding.

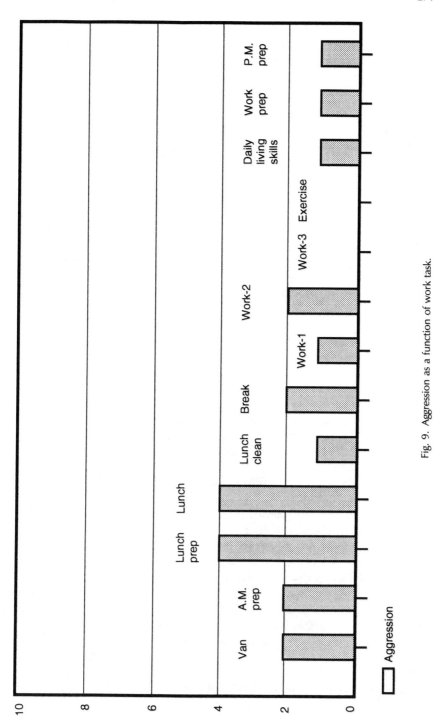

Fig. 9. Aggression as a function of work task.

12 weeks, aggression continued to be lower than during assessment. Additionally, despite the increase in aggression, anxious behaviors were maintained at the previously obtained lower rates indicating continued overall reductions in anxiety. Within 3 months, rates of aggression were back at near-zero levels. Second, in Week 53, as a result of some changes in program structure, a change was made in Oscar's daily schedule. This chage resulted in a single aggression, followed with a rapid return to zero rates of aggression (Figures 8 and 9).

## DISCUSSION

The case of Oscar is provided as a relatively straightforward example of the use of the EDM in the development of an applied functional analysis and related intervention strategies. This case serves to highlight the benefits of the use of the EDM in addressing a severely problematic behavior; that of a high-intensity aggression of relatively low-frequency (that is, in terms of data collection for assessment purposes). First, by reviewing the separate components of the EDM, an applied functional analysis or assessment process may be developed that addresses a variety of stimulus conditions that may be associated with the defined behavior. In Oscar's case, this resulted in the elimination of possible medical causation, the identification of possible environmental factors associated with the behavior (crowding), and the identification of the curricular conditions under which the behavior most frequently occurred (kitchen tasks).

Second, the EDM provides for the integration of separate strategies into one, comprehensive treatment package. In the case of Oscar, this resulted in a final package of strategies that included functional escape training, training in the use of task choices, continued emphasis on alternate response training (relaxation), and a functionally defined reinforcement system. In Oscar's case, differential reinforcement alone was not considered an appropriate option due to the intensity of aggression and the potential for harm. As previously noted, this required a potentially aversive component (restraint) being in effect throughout the EDM process. However, given the lack of any reductive effect of restraint, it could not be considered a functional aversive. Restraint, in this case, could more accurately be described as a crisis-management procedure that allowed for the EDM process to continue while ensuring the safety of Oscar and others.

Third, the EDM allows for (indeed, requires) direct line-staff input at all levels of assessment. Involvement of this type can have many advantages, including a sense of professional validation for observations and perceptions used as a basis for the assessment process and, increased staff compliance (as a result of a degree of "ownership" in the process) in data collection and assessment process.

Last, the ongoing nature of the EDM assessment process allows for the continuing assessment of stimulus conditions over extended periods of time. This may be extremely important in cases where the behavior is of relatively low frequency, and stable data may only be obtained over extended periods of assessment. Additionally, continuing assessment allows for the identification of secondary or changing stimulus conditions that may precipitate the behavior.

Some cautions, however, are in order regarding the use of the EDM assessment process. The EDM, as discussed here, is presented solely as a set of general guidelines. Utilization of this model is not presented as a total or sufficient condition for the implementation of any decelerative behavioral procedure. Programmatic options presented with each component are only examples and are not intended to represent the totality of treatment options available.

Further, the EDM does not stand alone. In the development of intervention strategies, consideration must be given to the individual for whom a strategy is being considered in terms of his/her past history with behavior contingencies, his/her possible responses to any procedures, individual likes and dislikes, and the nature of the behavior itself. Concerns for the protection of an individual's right to effective treatment and to live and work in an environment free from abuse and neglect must also be an active component of the decision-making process. Aversive treatment strategies are to be chosen from a hierarchy of intrusiveness so as to select the least intrusive option that is likely to be effective. Behavior management and human rights peer-review committees must be knowledgeably staffed and actively maintained. Informed consent, meeting the three requirements of competence, knowledge, and volition (DiLorenzo and Ollendick, 1986), must be obtained and may be withdrawn at any time. Finally, staff training and supervision must promote the development of the highest level of technical expertise and ethical behavior among all concerned (Lovaas & Favell, 1987).

Professionals in the human service field face a variety of challenges as they endeavor to make habilitative and educational decisions with and for clients. In no area are these decisions so potentially controversial as they are in the area of behavior reduction. One active step toward reducing this potential for controversy is the careful and individualized use of the applied functional analysis process. The EDM is one way of accomplishing this, in a manner that is feasible, effective, and easily adaptable for ongoing assessment and monitoring in the applied program setting.

ACKNOWLEDGMENTS

The authors would like to acknowledge the following individuals who contributed to both the development of the Eden Decision Model and this manuscript: Carol Markowitz, Anne S. Holmes, David Roussell, James Ball, Michael Alessandri, and the staff of Eden W.E.R.C.s. The authors would like to thank Andy Bondy and Michael Powers for their insightful comments on an earlier version of this manuscript. Last, but by no means least, we would like to express our sincere gratitude, appreciation and respect to the Eden Family of Programs' participants and their families. Requests of reprints should be sent to Peter F. Gerhardt, The Eden Programs, One Logan Drive, Princeton, New Jersey 08540.

## REFERENCES

Axelrod, S. (1987). Functional and structural analysis of behavior: Approaches leading to reduced use of punishment procedures? *Research in Developmental Disabilities, 8,* 165–178.

Azrin, N. H., Besalel, V. A., Jamner, J. P., & Caputo, J. N. (1988). Comparative study of behavior methods of treating severe self-injury. *Behavioral Residential Treatment, 3,* 119–152.

Azrin, N. H., & Holz, W. C. (1966). Punishment. In W. K. Honig (Ed.), *Operant behavior: Areas of research and application* (pp. 380–447). New York: Appleton-Century-Crofts.

Bailey, J. S., & Pyles, D. A. M. (1989). Behavioral diagnostics. In E. Cipani (Ed.), *The treatment of severe behavior disorders: Behavior analysis approaches* (pp. 85–107). Washington, DC: American Association on Mental Retardation.

Bijou, S. W., Peterson, R. F., Harris, F. R., Allen, K. E., & Johnson, M. S. (1969). Methodology for experimental studies of young children in natural settings. *The Psychological Record, 19,* 177–210.

Carr, E. G. (1977). The motivation of self-injurious behavior: A review of some of the hypothesis. *Psychological Bulletin, 84,* 800–816.

Carr, E. G., & Durand, V. M. (1985). Reducing behavior problems through functional communication training. *Journal of Applied Behavior Analysis, 18,* 111–126.

Carr, E. G., & Newsome, C. D. (1985). Demand related tantrums: Conceptualization and treatment. *Behavior Modification, 9,* 403–426.

DiLorenzo, T. M., & Ollendick, T. H. (1986). Behavior modification: Punishment. In R. P. Barrett (Ed.), *Severe behavior disorders in the mentally retarded: Nondrug approaches to treatment* (pp. 27–60). New York: Plenum.

Donnellan, A. H., Mirenda, P. L., Mesaros, R. A., & Fassbender, L. L. (1984). Analyzing the communicative functions of aberrant behavior. *The Journal of the Association for Persons with Severe Handicaps, 9,* 201–212.

Evans, I. M., & Meyer, L. H. (1985). *An educative approach to behavior problems: A practical decision model for interventions with severely handicapped learners.* Baltimore: Paul H. Brooks.

Foster, S. L., Bell-Dolan, D. J., & Burge, D. A. (1988). Behavioral observation. In A. S. Bellack & M. Hersen (Eds.), *Behavioral assessment: A practical handbook* (pp. 119–160). New York: Pergamon.

Gardner, W. I. (1989). But in the meantime: A client perspective of the debate over the use of aversive/intrusive therapy procedures. *The Behavior Therapist, 12,* 179–181.

Gerhardt, P., Holmes, D. L. Alessandri, M., & Goodman, M. (1992). Social policy on the use of aversive interventions: Empirical, ethical, and legal considerations. *Journal of Autism and Developmental Disorders, 21,* 265–277.

Green, C. W., Reid, D. H., White, L. K., Halford, R. C., Brittain, D. P., & Gardner, S. M. (1988). Identifying reinforcers for persons with profound handicaps: Staff opinion versus systematic assessment of preferences. *Journal of Applied Behavior Analysis, 21,* 31–43.

Griffith, R. G. (1986). Administrative considerations and responsibilities: Legal and ethical issues. In R. P. Barrett (Ed.), *Severe behavior disorders in the mentally retarded: Nondrug approaches to treatment* (pp. 359–394). New York: Plenum.

Groden, G. (1989). A guide for conducting a comprehensive behavioral analysis of a target behavior. *Journal of Behavior Therapy and Experimental Psychiatry, 20,* 163–169.

Guess, D., Helmstetter E., Turnbull, H. R. III, & Knowlton, S. (1987). Use of aversive procedures with individuals who are disabled: A historical review and critical analysis. *Monograph of the Association of Persons with Severe Handicaps, 2,* 1.

Gunsett, R. P., Mulick, J. A., Fernald, W. B., & Martin, J. L. (1989). Brief report: Indications for medical screening prior to behavioral programming for severely and profoundly mentally retarded clients. *Journal of Autism and Developmental Disorders, 19,* 167–172.

Harris, S. L., & Wolchik, S. A. (1979). Suppression of self stimulation: Three alternative strategies. *Journal of Applied Behavior Analysis, 12,* 185–198.

Hart, B., & Risley, T. (1976). Environmental programming: Implications for the severely handicapped. In H. Prehm & S. Deitz (Eds.), *Early intervention for the severely handicapped: Programming accountability* (pp. 197–221). Eugene: University of Oregon, College of Education.

Holmes, D. L., & Gerhardt, P. F. (1989). Punishment: The issues as we see them. *Links, 14,* 8–9.

Holmes, D. L., & Holmes, A. S. (Eds.) (1987). *The Eden Programs General Procedures Manual.* Princeton, NJ: Eden.

Iwata, B. (1987). *Aversive events and their role in the treatment of life threatening behavior.* Paper presented at the conference on Life Threatening Behavior: Aversive versus Nonaversive Intervention, Piscataway, NJ.

Iwata, B. A., Dorsey, M. F., Slifer, K. J., Bauman, K. E., & Richman, G. S. (1982). Toward a functional analysis of self injury. *Analysis and Intervention in Developmental Disabilities, 2,* 3–20.

Koegel, R. L., & Koegel, L. K. (1989). Community-referenced research on self-stimulation. In E. Cipani (Ed.), *Treatment of severe behavior disorders: Behavior Analysis Approaches* (pp. 129–150). Washington, DC: AAMR.

LaVigna, G. W., & Donnellan, A. M. (1986). *Alternatives to punishment: Solving problem behavior with nonaversive strategies.* New York: Irvington.

Lovaas, O. I., & Favell, J. E. (1987). Protection for clients undergoing aversive/restrictive interventions. *Education and Treatment of Children, 10,* 311–325.

Lovaas, O. I., Newsome, C., & Hickman, C. (1987). Self stimulatory behavior and perceptual reinforcement. *Journal of Applied Behavior Analysis, 20,* 45–68.

Matson, J. L., & DiLorenzo, T. M. (1984). *Punishment and its alternatives: A new perspective for behavior modification.* New York: Springer.

O'Neill, R. E., Horner, R. H., Albin, R. W., Storey, K., & Sprague, J. (1990). *Functional analysis of problem behavior: A practical assessment guide.* Sycamore, IL: Sycamore Publishing.

Pace, G. M., Ivancic, M. T., Edwards, G. L., Iwata, B. A., & Page, T. J. (1985). Assessment of stimulus preference and reinforcer value with profoundly retarded individuals. *Journal of Applied Behavior Analysis, 18,* 249–255.

Powers, M. D., & Handleman, J. H. (1984). *Behavioral assessment of severe developmental disabilities.* Rockville, MD: Aspen.

Schopler, E. (1990). Editorial: Basic disagreements with Autism Society of America. *Spectrum, 4,* 10–11.

Schopler, E., & Mesibov, G. B. (Eds.). (1983). *Autism in adolescents and adults.* New York: Plenum.

Schopler, E., Mesibov, G., & Baker, A. (1982). Evaluation of treatment for autistic children and their parents. *Journal of the American Academy of Child Psychiatry, 21,* 262–267.

Simpson, R. L., & Regan, M. (Eds.). (1986). *Management of autistic behavior: Information service for educators.* Rockville, MD: Aspen.

Simpson, R. L., Regan, M., Sasso, G., & Noll, M. B. (1986). Behavioral intervention techniques. In

R. Simpson & M. Regan (Eds.), *Management of autistic behavior: Information service for educators* (pp. 6.1–6.36). Rockville, MD: Aspen.

Touchette, P. E., MacDonald, R. F., & Langer, S. N. (1985). A scatter plot for identifying the stimulus control of a problem behavior. *Journal of Applied Behavior Analysis, 18,* 343–351.

Van Houten, R., Axelrod, S., Bailey, J. S., Favell, J. E., Foxx, R. M., Iwata, B. A., & Lovaas, O. I. (1988). The right to effective behavioral treatment. *Journal of Applied Behavior Analysis, 21,* 381–384.

Williams, B. F., Williams, R. L., & McLaughlin, T. F. (1989). The use of token economies with individuals who have developmental disabilities. In E. Cipani (Ed.), *The treatment of severe behavior disorders: Behavior analysis approaches* (pp. 3–18). Washington, DC: AAMR.

# Author Index

# Subject Index